Clinical Neuroanatomy

A Review with Questions and Explanations

THIRD EDITION

CLINICAL NEUROANATOMY

A Review with Questions and Explanations

THIRD EDITION

Richard S. Snell, MD, PhD
Emeritus Professor of Anatomy
George Washington University
School of Medicine and Health Sciences
Washington, D.C.

LIPPINCOTT WILLIAMS & WILKINS
A **Wolters Kluwer** Company
Philadelphia • Baltimore • New York • London
Buenos Aires • Hong Kong • Sydney • Tokyo

Editor: Rob Anthony
Managing Editor: Ulita Lushnycky
Marketing Manager: Aimee Sirmon
Production Manager: Susan Rockwell

351 West Camden Street
Baltimore, Maryland 21201-2436 USA

530 Walnut Street
Philadelphia, Pennsylvania 19106 USA

Printed in the United States of America

Library of Congress Cataloging-in-Publication Data
LOC data is available.

00 01 02
1 2 3 4 5 6 7 8 9 10

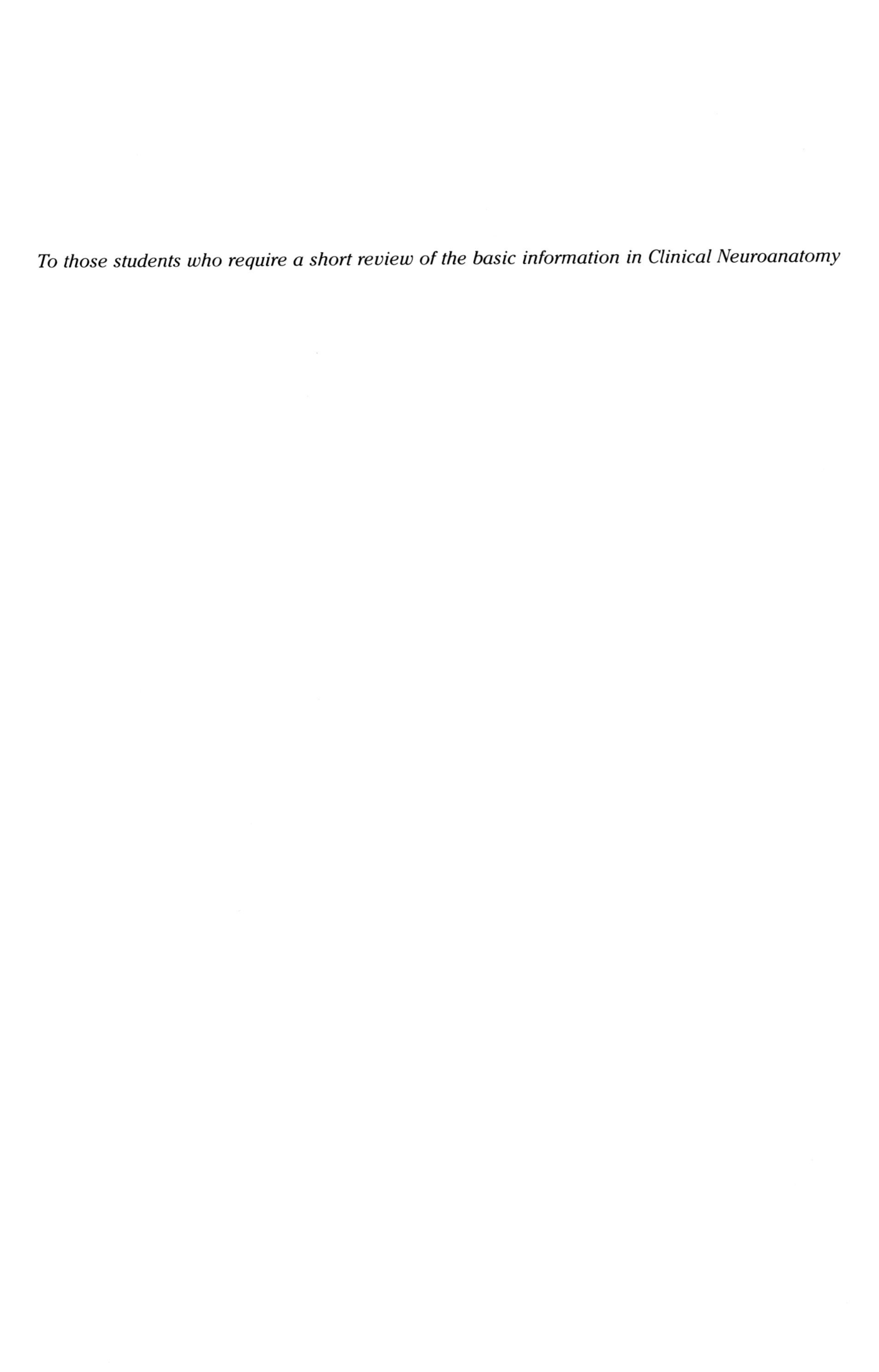

To those students who require a short review of the basic information in Clinical Neuroanatomy

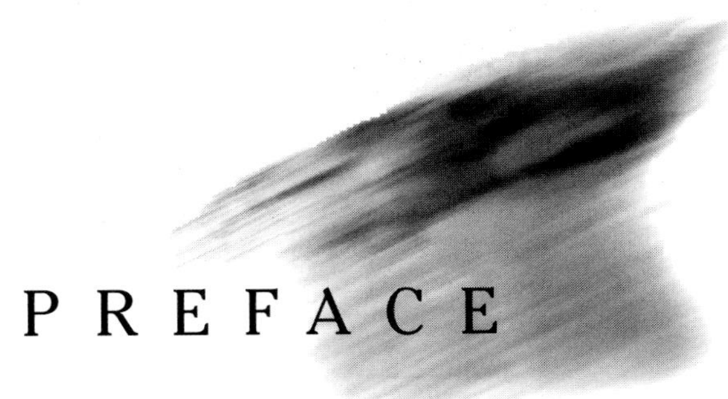

PREFACE

This book was written specifically for medical, dental, and allied health students who are preparing for examinations. The book can also be used during their clinical clerkships for a quick review of clinical neuroanatomy. It is also designed to meet the needs of residents who are about to embark on a Neurology or Neurosurgical Residency and need to review important basic material.

The clinical neuroanatomy is presented in a condensed form, with simple diagrams, radiographs, CTscans, MRIs, and a PETscan. At the end of each chapter are Review Questions, which are followed by answers and, where appropriate, brief explanations. Some of the questions in this edition are centered around clinical problems that require neuroanatomical or neurophysiological answers. For a more extensive review, this book may be used in conjunction with Clinical Neuroanatomy for Medical Students, Fifth Edition, also published by Lippincott Williams & Wilkins.

The book begins with an introductory chapter on the organization of the nervous system and the basic structure and function of neurons, nerve processes, synapses, and nerve fibers. This is followed by chapters dealing with the neuroglia, degeneration and regeneration of nervous tissue, peripheral nerves, and peripheral nerve endings. The different parts of the central nervous system and their connections are discussed. Other chapters deal with simplifying and describing the connections of the cranial nerves and the structure and function of the autonomic nervous system. Numerous tables have been used throughout the text to assist in the memorization of factual material.

The purpose of the Review Questions is threefold: 1) They focus students' attention on areas of importance; 2) They enable students to identify areas of weakness; and 3) When answered under examination conditions, they provide students with an effective form of self-evaluation.

In this new edition, the successful overall presentation has been retained. The Clinical Notes Sections have been updated and expanded, and the Review Questions are similar to those used in the USML Step 1 examinations.

ACKNOWLEDGMENTS

I sincerely thank Myra Feldman and Ira Alan Grunther, AMI, for their excellent artwork. I once again express my gratitude and appreciation to the publishers for their assistance throughout the preparation of this book.

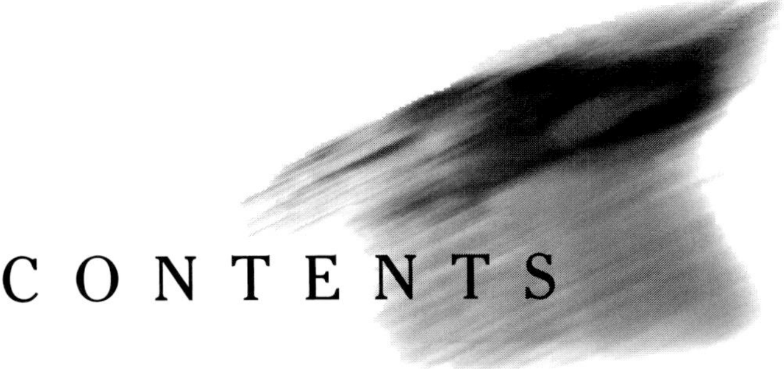

CONTENTS

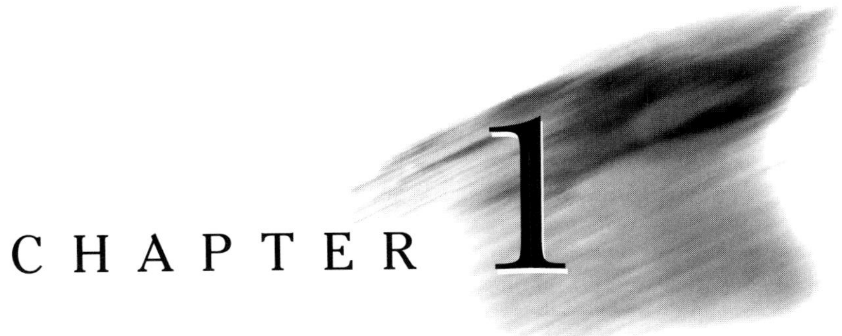

CHAPTER 1

Organization of the Nervous System and the Neurobiology of the Neuron

CHAPTER OUTLINE

SUGGESTED PLAN FOR REVIEW OF CHAPTER 1

1. Understand the organization of the nervous system and realize that nerve fibers can run from one part to another without interruption. Throughout this text emphasis is placed on understanding the spatial relationships of different parts of the nervous system. Once you have mastered this, it is easier to appreciate how nerve fibers travel from one part to another. If you also learn the functions of the parts, then it is much easier to learn the nervous connections between them. In other words, you begin to be able to visualize the connections in your mind's eye rather than having to learn facts like a parrot.
2. Learn the types of neurons and know examples of each type.
3. Review the cell biology of a neuron so that you may more easily understand the function of a nerve cell and its processes. Pay particular attention to the structure of the plasma membrane as it is related to its physiology.
4. Understand axon transport.
5. Synapses are very important, so learn the detail. Include in your review the different types of neurotransmitters and their actions (see p. 8).
6. Learn the structure of myelinated and nonmyelinated nerves. Understand how the physiology of conduction is related to the structure of nerve fibers.

NERVOUS SYSTEM

The nervous system and the endocrine system control the functions of the body. The nervous system exerts its control by means of specialized cells that rapidly pass signals to different parts of the individual. The nervous system receives input signals from the external and internal environments by means of sensory receptors. Once inside the nervous system, the signals are integrated with one another and either are transmitted to bring about muscle contraction or glandular activity or are stored in the memory for future use. Learning occurs as the result of the continual adaptation of the connections of the nervous system as the body is exposed to new sensations.

Organization

The nervous system is divided into two main parts, the **central nervous system**, consisting of the brain and spinal cord, and the **peripheral nervous system**, consisting of the cranial and spinal nerves and their ganglia (Box 1-1). The **autonomic nervous system** is an important subdivision of the nervous system, which innervates involuntary structures, such as the heart, smooth muscle, and glands.

The basic units of the nervous system are the nerve cells, which are specialized to conduct nerve impulses over long distances at great speeds. The **neuron** is the name given to the nerve cell and all its processes (Fig. 1-1). Neurons possess a **cell body** and processes called **neurites**. The long processes of a nerve cell are called **axons**, or **nerve fibers**; the short processes are **dendrites**. Unlike most other cells in the body, normal neurons in the mature individual do not undergo division and replication.

The central nervous system is composed of large numbers of neurons supported by specialized tissue called **neuroglia**. In the peripheral nervous system, the nerve fibers and the nerve cells in ganglia are supported by delicate areolar tissue.

The interior of the central nervous system is organized into **gray** and **white matter**. Gray matter consists of nerve cells embedded in neuroglia. White matter consists of nerve fibers embedded in neuroglia.

NEURONS

Types of Neurons

Neurons can be classified according to the number and mode of branching of the neurites (Fig. 1-1):

Unipolar neurons are those that have a single neurite that divides a short distance from the cell body into two branches, one proceeding to a peripheral structure and the other entering the central nervous system. Examples of this form of neuron are found in the posterior root ganglion.

Bipolar neurons possess an elongated cell body that gives rise to a single neurite at each end. Examples of this form of neuron are found in the retina and the sensory ganglia of the cochlear and vestibular nerves.

Multipolar neurons are those in which a number of neurites arise from the cell body. With the exception of the long process, the axon, the neurites are dendrites. Almost all the neurons of the central nervous system are of this type.

Neurons can also be classified by their size:

Golgi type I neurons have long axons that may be 1 meter long in extreme cases. The axons of these neurons form the long fiber tracts of the brain and spinal cord and the nerve fibers of peripheral nerves. The pyramidal cells of the cerebral cortex, the Purkinje cells of the cerebellar cortex, and the motor anterior gray column cells of the spinal cord are Golgi type I neurons.

Golgi type II neurons have a short axon that terminates near the cell body or have no axon. The short dendrites give these cells a star-shaped appearance. This type of

Box 1–1 Major Divisions of the Central and Peripheral Nervous Systems

Central nervous system
Brain
- Forebrain
  - Cerebrum
  - Diencephalon (between brain)
- Midbrain
- Hindbrain
  - Medulla oblongata
  - Pons
  - Cerebellum

Spinal cord
- Cervical segments
- Thoracic segments
- Lumbar segments
- Sacral segments
- Coccygeal segments

Peripheral nervous system
Cranial nerves and their ganglia
- 12 pairs that exit the skull through the foramina

Spinal nerves and their ganglia
- 31 pairs that exit the vertebral column through the intervertebral foramina
  - 8 Cervical
  - 12 Thoracic
  - 5 Lumbar
  - 5 Sacral
  - 1 Coccygeal

Table 1–1 Summary of the Classification of Neurons

Morphological Classification	Arrangement of Neurites	Location
Number, Length, Mode of Branching of Neurites		
Unipolar	Single neurite divides short distance from cell body	Posterior root ganglion
Bipolar	Single neurite emerges from either end of cell body	Retina, sensory cochlear, and vestibular ganglia
Multipolar	Many dendrites and one long axon	Fiber tracts of brain and spinal cord, peripheral nerves, and motor cells of spinal cord
Size of Neuron		
Golgi type I	Single long axon	Fiber tracts of brain and spinal cord, peripheral nerves, and motor cells of spinal cord
Golgi type II	Short axon that with dendrites resembles a star	Cerebral and cerebellar cortex

neuron greatly outnumbers the Golgi type I neurons, and they are found in large numbers in the cerebral and cerebellar cortex and in the retina.

The classification of neurons is summarized in Table 1-1.

Structure and Function of a Neuron

NERVE CELL BODY

The nerve cell body consists of a mass of cytoplasm in which a nucleus is embedded (Table 1-2) and is surrounded by a plasma membrane (Fig. 1-2). The cell body produces the organelles that are passed out into the axon and dendrites; it also synthesizes the transmitter substances that are transported in the axoplasm down the axon. The plasma membranes of the dendrites and cell body possess receptors that are stimulated by transmitter substances from other neurons. When the receptors are stimulated, electrical currents begin to flow through the membrane so that the resting potential of the dendrites or cell body is raised or lowered. The altered potential, which spreads along the nerve fiber as the nerve impulse, if great enough, will induce similar changes in rapid succession along the plasma membrane of the axon.

Nucleus

The nucleus is large and pale with widely dispersed fine chromatin granules. There is usually a prominent nucleolus.

Cytoplasm

The cytoplasm possesses granular and agranular endoplasmic reticulum and the following organelles and inclusions.

Nissl Substance

This granular material is composed of rough-surfaced endoplasmic reticulum. It is found throughout the cytoplasm of the cell body except the region where the axon emerges; this area is known as the **axon hillock**. It also extends into the proximal parts of the dendrites. The Nissl substance synthesizes protein.

Golgi Apparatus

This is composed of clusters of flattened cisternae and small vesicles made up of smooth-surfaced endoplasmic reticulum. It is found close to the nucleus. The Golgi apparatus adds carbohydrate to the protein molecules brought to it, packages products for export from the cell, and forms cell membranes.

Mitochondria

These are found scattered throughout the cytoplasm of the cell body and the dendrites and axons. They are vesicular structures having an outer membrane that surrounds the mitochondrion and an inner membrane that is folded to form cristae. Mitochondria are responsible for cellular respiration and are the chief sites for the formation of chemical energy.

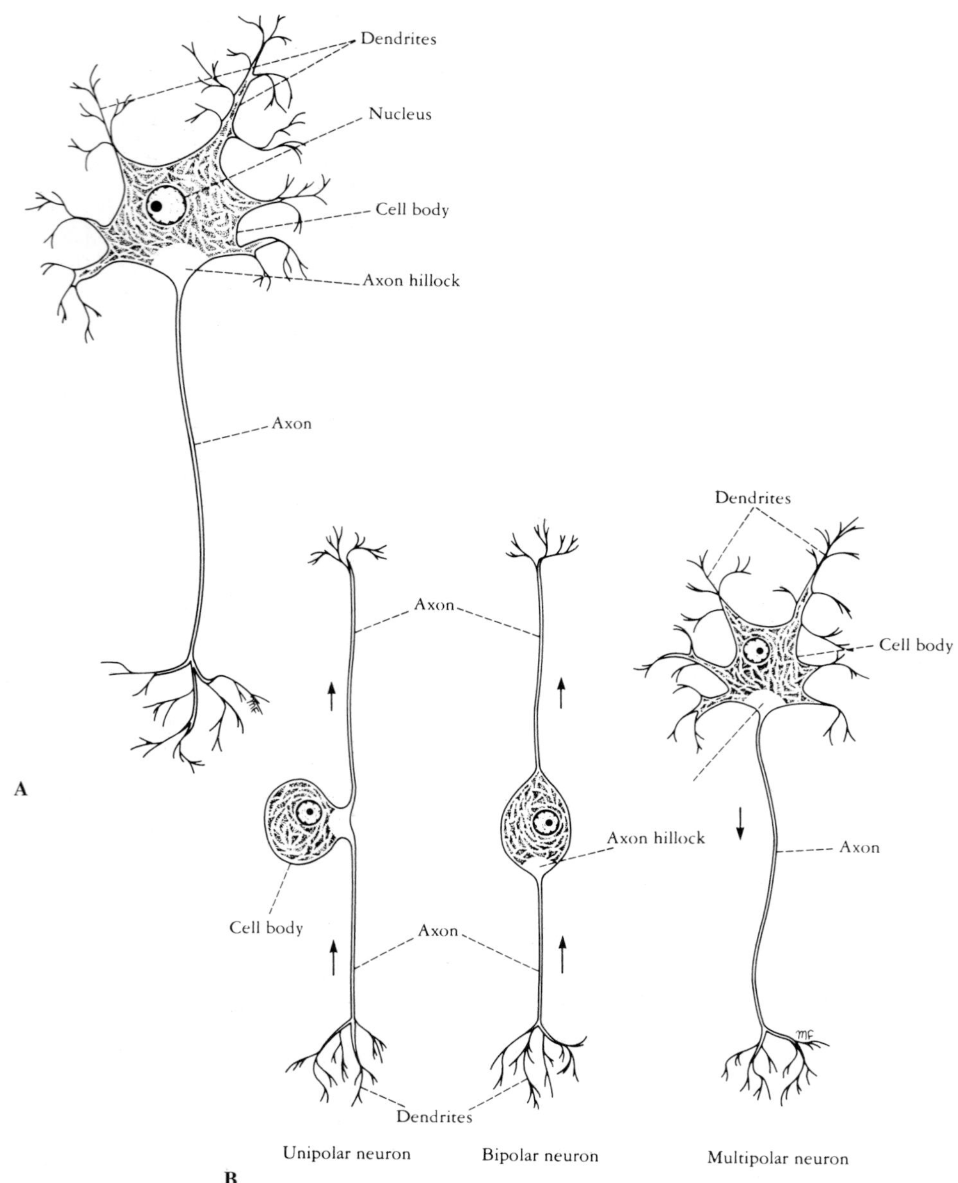

Figure 1–1 **A**. Neuron. **B**. Different types of neurons classified according to the number, length, and mode of branching of the neurites.

Neurofibrils

These are found running parallel to one another through the cell body and into the neurites. Each neurofibril consists of a bundle of microfilaments, each of which measures about 7 nm in diameter. The function of the filaments is not known, although the presence of actin and myosin within them would suggest that they may give contractile assistance to transport mechanisms.

Microtubules

These are found scattered in among the microfilaments and are found in the cell body and the neurites. Each tubule measures about 20 to 30 nm in diameter. Microtubules are thought to transport substances from one part of the neuron to another with the assistance of the microfilaments. A ratchet mechanism, consisting of proteins projecting out from the tubules, assisted by the contracting microfilaments, is thought to transport substances to and from the cell body.

Lysosomes

These are membrane-bound vesicles measuring about 8 nm in diameter. They are formed from the Golgi apparatus and serve as intracellular scavengers. They contain hydrolytic enzymes. Lysosomes exist in three forms: (1) **primary lysosomes,** which have just been formed; (2) **secondary lysosomes**, which contain partially digested material (**myelin**

Table 1–2 Summary of the Main Structures in a Nerve Cell Body

Structure	Shape	Appearance	Location	Function
Nucleus	Large, rounded	Pale, chromatin widely scattered; single prominent nucleolus; Barr body present in female	Centrally placed; displaced to periphery in cell injury	Controls cell activity
Cytoplasmic organelles				
Nissl substance	Granules of rough endoplasmic reticulum	Broad cisternae; ribosomes are basophilic	Throughout cytoplasm and proximal part of dendrites; absent from axon hillock and axon; fatigue and injury result in concentration at periphery	Synthesis of protein
Golgi apparatus	Wavy threads; clusters of flattened cisternae and small vesicles	Smooth endoplasmic reticulum	Close to the nucleus	Adds carbohydrate to protein molecule; packages products for transport to nerve terminals; forms cell membranes
Mitochondria	Spherical, rod-shaped	Double membrane with cristae	Scattered	Formation of chemical energy
Neurofibrils	Linear fibrils	Run parallel to each other; composed of bundles of microfilaments each 7 nm in diameter	Run from dendrites through cell body to axon	Assist in cell transport
Microtubules	Linear tubes	Run between neurofibrils; 20–30 nm in diameter	Run from dendrites through cell body to axon	Cell transport
Lysosomes	Vesicles	8 nm in diameter; three forms: primary, secondary, and residual bodies	Throughout cell	Cell scavengers
Centrioles	Paired hollow cylinders	Wall made up of bundles of microtubules	Confined to cytoplasm of cell body	Take part in cell division; maintain microtubules
Lipofuscin	Granules	Yellow, brown	Scattered through cytoplasm	Metabolic by-product
Melanin	Granules	Yellow, brown	Substantia nigra of midbrain	Related to formation of dopa

figures); and (3) **residual bodies**, in which the enzymes are inactive and which have evolved from secondary lysosomes.

Centrosome

This is found in immature nerve cells that are undergoing cell division. Occasionally they are found in mature nerve cells where their function may be associated with the formation of microtubules.

Lipofuscin

This is a yellowish-brown pigment found in the cytoplasm. It is a metabolic by-product that accumulates with age.

Melanin Granules

These are found in the cytoplasm of nerve cells in the substantia nigra of the midbrain. They may be associated with the catecholamine-synthesizing function of these cells.

Glycogen

This carbohydrate is seen as electron-dense rosettes in the cytoplasm and serves as a source of energy.

Lipid

This occurs as droplets in the cytoplasm and is a source of energy.

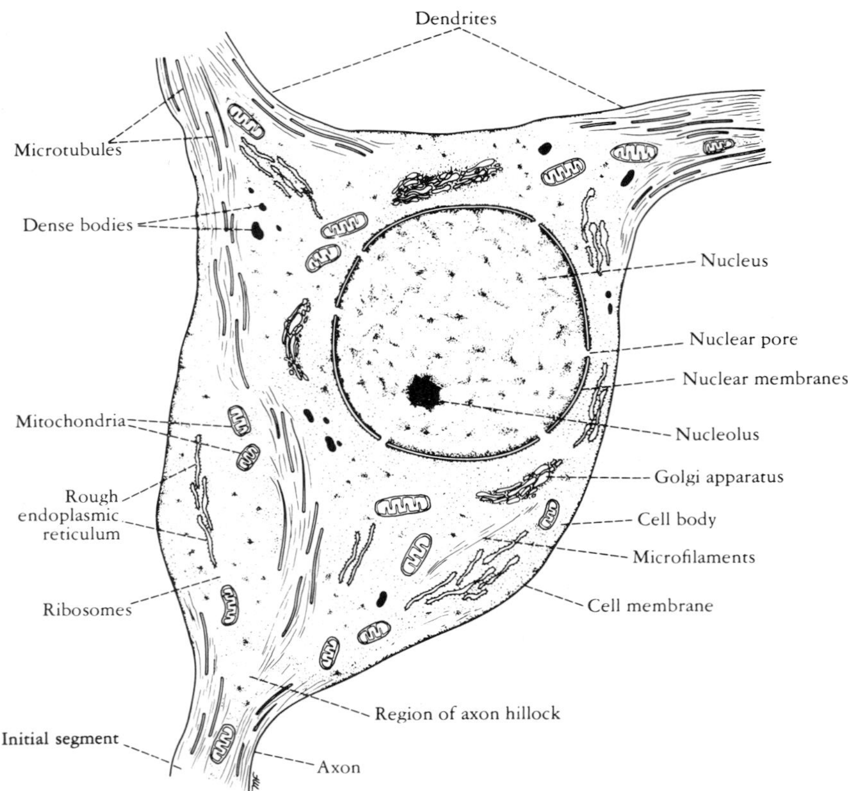

Figure 1–2 Fine structure of a neuron cell body.

Plasma Membrane

The plasma membrane is about 8 nm thick and separates the cytoplasm from the exterior. It is composed of an inner and outer layer of protein molecules, separated by a middle layer of lipid. Certain protein molecules lie within the lipid layer spanning its entire width. The molecules provide the membrane with hydrophilic channels through which inorganic ions may enter and leave the cell. Carbohydrate molecules are attached to the outside of the plasma membrane forming the cell coat, or **glycocalyx**.

The plasma membrane forms a semipermeable membrane that allows diffusion of certain ions through it, but restricts others. In the resting state (unstimulated state) the K^+ ions diffuse through the plasma membrane from the cell cytoplasm to the tissue fluid (Fig. 1-3). The permeability of the membrane to K^+ ions is much greater than the permeability to Na^+ ions, so that the passive efflux of K^+ is much greater than the influx of Na^+. This results in a steady potential difference of about −80 mV, which can be measured across the plasma membrane since the inside of the membrane is negative with respect to the outside. This potential is known as the **resting potential**.

Excitation of the Plasma Membrane of the Nerve Cell Body

Stimulation of a nerve cell by electrical, mechanical, or chemical means produces a rapid change in membrane permeability to Na^+ ions, which diffuse through the plasma membrane into the cell cytoplasm from the tissue fluid (Fig. 1-3). This results in the membrane becoming progressively depolarized. The sudden influx of Na^+ ions followed by the altered polarity produces the so-called **action potential**, which is approximately +40 mV. This potential is, however, very brief, lasting about 5 msec, for very quickly the increased membrane permeability for Na^+ ions ceases and that for K^+ ions increases, so that the K^+ ions start to flow from the cell cytoplasm and so return the localized area of the cell to the resting state.

Once generated, the action potential spreads over the plasma membrane, away from the site of initiation, and is conducted along the axon as the **nerve impulse**. This impulse is self-propagated, and its size and frequency do not alter (Fig. 1-6). Once the nerve impulse has spread over a given region of plasma membrane, another action potential cannot be elicited immediately. The duration of this nonexcitable state is referred to as the **refractory period**.

The greater the strength of the initial stimulus, the larger will be the initial depolarization and the greater the spread into the surrounding areas of the plasma membrane. If multiple excitatory stimuli are applied to the surface of a neuron, then the effect can be summated. For example, subthreshold stimuli may pass over the surface of the cell body and be **summated** at the root of the axon and so initiate an action potential.

Inhibitory stimuli are believed to produce their effect by causing an influx of Cl^- ions through the plasma membrane into the neuron, thus producing hyperpolarization and reducing the excitatory state of the cell.

Nerve Cell Processes

Nerve cell processes or neurites can be divided into dendrites and an axon (Fig. 1-2).

DENDRITES

These are the short processes of the cell body and are extensions of the cell body to increase the surface area for the reception of axons from other neurons. They conduct the nerve impulse toward the cell body. Dendrites often branch extensively, and in some neurons the smaller branches bear projections called **dendritic spines**.

AXON

This is the name of the longest process of the cell body. It arises from the axon hillock. It has a smooth surface and is uniform in diameter. Axons may be very short, as in many neurons of the central nervous system, or very long, as in peripheral nerves. The diameter of axons varies with different neurons. The plasmalemma bounding the axon is called the **axolemma**. The cytoplasm of the axon is called the **axoplasm**. The axoplasm possesses no Nissl substance or Golgi apparatus. Just before their termination, axons often branch extensively. The distal ends of the branches are commonly enlarged and are called **terminals or boutons terminaux**.

The **initial segment** of the axon is the first 50 to 100 µm after it leaves the axon hillock of the nerve cell body (Fig. 1-2). This is the most excitable part of the axon and is the site at which an action potential originates. It is important to remember that under normal conditions an action potential does not originate on the plasma membrane of the cell body, but always at the initial segment.

An axon always conducts impulses away from the cell body. The axons of sensory posterior root ganglion cells are an exception; here the long neurite, which is indistinguishable from an axon, carries the impulse toward the cell body (see unipolar neurons, p. 2).

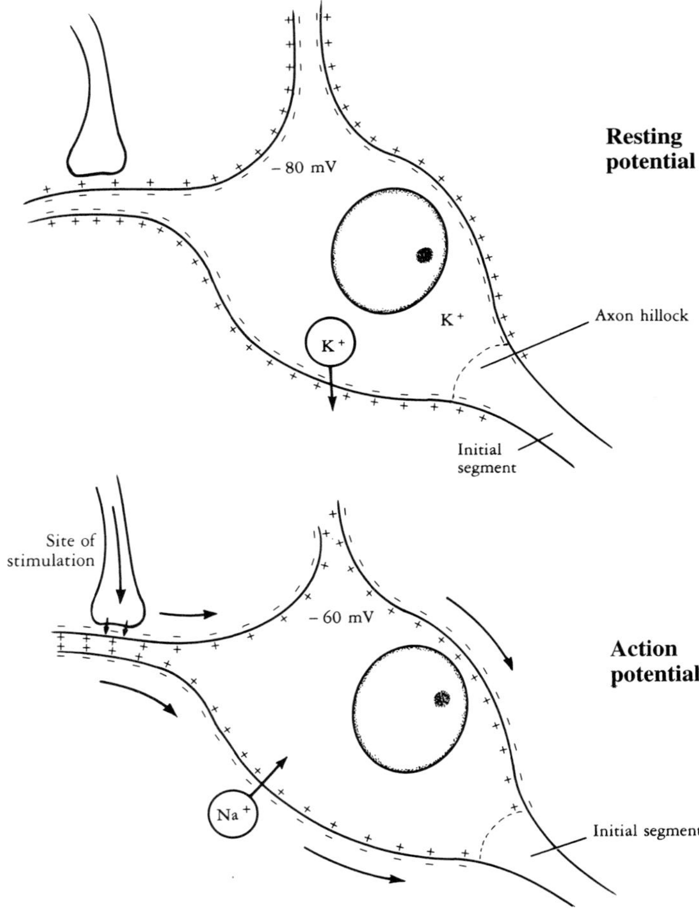

Figure 1–3 Creation of the action potential by the arrival of a stimulus from a single presynaptic terminal. Note that the action potential generated at the initial segment will only occur if the threshold for excitation is reached at the initial segment.

Axon Transport

Materials are transported from the cell body to the axon terminals by a process called **anterograde transport**, and to a lesser extent in the opposite direction, a process called **retrograde transport.**

Fast anterograde transport of 100 to 400 mm per day refers to the transport of proteins and neurotransmitter substances or their precursors. **Slow anterograde transport** of 1 to 3 mm per day refers to the transport of axoplasm and includes microfilaments and microtubules.

Retrograde transport explains how the cell bodies of nerve cells respond to changes in the distal end of the axons. Pinocytotic vesicles arising at the axon terminals can be returned quickly to the cell body. Worn-out mitochondria are returned to the cell body for breakdown by the lysosomes.

The microtubules and the microfilaments of the axoplasm are involved in the transport mechanism (see p. 4).

STRUCTURE AND FUNCTION OF SYNAPSES

The nervous system consists of a large number of neurons that are linked together to form functional conducting pathways. The site where two neurons come into close proximity and functional interneuronal communication occurs is called a **synapse.** The definition has also come to include the site where a neuron comes into close proximity with a skeletal muscle cell and where communication occurs.

The most common synapse is that which occurs between an axon of one neuron and the dendrite or cell body of a second neuron. The axon may have a terminal expansion (bouton terminaux) or a series of expansions (bouton de passage) so that the axon makes several contacts as it passes through the dendritic tree. In other types, the axon synapses on the proximal segment (initial segment) of another axon, or there may be synapses between terminal expansions from different neurons. Depending on the site of the synapse, they are called **axodendritic, axosomatic,** or **axoaxonic**.

Synapses are of two types: chemical and electrical. Most synapses are chemical, in which a chemical substance, the **neurotransmitter**, passes across the narrow space between the cells and becomes attached to a protein molecule in the postsynaptic membrane called the **receptor**.

It is now recognized that in most chemical synapses there are several neurotransmitters. One neurotransmitter is usually the principal activator and acts directly on the postsynaptic membrane, while the other transmitters function as modulators and modify the activity of the principal transmitter.

Chemical Synapses

ULTRASTRUCTURE OF CHEMICAL SYNAPSES

The apposed surfaces of the terminal axonal expansion and the neuron are termed the **presynaptic** and **postsynaptic membranes**, respectively, and are separated by a **synaptic cleft** 20 nm wide. The presynaptic and postsynaptic membranes are thickened, and the underlying cytoplasm shows increased density. On the presynaptic side, the dense cytoplasm is broken up into groups, and on the postsynaptic side, the density often extends into a **subsynaptic web**. Close to the presynaptic membrane are presynaptic vesicles, mitochondria, and lysosomes in the cytoplasm. On the postsynaptic side of the synapse, the cytoplasm often contains parallel cisternae.

The presynaptic terminal contains many small presynaptic vesicles that contain the neurotransmitter(s). The vesicles fuse with the presynaptic membrane and discharge the neurotransmitter(s) into the synaptic cleft by a process of exocytosis.

NEUROTRANSMITTERS AT CHEMICAL SYNAPSES

The presynaptic vesicles and the mitochondria play a key role in the release of neurotransmitter substances. The vesicles contain the neurotransmitter substance that is released into the synaptic cleft, and the mitochondria provide adenosine triphosphate (ATP) for the synthesis of new transmitter substance.

The majority of neurons produce and release only one principal transmitter at all their nerve endings. For example, acetylcholine is widely used as a transmitter by different neurons in the central and peripheral parts of the nervous system, whereas dopamine is released by neurons in the substantia nigra. Glycine, another transmitter, is found principally in synapses in the spinal cord.

The following are chemical substances known to act as neurotransmitters and there are probably many more yet to be discovered: acetylcholine, norepinephrine, epinephrine, dopamine, glycine, serotonin, gamma-aminobutyric acid (GABA), enkephalins, substance P, and glutamic acid.

Action of Neurotransmitters

All neurotransmitters are released from their nerve endings by the arrival of the nerve impulse (action potential). This results in an influx of calcium ions, which causes the synaptic vesicles to fuse with the presynaptic membrane. The neurotransmitters are then ejected into the synaptic cleft. Once in the cleft they achieve their objective by raising or lowering the resting potential of the postsynaptic membrane for a brief period.

The receptor proteins on the postsynaptic membrane bind the transmitter substance and undergo an immediate conformational change that opens the ion channel, generating an immediate but brief excitatory postsynaptic potential (EPSP) or an inhibitory postsynaptic potential (IPSP). Examples of this type of excitation are seen with acetylcholine (nicotinic) and L-glutamate or examples of inhibition with GABA (Table 1-3). Other receptor proteins bind the transmitter substance and activate a second messenger system, usually through a molecular transducer, a G-protein. These receptors have a longer latent period and the response may last several minutes or longer. Acetylcholine (muscarinic), serotonin, histamine, neuropeptides, and adenosine are good examples of this type of transmitter (these types of transmitters are often referred to as **neuromodulators,** see below).

Table 1–3 Examples of Principal Neurotransmitters and Neuromodulators

Chemical Mediator	Function	Receptor Mechanism	Ionic Mechanism	Examples	Location
Principal neurotransmitter	Rapid excitation or rapid inhibition	Opens ion channel	Opens cation channel for Na (fast EPSP) or opens anion channel for Cl (fast IPSP)	Acetylcholine (nicotinic), GABA, L-glutamate	Main sensory and motor systems
Neuromodulator	Modulation and modification of activity of postsynaptic neuron	G-protein coupled receptors	Opens or closes K or Ca channels (slow IPSP and slow EPSP)	Acetylcholine (muscarinic), GABA, L-glutamate	

EPSP = excitatory postsynaptic potential; IPSP = inhibitory postsynaptic potential; GABA = gamma-aminobutyric acid.

The excitatory and inhibitory effects on the postsynaptic membrane of the neuron depend on the summation of the postsynaptic responses at the different synapses. If the overall effect is one of depolarization, the neuron will be excited and an action potential will be initiated at the initial segment of the axon and a nerve impulse will travel along the axon. If, on the other hand, the overall effect is one of hyperpolarization, the neuron will be inhibited and no nerve impulse will arise.

Distribution of Neurotransmitters

The distribution of the neurotransmitters varies in different parts of the nervous system. For example, **acetylcholine** is found at the neuromuscular junction (see p. 50), in autonomic ganglia, and at parasympathetic nerve endings. In the central nervous system, the motor neuron collaterals to the Renshaw cells are cholinergic. In the hippocampus, the ascending reticular pathways, and the afferent fibers for the visual and auditory systems, the neurotransmitters are also cholinergic.

Norepinephrine is found at sympathetic nerve endings. In the central nervous system, it is found in high concentration in the hypothalamus. **Dopamine** is found in high concentration in different parts of the central nervous system, for example, in the basal ganglia.

Fate of Neurotransmitters

The effect produced by a neurotransmitter is limited by its destruction or reabsorption. For example, the effect of acetylcholine is limited by its destruction in the synaptic cleft by the enzyme **acetylcholinesterase (AChE).** However, with the **catecholamines** the effect is limited by the return of the transmitter to the presynaptic nerve ending.

NEUROMODULATORS AT CHEMICAL SYNAPSES

In many synapses, certain substances other than the principal neurotransmitters are ejected from the presynaptic membrane into the synaptic cleft. These are capable of modulating and modifying the activity of the postsynaptic neuron and are called **neuromodulators**.

Action of Neuromodulators

One neuromodulator or more may coexist with the principal neurotransmitter at a single synapse. Usually, the neuromodulators are in separate presynaptic vesicles, but this is not always the case. Whereas the principal neurotransmitters, when released into the synaptic cleft, have a rapid, brief effect on the postsynaptic membrane, the neuromodulators on release into the cleft do not have a direct effect on the postsynaptic membrane. Rather they enhance, prolong, inhibit, or limit the effect of the principal neurotransmitter on the postsynaptic membrane. The neuromodulator acts through a second messenger system, usually through a molecular transducer, a G-protein, and alters the response of the receptor to the neurotransmitter. In a given area of the nervous system, many different afferent neurons may release several different neuromodulators that are picked up by the postsynaptic neuron. Such an arrangement can lead to a wide variety of responses depending on the input from the afferent neurons.

Electrical Synapses

Most synapses in the nervous system are chemical. Electrical synapses are gap junctions that contain channels extending from the cytoplasm of the presynaptic neuron to that of the postsynaptic neuron. There is no chemical transmitter, and the neurons communicate electrically. The bridging channels permit the flow of ionic current from one cell to the other with the minimum of delay. In electrical synapses the rapid spread of activity from one neuron to another ensures that a group of neurons performing an identical function act together. Electrical synapses also have the advantage that they are bidirectional, which the chemical synapses are not.

STRUCTURE AND FUNCTION OF NERVE FIBERS

A nerve fiber is an axon (or a dendrite) of a nerve cell. Two types of nerve fibers exist in the central and peripheral parts of the nervous system: myelinated and nonmyelinated fibers.

Myelinated Nerve Fibers

A myelinated nerve fiber is one that is surrounded by a myelin sheath (Fig. 1-4). The myelin sheath is not part of the neuron but is formed by a supporting cell. The supporting cell in the central nervous system is the oligodendrocyte and in the peripheral nervous system is the Schwann cell.

The myelin sheath is segmented, the segments being separated at regular intervals by the nodes of Ranvier. In the central nervous system, each oligodendrocyte can form and maintain myelin sheaths for as many as 60 nerve fibers (axons). In the peripheral nervous system, there is only one Schwann cell for each segment of a single nerve fiber.

Myelination of Peripheral Nerve Fibers

This process begins during late fetal development and during the first postnatal year. The nerve fiber first grooves the side of a Schwann cell and then sinks further into the cell. In this manner the plasma membrane of the Schwann cell forms a **mesaxon**, which suspends the axon within the cell. The Schwann cell now rotates on the axon so that the plasma membrane becomes wrapped repeatedly around the axon in a spiral. The cytoplasm recedes from the spirals into the Schwann cell body, and the cytoplasmic surfaces of the plasma membrane in the elongating mesaxon come into apposition to form the **major dense lines** seen on

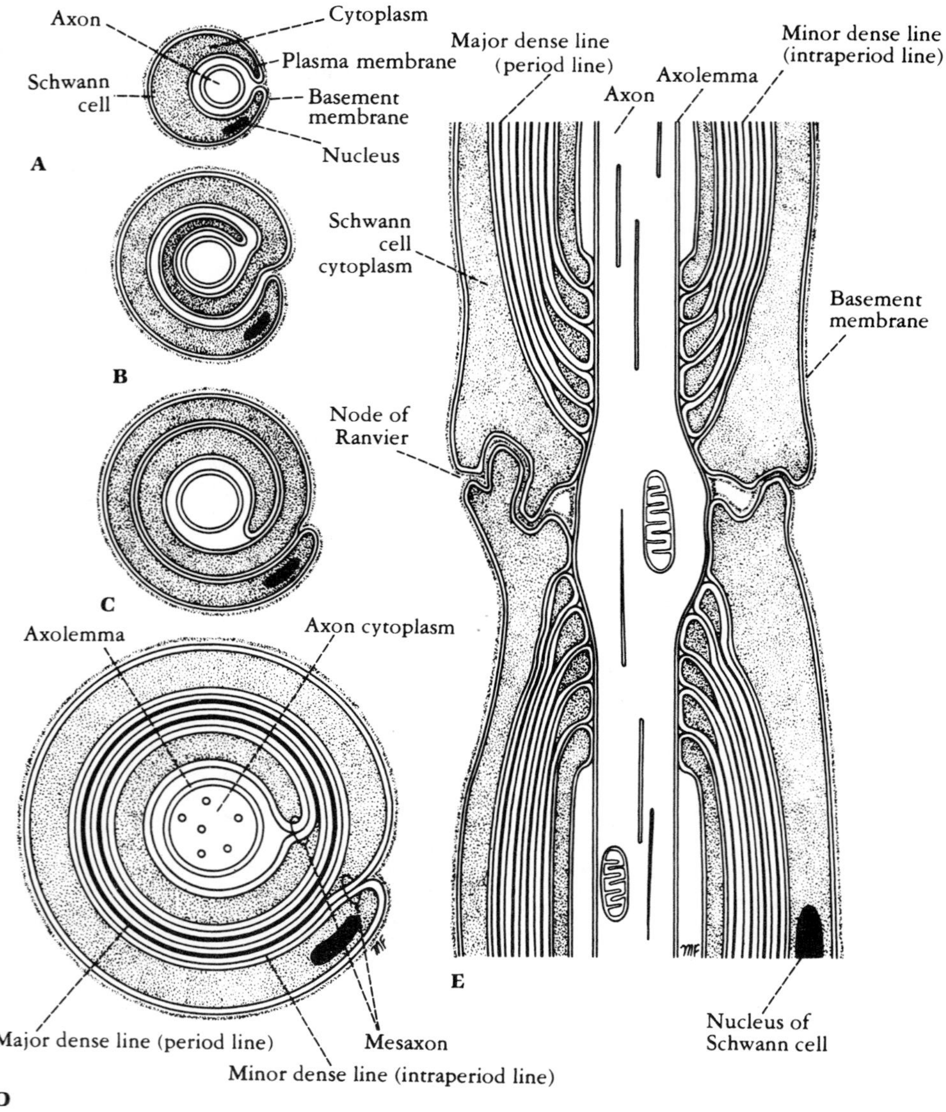

Figure 1–4 **A–D.** Cross sections of a myelinated nerve fiber showing the different stages in the formation of myelin. **E.** Longitudinal section of a mature myelinated nerve fiber showing a node of Ranvier.

electron micrographs of transverse sections. The external surfaces of the plasma membrane of the mesaxon also come together to form the **minor dense lines**. The fused outer protein layers of the outer plasma membranes form a thin **intraperiod line**. At the node of Ranvier, two adjacent Schwann cells terminate and the plasma membrane of the axon is exposed.

Myelination of Central Nerve Fibers

Myelination begins during late fetal development and the process continues after birth. The pyramidal tracts and the fasciculus gracilis and fasciculus cuneatus, for example, are not completely myelinated at birth.

The plasma membrane of the oligodendrocyte becomes wrapped around the axon to form the myelin (Fig. 1-5). The nodes of Ranvier are situated in the intervals between adjacent oligodendrocytes. A single oligodendrocyte may be connected to the myelin sheaths of as many as 60 nerve fibers. It is believed that myelination in the central nervous system takes place by the growth in length of the process of the oligodendrocyte, the process wrapping itself around the axon.

Nonmyelinated Peripheral Nerve Fibers

These are usually small-diameter nerve fibers (less than 1 mm in diameter). Each axon indents the plasma membrane of the Schwann cell so that it lies within a trough. Fifteen or more axons may lie within their own troughs on a single Schwann cell; sometimes an axon will share a trough. In some Schwann cells the troughs may be deep so that a mesaxon is formed from the Schwann cell plasma membrane. The Schwann cells lie close to one another along the length of the axons and there are no nodes of Ranvier. In regions where there are synapses or where transmission occurs, the axon emerges from the trough of the Schwann cell, thus exposing the axon.

Nonmyelinated Central Nerve Fibers

These fibers run in small groups and are not particularly related to the oligodendrocytes.

Conduction in Nerve Fibers

In the resting unstimulated state, a nerve fiber is polarized so that the interior is negative to the exterior. The potential difference across the axolemma is about −80 mV and is called the **resting membrane potential**. As explained previously, this so-called resting potential is produced by the diffusion of sodium and potassium ions through the plasma membrane and is maintained by the sodium-potassium pump. The pump involves active transport across the membrane and requires ATP to provide the energy.

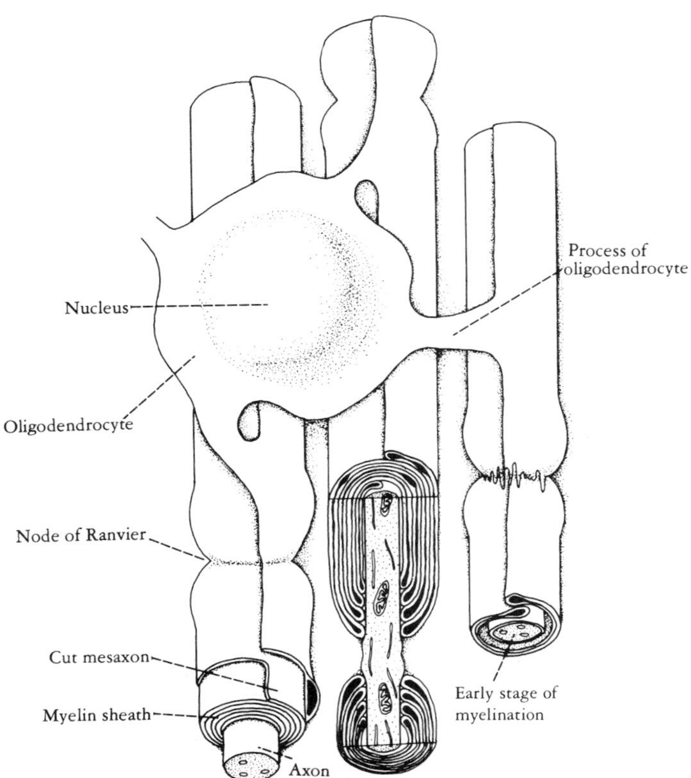

Figure 1–5 Oligodendrocyte and myelinated nerve fibers in the central nervous system.

A nerve impulse (action potential) is initiated at the initial segment of the axon. A nerve impulse is a self-propagating wave of electrical negativity that passes along the surface of the plasma membrane (axolemma). The wave of electrical negativity is initiated by an adequate stimulus being applied to the surface of the neuron. Under normal circumstances this occurs at the initial segment of the axon, which is the most sensitive part of the neuron. The stimulus alters the permeability of the membrane to Na^+ ions at the point of stimulation. Now Na^+ ions rapidly enter the axon (Fig. 1-6). The positive ions outside the axolemma quickly decrease to zero. The membrane potential therefore is reduced to zero and is **depolarized**. A typical resting potential is −80 mV, with the outside of the membrane positive to the inside; the action potential is about +40 mV, with the outside of the membrane negative to the inside.

The negatively charged point on the outside of the axolemma now acts as a stimulus to the adjacent positively charged axolemma, and in less than 1 msec the polarity of the adjacent resting potential is reversed (Fig. 1-6). The action potential now has moved along the axolemma from the point originally stimulated to the adjacent point on the membrane. It is in this manner that the action potential travels along the full length of a nerve fiber.

As the action potential moves along the nerve fiber, the entry of the Na^+ ions into the axon ceases and the permeability of the axolemma to K^+ ions increases. Now K^+ ions rapidly diffuse outside the axon (since the concentration is

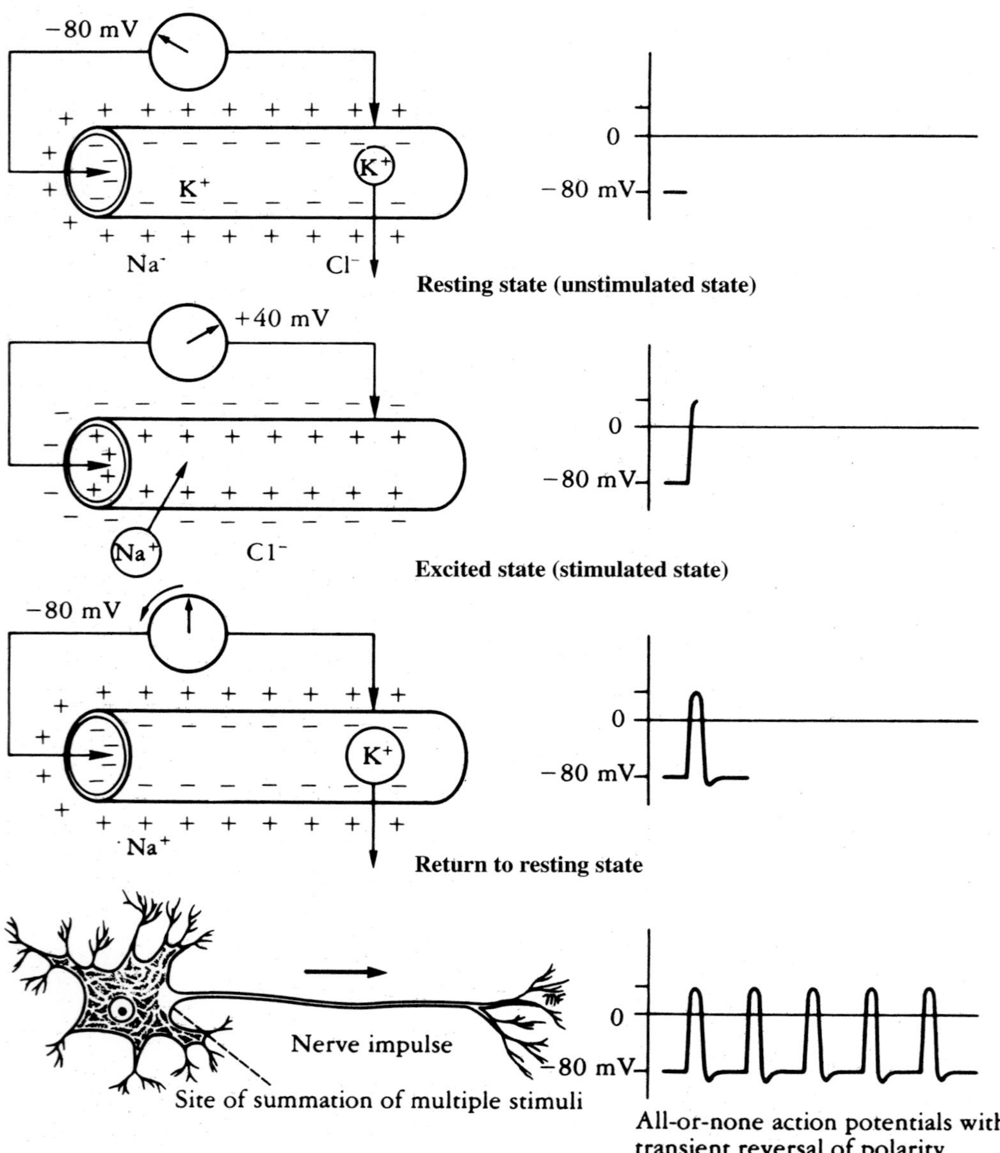

Figure 1–6 Ionic and electrical changes that occur in a nerve fiber when it is stimulated.

much higher within the axon than outside) so that the original resting membrane potential is restored. The permeability of the axolemma now decreases and the status quo is restored by the active transport of the Na^+ ions out of the axon and the K^+ ions into the axon. The outer surface of the axolemma is again electrically positive compared to the inner surface.

For a short time after the passage of a nerve impulse along a nerve fiber, while the axolemma is still depolarized, a second stimulus, however strong, is unable to excite the nerve. This period of time is known as the **absolute refractory period**. This period is followed by a further short interval during which the excitability of the nerve gradually returns to normal. This latter period is called the **relative refractory period**. It is clear from this that the refractory period makes a continuous excitatory state of the nerve impossible and it limits the frequency of the impulses.

Sodium and Potassium Channels

The so-called sodium channels and potassium channels through which physiologists believe the sodium and potassium ions diffuse through the plasma membrane have not been identified. Some of the protein molecules that extend through the full thickness of the plasma membrane may serve as channels. Each channel is thought to be controlled by an electrically charged gate that can open or close the channel.

In the nonstimulated state, the gates of the potassium channels are wider open than those of the sodium channels, which are nearly closed. This allows the potassium ions to diffuse out more readily than the sodium ions can diffuse in. In the stimulated state, the gates of the sodium channels are at first wide open; then the gates of the potassium channels are opened and the gates of the sodium channels are nearly closed again. It is thus seen that it is the opening and closing of the sodium and potassium channels that is thought to produce the depolarization and repolarization of the plasma membrane.

The absolute refractory period, which occurs at the onset of the action potential when a second stimulus is unable to produce a further electrical change, is thought to be due to the inability to get the sodium channels open. During the relative refractory period, when a very strong stimulus can produce an action potential, presumably the sodium channels are opened.

Conduction Velocity in Nerve Fibers

The conduction velocity of an axon is much greater in large-diameter axons than in small-diameter axons. In nonmyelinated axons, the action potential passes continuously along the axolemma, progressively exciting neighboring areas of membrane (Fig. 1-7). In myelinated axons, the presence of a myelin sheath serves as a perfect insulator and prevents the flow of ions to any extent. However, at the nodes of Ranvier there is no myelin, and ionic flow is possible. Consequently, in a myelinated axon, the action potential is conducted from node to node, i.e., it jumps from node to node, a process called **saltatory conduction** (Fig. 1-7).

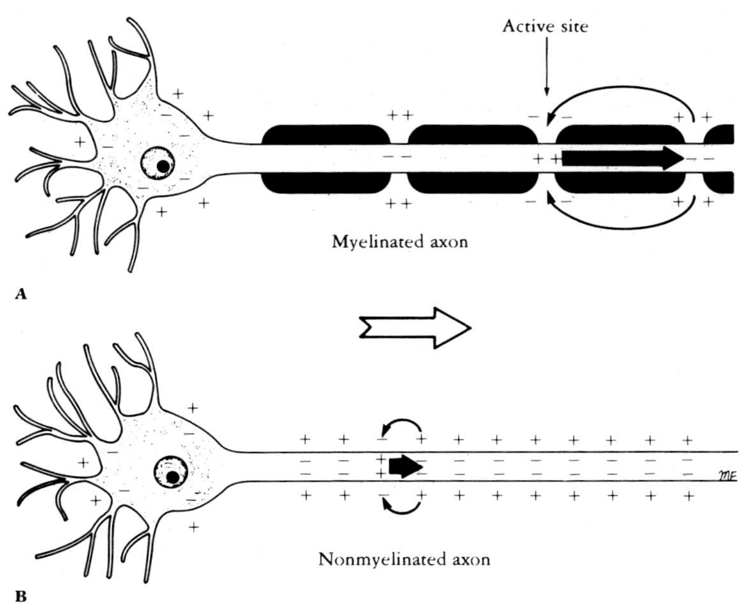

Figure 1–7 **A.** Stimulated myelinated axon (saltatory conduction). **B.** Stimulated nonmyelinated axon.

The action potential at one node sets up a current in the surrounding tissue fluid that quickly produces depolarization at the next node. This jumping of the depolarization process along the length of the axon in myelinated fibers is a much more rapid mechanism than is found in nonmyelinated fibers. Furthermore, since the ionic exchange across the axolemma is practically restricted to the nodes, less energy is required to conduct the nerve impulse.

The conduction velocity in large myelinated fibers may be as high as 120 meters per second and as small as 0.5 meter per second in small unmyelinated fibers.

Clinical Notes

Reaction of a Neuron to Injury

The first reaction of a nerve cell to injury is loss of function. Whether the cell recovers or dies will depend on the severity and duration of the damaging agent. If death occurs quickly, from lack of oxygen, no morphological changes will be immediately apparent. Morphological evidence of cell injury requires a minimum of 6–12 hours of survival. The nerve cell becomes swollen and rounded off, the nucleus swells and is displaced toward the periphery of the cell, and the Nissl granules become dispersed toward the periphery of the cytoplasm. At this stage the neuron could recover. If the kind of neuronal injury were not so severe as to cause death, the reparative changes would start to appear. The cell would resume its former size and shape, the nucleus would return to the center of the cell body, and the Nissl granules would take up their normal position.

Tumors of Neurons

When considering tumors of the nervous system, one must not forget that the nervous system is made up of many different types of tissues. In the central nervous system there are neurons, neuroglia, blood vessels, and meninges and in the peripheral nervous system there are neurons, Schwann cells, connective tissue, and blood vessels. Tumors of neurons in the central nervous system are rare but tumors of peripheral neurons are not uncommon.

Synaptic Blocking Agents

Ganglionic blocking agents may be divided into three groups, depending on their mechanism of action. The first group of agents, which include the **hexamethonium** and **tetraethylammonium salts**, resemble acetylcholine at the postsynaptic membrane; they thus inhibit transmission across a synapse. The second group of agents, which include **nicotine,** have the same action as acetylcholine on the postsynaptic membrane but they are not destroyed by the cholinesterase. This results in a prolonged depolarization ot the postsynaptic membrane, so that it is insensitive to further stimulation by acetylcholine. Unfortunately, this depolarization block is associated with initial stimulation and therefore these drugs are not suitable for clinical use. The third group of agents, which include **procaine**, inhibit the release of acetylcholine from the preganglionic fibers.

In the central nervous system the motor neuron collaterals to the Renshaw cells have been shown to liberate acetylcholine at their endings. Many synapses in the central nervous system are also cholinergic. Cholinergic blocking agents used in the peripheral nervous system have little or no effect on the cholinergic synapses of the central nervous system because they are unable to cross the blood-brain barrier in significant concentrations. **Atropine, scopolamine,** and **diisopropylphosphorofluoridate (DPF)** can effectively cross the barrier and their effects on human behavior have been extensively studied. Similarly, it is believed that many psychotropic drugs bring about changes in the activities of the central nervous system by influencing the release of catecholamines at synaptic sites. The **phenothiazines,** for example, are thought to block dopamine receptors on postsynaptic neurons.

Action of Local Anesthetics on Nerve Conduction

When applied locally to a nerve fiber, local anesthetics block nerve conduction. They interfere with the transient increase in permeability of the axolemma to Na^+, K^+, and other ions. The sensitivity to local anesthetics is greatest in small nerve fibers; small fibers are also slower to recover.

Axonal Transport and the Spread of Disease

Rabies, which is an acute viral disease of the central nervous system, is transmitted by the bite of an infected animal. The virus travels to the central nervous system by way of axonal transport in both sensory and motor nerves.

Herpes simplex and **herpes zoster** are viral diseases that also spread by axonal transport to different parts of the body.

In **poliomyelitis**, axonal transport is believed to play a role in the spread of the virus from the gastrointestinal tract to the motor cells of the anterior gray horns of the spinal cord and the brainstem.

Blood Nerve Barrier

As in the central nervous system, the peripheral nerve fibers are protected by a blood-nerve barrier. This barrier occurs in the endoneurial capillary walls where the endothelial cells are nonfenestrated and are held together with tight junctions; the capillaries are also surrounded by a continuous basal lamina.

REVIEW QUESTIONS

Directions: Each of the numbered items in this section is followed by answers that are positively phrased. Select the ONE lettered answer that is an EXCEPTION.

1. The following statements concerning the nervous system are correct **except:**
   (a) The gray matter consists of nerve cells embedded in neuroglia
   (b) The white matter consists of nerve fibers embedded in neuroglia
   (c) Golgi type 11 neurons have short axons
   (d) Golgi type 1 neurons greatly outnumber Golgi type 11 neurons
   (e) The processes of a nerve cell body are called neurites
2. The following statements concerning the cytology of a nerve cell body are correct **except:**
   (a) The Nissl substance is composed of smooth-surfaced endoplasmic reticulum
   (b) The Nissl substance synthesizes protein
   (c) Melanin granules are found in the cytoplasm of nerve cells in the substantia nigra of the midbrain
   (d) Microtubules are thought to play a role in the transport of substances from one part of the neuron to another
   (e) Lipofuscin granules are found in some nerve cells in the elderly
3. The following statements concerning the nervous system are correct **except:**
   (a) An example of a unipolar neuron is seen in a posterior root ganglion
   (b) An example of a bipolar neuron is found in the sensory ganglion of the cochlear nerve
   (c) A dendrite conveys a nerve impulse toward the nerve cell body
   (d) The dendritic spines are small projections of the plasma membrane and are artifacts produced by the process of fixation of the neuron
   (e) Most dendrites narrow as they extend out from the nerve cell body
4. The following statements concerning neurobiology are correct **except:**
   (a) Microfilaments contain actin and myosin and probably assist in nerve cell transport
   (b) The volume of cytoplasm within the nerve cell body is often much less than that in the axon and dendrites
   (c) Mitochondria present in the axons provide ATP for the synthesis of transmitter substances
   (d) The subsynaptic web lies beneath the postsynaptic membrane
   (e) The synaptic cleft measures about 200 nm wide
5. The following statements concerning axons are correct **except:**
   (a) They may be extremely long compared to dendrites
   (b) When of large diameter they are myelinated
   (c) Recurrent collaterals do not function in feedback inhibition
   (d) The ending may be either a synapse or a motor end-plate
6. The following features concerning an axon are correct **except:**
   (a) Usually one per neuron
   (b) May be myelinated
   (c) Cylindrical in shape
   (d) Usually short with acute angle branching
   (e) Smooth contour without many synapses
7. The following statements concerning an axon are correct **except:**
   (a) The action potential is produced by the influx of Na^+ ions into the axoplasm
   (b) The initial segment of the axon is the first millimeter after it leaves the cell body
   (c) The spread of the action potential along the plasma membrane of the axon is known as the nerve impulse
   (d) The axon hillock is situated at the point where the axon leaves the cell body of the neuron
8. Axons can be traced along their pathways in the central nervous system by using methods that rely on the following facts **except:**
   (a) Retrograde transport of proteins
   (b) Degeneration of an axon cut off from the cell body of origin
   (c) Anterograde transport of newly synthesized proteins
   (d) The presence of Nissl substance in the axon
9. The following statements concerning the plasma membrane of a neuron are correct **except:**
   (a) The plasma membrane channels are protein molecules that extend through the full thickness of the membrane
   (b) The resting potential is brought about by the diffusion of sodium and potassium ions through the membrane
   (c) In the resting state, the resting potential is about –80 mV
   (d) In the resting state, the inside of the membrane is negative with respect to the outside
   (e) In the stimulated state the gates of the sodium channels are at first closed

Directions: Each of the incomplete statements in this section is followed by completions of the statement. Select the ONE lettered completion that is BEST in each case.

10. The large anterior horn cells of the spinal cord are:
    (a) upper motor neurons
    (b) inhibitory
    (c) Golgi type II
    (d) Alpha efferent
    (e) bipolar
11. The recycling of membranes of synaptic vesicles (that have released their neurotransmitter into the synaptic cleft) involves the:
    (a) breakdown of clear vesicles
    (b) presynaptic membrane
    (c) breakdown of coated vesicles
    (d) postsynaptic membrane

12. To qualify as a neurotransmitter, a substance:
    (a) must be an amino acid or a peptide
    (b) should have no method of inactivation or disposal
    (c) should reproduce the effect of neural presynaptic stimulation
    (d) must be shown to be synthesized outside the neuron
13. The release of a neurotransmitter involves:
    (a) the fusion of vesicles with the postsynaptic membrane
    (b) a decrease in the presynaptic permeability to Ca^{++}
    (c) the rupture of the vesicles within the axon
    (d) the piercing of the postsynaptic membrane by the vesicles
    (e) the arrival of an action potential at the axon terminal
14. In most typical synapses, many small vesicles containing neurotransmitter substances are found in the:
    (a) dendrite
    (b) soma of the neuron
    (c) bouton
    (d) axon
    (e) synaptic cleft
15. In a typical multipolar motor neuron, the part of the neuron providing the greatest surface area for synaptic reception is the:
    (a) axon
    (b) cell body
    (c) dendritic processes
    (d) all of the above
    (e) none of the above
16. The pyramidal tracts myelinate:
    (a) at the third month of fetal life
    (b) at puberty
    (c) at the sixth month of fetal life
    (d) at birth and the process is not complete until the second or third year
    (e) at the eighth month of fetal life
17. The major dense line in the myelin sheath of an axon is associated with the:
    (a) inner mesaxon
    (b) basal lamina
    (c) apposition of the outer cytoplasmic surface of the plasma membrane in the mesaxon
    (d) fusion of the inner cytoplasmic surface of the plasma membrane in the mesaxon
    (e) outer cytoplasmic layer of the plasma membrane
18. The interruption of the individual myelin sheath segments along a peripheral axon is called:
    (a) an ionic channel
    (b) a paranode region
    (c) a major dense line
    (d) a node of Ranvier
19. The larger the diameter of a myelinated axon the:
    (a) thinner is its axolemma
    (b) greater is its conduction velocity
    (c) greater is its sensitivity to local anesthetic blockade
    (d) greater is its sensitivity to painful stimulation of the skin

Directions: Read the case histories then answer the questions. You will be required to select ONE BEST lettered answer. A 25-year-old man severely lacerated his right index finger while sharpening a knife on a grinding machine. The laceration was sutured after a local anesthetic was used to completelly block conduction in the nerves supplying the finger.

20. Which of the following types of nerve fibers does the local anesthetic block **first?**
    (a) Large pain sensory fibers
    (b) Small, deep pain sensory fibers
    (c) Vibration sensory fibers
    (d) Sensory touch fibers
21. Which of the following nerve fibers recover first as the effect of the anesthetic wears off?
    (a) Alpha A fibers
    (b) C fibers
    (c) B fibers
    (d) Beta A fibers
    (e) Delta A fibers

A 12-year old girl was fondling a wild racoon in her garden and the animal bit her. The racoon was later found to be rabid.

22. By which of the following pathways is the virus transported from the bite to the central nervous system?
    (a) Lymphatic vessels
    (b) Bloodstream
    (c) Axonal transport in both sensory and motor nerves
    (d) Along the epineurium
    (e) Through the spaces of the endoneurium

ANSWERS AND EXPLANATIONS

1. D
2. A. Nissl substance is composed of rough-surfaced endoplasmic reticulum
3. D. Dendritic spines are structural projections of the plasma membrane of the dendrite and serve to increase the receptive area of the dendrite
4. E. The synaptic cleft measures about 20-30 nm wide
5. C. In certain areas of the central nervous system (e.g., the thalamus and cerebral cortex), recurrent collateral branches of an axon exert inhibitory influences on the neuron that gave rise to the axon.
6. D. Dendrites are usually short with acute angle branching.
7. B. The initial segment of the axon is restricted to the first 50 to 100 μm after it leaves the nerve cell body.

8. D. A. Retrograde transport of proteins. Horseradish peroxidase is injected into the region of the axon under investigation. The enzyme is absorbed into the axon and travels by retrograde transport to the cell body of the axon. B. An axon or a dendrite when cut off from its cell body undergoes degeneration and this process may be studied microscopically (see Chap. 3). C. Anterograde transport of newly synthesized proteins. A radioactively labelled amino acid is injected into the region of the nerve cell body. It becomes incorporated into the proteins within the cell body and is transported anterogradely to the axon terminals. D. Nissl granules are not present in the axon but are confined to the nerve cell body (except the area of the axon hillock) and the proximal parts of the dendrites.
9. E. In the stimulated state of a neuron, the gates of the sodium channels are wide open.
10. D. A. The large anterior horn cells of the spinal cord are lower motor neurons. B. They are not inhibitory. C. They are Golgi type I cells. E. They are multipolar.
11. B. A. The recycling of membranes of synaptic vesicles may involve the formation of clear presynaptic vesicles. C. The process may involve the formation of coated presynaptic vesicles. D. The process does not involve the postsynaptic membrane.
12. C. A. A neurotransmitter can be an amino acid, a peptide or an amine. Examples of an amine as a neurotransmitter are norepinephrine, epinephrine, dopamine, and serotonin. B. They must have a well defined method of inactivation or disposal. D. They should be shown to be synthesized within the neuron.
13. E. A. The release of neurotransmitters involves the fusion of the vesicles with the presynaptic membrane. B. An increase in the presynaptic permeability to Ca^{++}. C. A rupture of the presynaptic vesicles into the cleft of the synapse. D. The postsynaptic membrane is not pierced by the vesicles.
14. C
15. C. The dendritic processes and their spines provide an enormous surface area for synaptic contact.
16. D. The pyramidal tracts start to myelinate at birth and are not complete until the second or third year.
17. D. For details concerning the process of myelination, see pages 10 and 11.
18. D
19. B. The axolemma is of uniform thickness irrespective of the diameter of the axon; the larger the diameter of the axon, the less sensitive it is to local anesthetic agents; small-diameter nerve fibers (delta type A fibers) conduct painful impulses from the skin.
20. B. In a mixed peripheral nerve, the smallest-diameter nerve fibers are blocked first by the local anesthetic and the largest-diameter fibers are the last to be blocked.
21. A. In a mixed peripheral nerve, the largest-diameter nerve fibers are the first to recover from a local anesthetic and the smallest fibers are the last to recover. (See Table 4-1 for classification of nerve fibers.)
22. C

CHAPTER 2

Neurobiology of Neuroglia

CHAPTER OUTLINE

SUGGESTED PLAN FOR REVIEW OF CHAPTER 2

1. Understand that the neuroglial cells far outnumber the nerve cells in the central nervous system and that they provide support for the nerve cells.
2. Learn the structure and function of each of the four types of neuroglial cells and know where each type is located.
3. Understand the difference between active and inactive microglial cells.
4. Be able to define what is meant by ependymocytes, tanycytes, and choroidal epithelial cells.
5. Understand the extracellular space in the central nervous system and learn where it opens into.
6. Be able to define the blood-brain barrier.

INTRODUCTION

The neurons of the central nervous system are supported by nonexcitable cells called **neuroglial cells** (Fig. 2-1). Neuroglial cells are generally smaller than neurons and outnumber them 5 to 10 times. There are four types: (1) astrocytes, (2) oligodendrocytes, (3) microglia, and (4) ependyma.

ASTROCYTES

Astrocytes have small cell bodies with numerous branching processes. Many of the processes end as expansions on capillary blood vessels (perivascular feet), on ependymal cells, and on the pia mater. Large numbers of astrocytic processes are interwoven at the outer and inner surfaces of

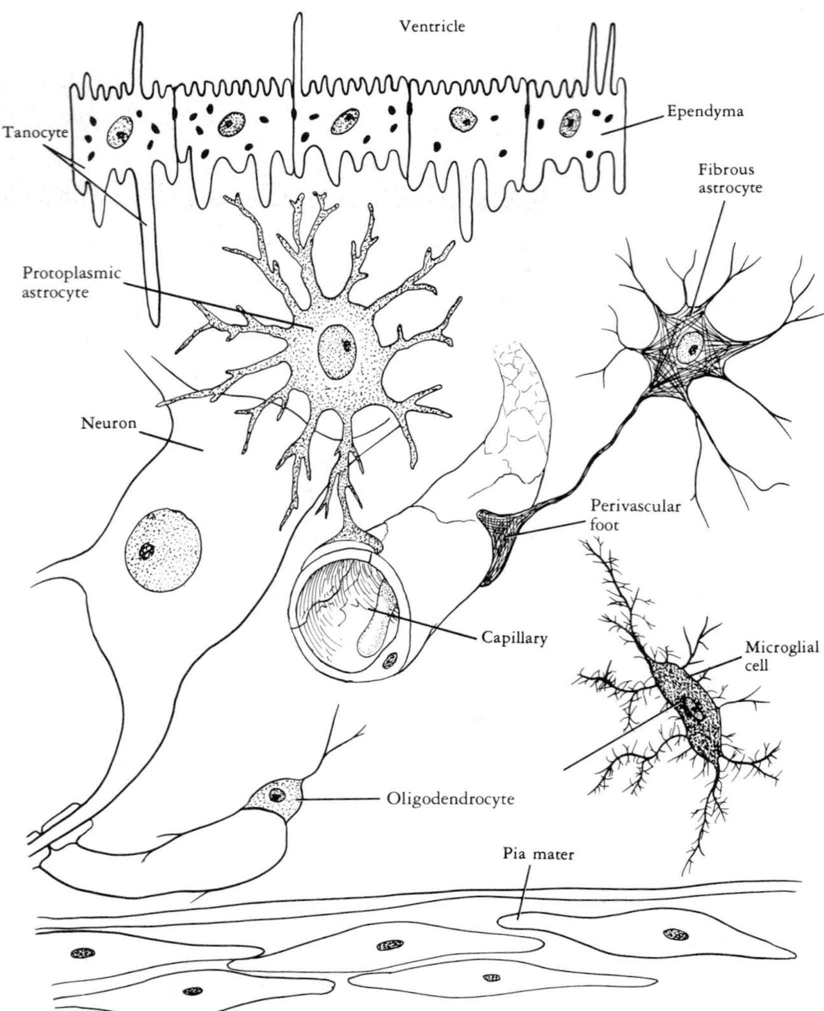

Figure 2–1 Different types of neuroglial cells.

the central nervous system, where they form the **outer** and **inner glial limiting membranes**. Thus the outer glial limiting membrane is found beneath the pia mater and the inner glial limiting membrane is situated beneath the ependyma lining the ventricles of the brain and the central canal of the spinal cord.

Large numbers of astrocytes are found around the initial segment of most axons and in the bare segments of axons at the nodes of Ranvier. Axon terminals at many sites are separated from other nerve cells and their processes by an envelope of astrocytic processes. Two types of astrocytes can be identified, fibrous and protoplasmic.

Fibrous astrocytes are found mainly in the white matter where their long processes pass between the nerve fibers. The cell bodies and their processes contain many filaments in their cytoplasm.

Protoplasmic astrocytes are found mainly in the gray matter where their short branching processes pass between the nerve cell bodies. The cytoplasm of these cells contains fewer filaments than that of the fibrous astrocytes.

Functions of Astrocytes

1. They form a supporting framework for the neurons, and in the embryo they serve as a scaffolding for the migration of immature neurons.
2. They cover the synaptic contacts between neurons and may serve as insulators preventing axon terminals from influencing neighboring and unrelated neurons.
3. They absorb glutamate and gamma-aminobutyric acid (GABA) secreted by the nerve terminals, thus limiting the influence of these neurotransmitters.
4. They absorb excess K + ions in the extracellular fluid.
5. They store glycogen within their cytoplasm. The glycogen can be broken down into glucose and released to surrounding neurons in response to norepinephrine.

6. They serve as phagocytes by taking up degenerating synaptic axon terminals.
7. Following the death of neurons due to disease, they proliferate and fill in the spaces previously occupied by the neurons, a process called **replacement gliosis**.
8. Metabolites may be transported from blood capillaries by the astrocytes to the neurons through their perivascular feet. The fact that astrocytes are linked together by gap junctions would enable ions to pass from one cell to another without entering the extracellular space.
9. They may produce substances that have a trophic influence on neighboring neurons.

OLIGODENDROCYTES

Oligodendrocytes have small cell bodies and a few delicate processes; there are no filaments in their cytoplasm. Oligodendrocytes are found in rows along myelinated nerve fibers and surround nerve cell bodies. The processes of a single oligodendrocyte join the myelin sheaths of several more fibers. However, only one process joins the myelin between two adjacent nodes of Ranvier. Unlike Schwann cells in the peripheral nervous system, oligodendrocytes and their associated axons are not surrounded by a basement membrane.

Functions of Oligodendrocytes

1. They are responsible for the formation of the myelin sheath of nerve fibers in the central nervous system, much as the myelin of peripheral nerves is formed from Schwann cells. Because oligodendrocytes have several processes, unlike Schwann cells, they can each form several internodal segments of myelin on the same or different axons. A single oligodendrocyte can form as many as 60 internodal segments.
2. Oligodendrocytes that surround nerve cell bodies (satellite oligodendrocytes) probably have a similar function to the satellite or capsular cells of peripheral sensory ganglia. They are thought to influence the biochemical environment of neurons.

MICROGLIA

Microglial cells are the smallest of the neuroglial cells; they are scattered throughout the central nervous system. Their small cell bodies give rise to branching processes with spinelike projections. They migrate into the nervous system during fetal life.

Functions of Microglia

In the normal central nervous system, the microglia are inactive and the cells are sometimes called **resting microglial cells**. In inflammatory and degenerative lesions of the nervous system, the microglial cells become active and proliferate and become phagocytic. These active cells are joined by monocytes that migrate into the tissue from the blood capillaries and form new microglial cells.

EPENDYMA

Ependymal cells are cuboidal and possess microvilli and cilia. They form a single layer that lines the cavities of the brain and the central canal of the spinal cord.

There are three groups of ependymal cells:

1. **Ependymocytes**, which line the ventricles of the brain and the central canal of the spinal cord and are in contact with the cerebrospinal fluid. Their adjacent surfaces have gap junctions, but the cerebrospinal fluid is in free communication with the intercellular spaces of the central nervous system.
2. **Tanycytes**, which line the floor of the third ventricle overlying the median eminence of the hypothalamus. These cells have processes that have end feet on blood capillaries.
3. **Choroidal epithelial cells**, which cover the surfaces of the choroid plexuses. The sides and bases of these cells are thrown into folds, and near their luminal surfaces the cells are held together by tight junctions that encircle the cells. The tight junctions prevent the leakage of cerebrospinal fluid into the underlying tissues.

Functions of Ependymal Cells

1. The cilia of the ependymal cells assist in the circulation of the cerebrospinal fluid within the cavities of the brain and the central canal of the spinal cord.
2. Tanycytes are believed to transport chemical substances from the cerebrospinal fluid into the capillaries of the median eminence of the hypothalamus and thus may via the hypophyseal portal system influence the control of the anterior lobe of the pituitary gland.
3. The choroidal epithelial cells have a secretory function and take part in the formation of cerebrospinal fluid.
4. The microvilli on the free surfaces would indicate that they also have an absorptive function.

Table 2-1 summarizes the structure, location, and function of the different neuroglial cells.

EXTRACELLULAR SPACE

The extracellular space is the narrow interval that exists between the neurons, the neuroglial cells, and the blood capillaries and is filled with tissue fluid. The extracellular space is in almost direct continuity with the cerebrospinal fluid in the subarachnoid space externally and the cerebrospinal fluid in the ventricles of the brain and the central canal of the spinal cord internally. The extracellular space thus provides a pathway for the exchange of ions and molecules between the blood and the neurons and glial cells. The plasma membrane of the endothelial cells of most capillaries is impermeable to many chemicals, and this forms the blood-brain barrier. The tight junctions of the endothelial cells of the blood capillaries are responsible for the **blood-brain barrier.**

Table 2–1 Summary of Structural Features, Location, and Function of the Different Neuroglial Cells

Neuroglial Cell	Structure	Location	Function
Astrocytes			
Fibrous	Small cell bodies, long slender processes, cytoplasmic filaments, perivascular feet	White matter	Form a supporting framework, are electrical insulators, limit spread of neurotransmitters, take up K ions, store glycogen, have a phagocytic function, take place of dead neurons, are a conduit for metabolites or raw materials, produce trophic substances
Protoplasmic	Small cell bodies, short thick processes, many branches, few cytoplasmic filaments, perivascular feet	Gray matter	
Oligodendrocytes	Small cell bodies, few delicate processes, no cytoplasmic filaments	In rows along myelinated nerves, surround neuron cell bodies	Form myelin in CNS, influence biochemistry of neurons
Microglia	Smallest of neuroglial cells, wavy branches with spines	Scattered throughout CNS	Are inactive in normal CNS, proliferate in disease and phagocytose, joined by blood monocytes
Ependyma			
Ependymocytes	Cuboidal or columnar in shape with cilia and microvilli, gap junctions	Line ventricles, central canal	Circulate CSF, absorb CSF
Tanycytes	Long basal processes with end feet on capillaries	Line floor of third ventricle	Transport substances from CSF to hypophyseal-portal system
Choroidal epithelial cells	Sides and bases thrown into folds, tight junctions	Cover surfaces of choroid plexuses	Produce and secrete CSF

CNS = central nervous system; CSF = cerebrospinal fluid.

Clinical Notes

Reactions of Neuroglia to Injury

Gliosis

Gliosis is the hyperplasia and hypertrophy of astrocytes that occur in reaction to injury to the central nervous system, whether caused by physical trauma or by vascular occlusion.

Demyelination

This occurs if there is severe injury to the oligodendrocytes.

Microglial Cells and Disease

Microglial cells proliferate and are actively phagocytic in response to inflammatory and degenerative lesions. They are active in multiple sclerosis, dementia in AIDS, Parkinson's disease and Alzheimer's disease.

Cerebral Edema

Cerebral edema is an abnormal increase in the water content of the tissues of the central nervous system which can follow head injuries, cerebral infections, or tumors. The fluid can accumulate in the neurons, neuroglia, and the extracellular space.

Blood-Brain Barrier and Trauma

Direct trauma or inflammatory or chemical toxins can cause the breakdown of the blood-brain barrier, allowing free diffusion of large molecules from the blood into the nervous tissue.

Blood-Brain Barrier and Drugs

Penicillin, which is toxic to the central nervous tissue can only cross the barrier in small amounts, whereas chloramphenicol and tetracyclines readily cross the barrier.

Tumors of Neuroglia

Tumors of neuroglia account for 40 to 50 percent of intracranial tumors. Such tumors are referred to as **gliomas.** Tumors of astrocytes are those most commonly encountered and include **astrocytomas** and **glioblastomas.** Apart from the ependymomas, tumors of the neuroglia are highly invasive.

REVIEW QUESTIONS

Directions: Each of the incomplete statements in this section is followed by completions of the statement. Select the ONE lettered completion that is BEST in each case.

1. The fibrous astrocytes:
   (a) have large cell bodies
   (b) are found mainly in the gray matter
   (c) contain many filaments in the cytoplasm of their cell bodies and their processes
   (d) do not contribute to the inner glial membrane
   (e) do not undergo hypertrophy or hyperplasia in gliosis
2. The oligodendrocytes:
   (a) are found in rows along nonmyelinated nerve fibers
   (b) are responsible for the formation of myelin in the central nervous system

(c) do not surround nerve cell bodies
(d) have large cell bodies
(e) are not found in rows along myelinated nerve fibers

3. The microglial cells:
(a) are metabolically very active in the normal nervous system
(b) have no branching processes
(c) are developmentally thought to be derived from ectoderm
(d) in an inflammatory lesion are formed from blood monocytes
(e) are larger than astrocytes

Directions: Each of the numbered items in this section is followed by answers that are positively phrased. Select the ONE lettered answer that is an EXCEPTION.

4. The following statements concerning ependymal cells are correct **except:**
(a) They possess cilia
(b) They are in contact with the cerebrospinal fluid
(c) They do not possess microvilli
(d) They are cuboidal
(e) Many of them have long basal processes

5. The following statements concerning astrocytes are correct **except:**
(a) They form perivascular feet
(b) Their processes are found in large numbers around the bare axolemma at the node of Ranvier
(c) They play no part in replacement gliosis
(d) They may function as electrical insulators around neurons
(e) They take part in the absorption of GABA secreted by nerve terminals

6. The following statements concerning the extracellular space in the nervous system are correct **except:**
(a) The space surrounds the neurons and the glial cells
(b) The space communicates with the ventricles of the brain and the central canal of the spinal cord
(c) The space in the central nervous system does not communicate with the synaptic cleft between neurons
(d) The space is filled with fluid that does not drain into lymph vessels
(e) The space is capable of containing an antibiotic in solution

7. The following general statements concerning neuroglia are correct **except:**
(a) One cytoplasmic process of an oligodendrocyte provides the myelin for one internode
(b) Tanycytes are special ependymal cells that line the third ventricle
(c) Tanycytes are involved in the control of endocrine glands
(d) Choroidal epithelial cells form a covering for the choroid plexuses and play no part in the formation of the cerebrospinal fluid
(e) Choroidal epithelial cells are joined together by tight junctions

Directions: Read the case history then answer the question. You will be required to select ONE BEST lettered answer.
A 31-year-old man was admitted to a hospital with a diagnosis of encephalitis. For treatment, the patient was given large doses of penicillin administered by intravenous drip.

8. Which of the following statements is **incorrect:**
(a) Most of the brain tissue is separated from the blood stream by the blood-brain barrier
(b) The tight junctions of the endothelial cells of the blood capillaries are responsible for the blood-brain barrier
(c) Penicillin molecules readily pass through the blood-brain barrier
(d) Chloramphenicol easily passed through the blood-brain barrier
(e) Penicillin in high concentrations is toxic to the central nervous system

ANSWERS AND EXPLANATIONS

1. C. A. Fibrous astrocytes have small cell bodies. B. They are found mainly in the white matter. D. They do contribute to the inner glial membrane. E. They undergo hypertrophy and hyperplasia in gliosis.
2. B. A. Oligodendrocytes are not found in rows along unmyelinated nerve fibers in the central nervous system. C. They do surround nerve cell bodies in the central nervous system. D. They have small cell bodies. E. They are found in rows along myelinated nerve fibers in the central nervous system.
3. D. A. Microglial cells are inactive cells in the normal nervous system. B. They have branching processes. C. They are derived from mesoderm. E. They are the smallest neuroglial cells.
4. C. Ependymal cells do possess microvilli, which have an absorptive function.
5. C
6. C. The extracellular space does communicate with the synaptic cleft between two neurons.
7. D. Choroidal epithelial cells have a secretory function and take part in the formation of cerebrospinal fluid.
8. C. Penicillin, which is toxic to the central nervous system, can only cross the blood-brain barrier in small doses.

CHAPTER 3

Degeneration and Regeneration of Nervous Tissue

CHAPTER OUTLINE

SUGGESTED PLAN FOR REVIEW OF CHAPTER 3

1. This material is important for clinical practice so the details outlined must be known.
2. The process of degeneration is rapid whereas regeneration is a slow process. Regeneration is only attempted in the central nervous system but quickly ceases.
3. Degeneration: Learn the changes that take place in the nerve fibers and then the changes that take place in the nerve cell bodies. Note that the process is similar in both the peripheral and central nervous systems. However, note the differences.
4. Regeneration in peripheral nerves: Learn the detailed histology of this process in the nerve fibers and then learn the changes that occur in the nerve cells during recovery.

SUGGESTED PLAN FOR REVIEW OF CHAPTER 3 (*continued*)

5. Attempted regeneration of nerve fibers in the central nervous system: Because today so much research is being devoted to investigating why regeneration in the central nervous system ceases within 2 weeks, the attempted histological changes that do occur must be learned.
6. Be able to define the following terms: wallerian degeneration, band fiber, retrograde degeneration, anterograde transneuronal degeneration, chromatolysis, and neuroma.
7. Understand plasticity of the central nervous system.

INTRODUCTION

The survival of the cytoplasm of a neuron depends on its being connected, however indirectly, with the nucleus. The nucleus plays a key role in the synthesis of proteins, which pass into the cell processes and replace proteins that have been metabolized by the cell activity. Thus, the cytoplasm of axons and dendrites will undergo degeneration quickly if these processes are separated from the nerve cell body.

In contrast to the rapid onset of degeneration, the process of regeneration may take several months. Regeneration in the peripheral nervous system may be very successful. However, in the central nervous system, regeneration is attempted but the process ceases after about 2 weeks.

DEGENERATION OF NERVES IN THE PERIPHERAL NERVOUS SYSTEM

When a nerve is cut, the axon is no longer in continuity with the nerve cell body and the distal segment undergoes simultaneous degeneration from the site of the lesion to its termination. Degeneration also extends proximally for a short distance as far as the first node of Ranvier. The process of degeneration is called **wallerian degeneration**.

During the first day the axon becomes swollen and irregular, and by the third or fourth day it becomes broken up into fragments (Fig. 3-1). Meanwhile the myelin sheath slowly breaks down and degenerates completely. The surrounding Schwann cells proliferate and fill the endoneurial sheath. The axonal and myelin debris is phagocytosed by the Schwann cells and tissue macrophages. The Schwann cells now become arranged in parallel cords within the persistent basement membrane. Each endoneurial sheath and the contained cords of Schwann cells are known as a **band fiber**. If regeneration does not occur, the axon and the Schwann cells are replaced by fibrous tissue produced by local fibroblasts.

Accompanying injury to the axon, changes may take place in the cell body, and are referred to as **retrograde degeneration**. The first changes that take place occur within the first 2 days following injury and reach their maximum within 2 weeks. The Nissl material breaks up and becomes fine and granular and dispersed throughout the cytoplasm, a process known as **chromatolysis**. The nucleus moves from its central position toward the periphery of the cell, and the cell body swells and becomes rounded due to osmotic changes. The amount of chromatolysis and swelling of the cell is greatest when the injury to the axon is close to the cell body. Synaptic contacts with the plasma membrane on injured motor neurons withdraw and processes of astrocytes enter the synaptic clefts. Sometimes death of the neuron occurs, while on other occasions, when there is only minor injury to the distal end of the axon, very little change may take place in the cell body.

DEGENERATION OF NERVES IN THE CENTRAL NERVOUS SYSTEM

In the brain and spinal cord, degeneration of the axons and myelin sheaths follows a similar pattern to that seen in the peripheral nerves. The debris is removed by the phagocytic activity of the microglial cells. Most of the latter cells are monocytes that have emigrated from the blood vessels. The phagocytic process in the central nervous system takes place more slowly than in the peripheral nervous system. The part played by the oligodendrocytes in this process is not known. The changes that take place in the nerve cell bodies in the central nervous system following injury are similar to those seen in the peripheral nervous system. However, chromatolysis is rarely seen and cell death is common.

After the debris has been removed by the microglial cells, the local astrocytes proliferate and replace the neuron with astrocytic processes and collagen fibers.

REGENERATION OF NERVES IN THE PERIPHERAL NERVOUS SYSTEM

The following regenerative processes take place if the proximal and distal stumps of the severed nerve area are in close apposition. The Schwann cells proliferate and fill in the space within the endoneurial tubes of the proximal stump as far proximally as the next node of Ranvier and in the distal stump as far distally as the end-organs. Any small gap that exists between the proximal and distal stumps is filled in by proliferating Schwann cells.

Each proximal axon end sends out many fine filaments with bulbous tips. These grow along the clefts between the Schwann cells and cross from the proximal to the distal nerve stump. Many filaments enter the proximal end of each

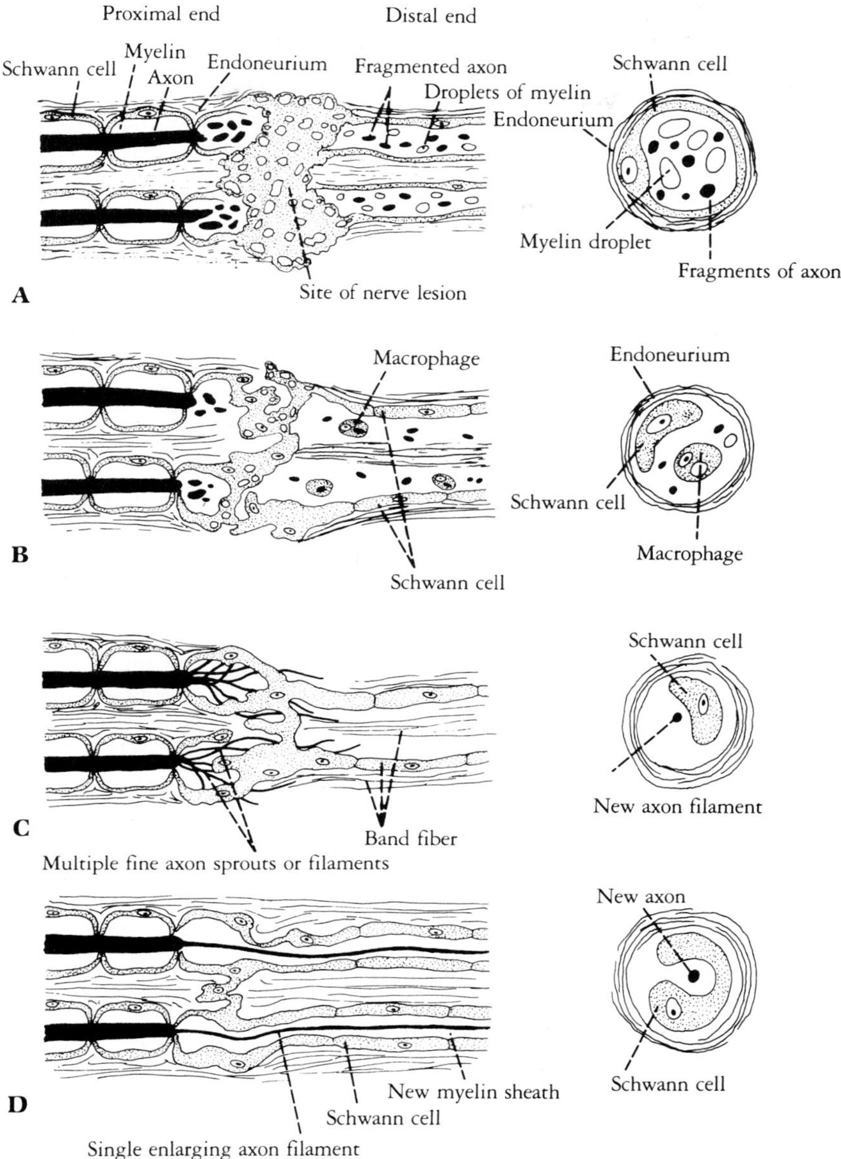

Figure 3–1 Process of degeneration and regeneration in a divided nerve.

endoneurial tube and grow distally in contact with the Schwann cells. Filaments from many different axons may enter a single endoneurial tube. However, only one filament persists, the remainder degenerating. The remaining filament now grows distally to reinnervate a motor or sensory end-organ and increases in diameter to about 80 percent of its original diameter. Autonomic axons regenerate in a similar manner.

As soon as the axon has reached the end-organ, the adjacent Schwann cells start to lay down a myelin sheath. This process starts at the site of the nerve injury and extends in a distal direction. By this means, the nodes of Ranvier are formed.

The rate of growth of the regenerating axon in a peripheral nerve is of the order of 2 to 4 mm daily. From a practical standpoint, if we include the delay incurred by the axons as they cross the site of injury, an overall regeneration rate of 1.5 mm daily should be remembered.

In a mixed peripheral nerve containing motor, sensory, and autonomic nerve fibers, the results after regeneration are less satisfactory than following the recovery from a lesion of a pure motor or a pure sensory nerve. The explanation is that regenerating fibers from the proximal stump may be directed to an incorrect destination in the distal stump, i.e., motor fibers entering sensory endings or vice versa, or motor fibers supplying incorrect muscles. Even if by chance the regenerating axon should reach the correct end-organ, the conduction velocity will not be as fast as that of the original axon, since the diameter reaches only about 80 percent of its original diameter.

In crush nerve injuries, where the axon is divided but the endoneurial sheath remains intact, the result of regeneration may be very satisfactory. If a peripheral nerve is divided and the ends are not sutured together, the ends may retract, leaving a gap of several millimeters. Under these circumstances, the gap becomes filled with fibrous tissue, or adjacent structures, such as muscles, may bulge into the gap. The outgrowing axonal filaments grow out into the surrounding connective tissue and form a tangled mass or **neuroma**. None of the filaments may enter the distal stump and no recovery takes place.

Accompanying the regenerative changes in the axon, the nerve cell body shows evidence of returning to normal. The nucleolus moves to the periphery of the nucleus and there is a reconstitution of the original Nissl structure, indicating that RNA and protein synthesis is being accelerated in preparation for the regeneration of the axon. There is a decrease in the swelling of the cell body and a return of the nucleus to its central position.

REGENERATION OF NERVES IN THE CENTRAL NERVOUS SYSTEM

In the central nervous system there is an attempt at regeneration of the axons, as seen by the sprouting of the axons and the formation of filaments. However, the process ceases after about 2 weeks. Long distance regeneration is rare and the injured axons make few new synapses. There is no evidence that restoration of function takes place. The reason for this is not understood, although the following suggestions have been made: (1) the absence of endoneurial tubes in the central nervous system, which may be necessary to guide the regenerating axons; (2) the failure of oligodendrocytes to serve in the same manner as Schwann cells; (3) the laying down of connective tissue (scar tissue) by astrocytes; and (4) the absence of nerve growth factors in the central nervous system or the presence of nerve growth inhibiting factors that may be produced by the neuroglial cells. Recent research has shown that if Schwann cells are transplanted into the central nervous system, axon sprouting and elongation are promoted.

The failure of axons to regenerate in the brain and spinal cord following injury means that permanent disability will follow.

TRANSNEURONAL DEGENERATION

In the central nervous system if one group of neurons is injured, then a second group farther along the pathway, serving the same function, may also show degenerative changes. This phenomenon is called **anterograde transneuronal degeneration**. For example, if the axons of the ganglion cells of the retina are cut, not only do the distal ends of the axons that pass to the lateral geniculate bodies undergo degeneration, but the neurons in the lateral geniculate bodies with which these axons form synapses also undergo degeneration. In some instances, a third set of neurons may be involved in the degenerative process in the visual cortex.

NEURON DEGENERATION ASSOCIATED WITH SENESCENCE

It has been estimated that in old age a person may have lost up to 20 percent of the original number of neurons. This may account to some extent for the loss of efficiency of the nervous system that is associated with old age.

CLINICAL NOTES

PLASTICITY OF THE CENTRAL NERVOUS SYSTEM FOLLOWING INJURY

Axon regeneration in the brain and spinal cord is minimal following a lesion and yet considerable functional recovery often occurs. This is especially the case when the lesions are small. Several explanations exist for the functional improvement, and more than one mechanism may be involved.

1. Following a lesion, the function of adjacent nerve fibers may be interrupted as the result of compression by edema fluid. Once the edema subsides, a substantial recovery may take place.
2. Nonfunctioning neurons may take over the function of damaged neurons.
3. Following a lesion to branches of a nerve, all the neurotransmitter may pass down the remaining branches, producing a greater effect.
4. Following a lesion of an afferent neuron, an increased number of receptor sites may develop on a postsynaptic membrane. This may result in the second neuron responding to neurotransmitter substances from neighboring neurons.
5. The damaged nerve fiber proximal to the lesion may form new synapses with neighboring normal neurons.
6. The normal neighboring nerve fibers may give off branches distal to the lesion, which then follow the pathway previously occupied by the damaged fibers.
7. If a particular function, as for example the contraction of voluntary muscle, is served by two nervous pathways in the central nervous system and one pathway is damaged, the remaining undamaged pathway may take over the entire function. Thus it is conceivable that if the corticospinal tract is injured, the corticoreticulospinal tract may take over the major role of controlling the muscle movement.

8. It is possible with intense physiotherapy for patients to be trained to use other muscles to compensate for the loss of paralyzed muscles.

Atrophy of Voluntary Muscle and Other End-Organs Following Peripheral Nerve Degeneration

Voluntary muscle undergoes degenerative changes following motor nerve section. First, there is an altered response to acetylcholine, followed by gradual wasting of the sarcoplasm, and finally loss of the fibrils and striations, Eventually the muscle completely atrophies and is replaced by fibrous tissue. Reinnervation of the muscle halts its degeneration, and if the muscle atrophy is not too advanced, normal structure and function return.

Return of Normal Function after Peripheral Nerve Injury

The satisfactory regeneration of axons and the return of normal function depend on the following factors:

1. In crush nerve injuries, where the axon is divided or its blood supply has been interfered with but the endoneurial sheaths remain intact, the regenerative process may be very satisfactory.
2. In nerves that have been completely severed there is much less chance of recovery, because the regenerating fibers from the proximal stump may be directed to an incorrect destination in the distal stump, that is cutaneous fibers entering incorrect nerve endings or motor nerves supplying incorrect muscles.
3. If the distance between the proximal and distal stumps of the completely severed nerve is greater than a few millimeters or the gap becomes filled with proliferating fibrous tissue or is simply filled by adjacent muscles that bulge into the gap, then the chances of recovery are very poor. The outgrowing axonal sprouts escape into the surrounding connective tissue and form a tangled mass or **neuroma.** In these cases, early close surgical approximation of the severed ends, if possible, greatly facilitates the chances of recovery.
4. When mixed nerves (those containing sensory, motor, and autonomic fibers) are completely severed, the chances of a good recovery are very much less than when the nerve is purely sensory or purely motor. The reason for this is that the regenerating fibers from the proximal stump may be guided to an incorrect destination in the distal stump; for example, cutaneous fibers may enter motor endoneurial tubes and vice versa.
5. Inadequate physiotherapy to the paralyzed muscles will result in their degenerating before the regenerating motor axons have reached them.
6. The presence of infection at the site of the wound will seriously interfere with the process of regeneration.

Specific Spinal Nerve Injuries

While a detailed description of the neurological deficits following the many spinal nerve injuries seen in clinical practice is beyond the scope of this book, it is appropriate to include a table that summarizes the important features found in cervical and lumbosacral root syndromes (Table 3-1). Also included are tables that summarize the branches of the brachial plexus (Table 3-2), lumbar and sacral plexuses (Table 3-3), and their distribution. These tables will assist you in determining the specific nerve lesion associated with a particular motor or sensory deficit in the upper or lower limbs.

Cranial nerve injuries are considered in Chapters 18, 19, and 20.

Table 3–1 Summary of Important Features Found in Cervical and Lumbosacral Root Syndromes

Root Injury	Dermatome Pain	Muscles Supplied	Movement Weakness	Reflex Involved
C5	Lower lateral upper part of arm	Deltoid and biceps	Shoulder abduction, elbow flexion	Biceps
C6	Lateral part of forearm	Extensor carpi radialis longus and brevis	Wrist extensors	Brachioradialis
C7	Middle finger	Triceps and flexor carpi radialis	Extension of elbow and flexion of wrist	Triceps
C8	Medial part of forearm	Flexor digitorum superficialis and profundus	Finger flexion	None
L1	Groin	Iliopsoas	Hip flexion	Cremaster
L2	Anterior part of thigh	Iliopsoas, sartorius, hip adductors	Hip flexion, hip adduction	Cremaster
L3	Medial part of knee	Iliopsoas, sartorius, quadriceps, hip adductors	Hip flexion, knee extension, hip adduction	Patellar
L4	Medial part of calf	Tibialis anterior, quadriceps	Foot inversion, knee extension	Patellar
L5	Lateral part of lower leg and dorsum of foot	Extensor hallucis longus, extensor digitorum longus	Toe extension, ankle dorsiflexion	None
S1	Lateral edge of foot	Gastrocnemius, soleus	Ankle plantar flexion	Ankle jerk
S2	Posterior part of thigh	Flexor digitorum longus, flexor hallucis longus	Ankle plantar flexion, toe flexion	None

Table 3–2 Summary of the Branches of the Brachial Plexus and Their Distribution

Branches	Distribution
Roots	
Dorsal scapular nerve (C5)	Rhomboid minor, rhomboid major, levator scapulae muscles
Long thoracic nerve (C5, C6, C7)	Serratus anterior muscle
Upper trunk	
Suprascapular nerve (C5, C6)	Supraspinatus and infraspinatus muscles
Nerve to subclavius (C5, C6)	Subclavius
Lateral cord	
Lateral pectoral nerve (C5, C6, C7)	Pectoralis major muscle
Musculocutaneous nerve (C5, C6, C7)	Coracobrachialis, biceps brachii, brachialis muscles; supplies skin along lateral border of forearm when it becomes the lateral cutaneous nerve of forearm
Lateral root of median nerve C(5), C6, C7	See Medial root of median nerve
Posterior cord	
Upper subscapular nerve (C5, C6)	Subscapularis muscle
Thoracodorsal nerve (C6, C7, C8)	Latissimus dorsi muscle
Lower subscapular nerve (C5, C6)	Subscapularis and teres major muscles
Axillary nerve (C5, C6)	Deltoid and teres minor muscles; upper lateral cutaneous nerve of arm supplies skin over lower half of deltoid muscle
Radial nerve (C5, C6, C7, C8, T1)	Triceps, anconeus, part of brachialis, brachioradialis, extensor carpi radialis longus; via deep radial nerve branch supplies extensor muscles of forearm: supinator, extensor carpi radialis brevis, extensor carpi ulnaris, extensor digitorum, extensor digiti minimi, extensor indicis, abductor pollicis longus, extensor pollicis longus, extensor pollicis brevis; skin, lower lateral cutaneous nerve of arm, posterior cutaneous nerve of arm, and posterior cutaneous nerve of forearm; skin on lateral side of dorsum of hand and dorsal surface of lateral 3½ fingers; articular branches to elbow, wrist, and hand
Medial cord	
Medial pectoral nerve (C8, T1)	Pectoralis major and minor muscles
Medial cutaneous nerve of arm joined by intercostal brachial nerve from second intercostal nerve (C8, T1, T2)	Skin of medial side of arm
Medial cutaneous nerve of forearm (C8, T1)	Skin of medial side of forearm
Ulnar nerve (C8, T1)	Flexor carpi ulnaris and medial half of flexor digitorum profundus, flexor digiti minimi, opponens digiti minimi, abductor digiti minimi, adductor pollicis, third and fourth lumbricals, interossei, palmaris brevis, skin of medial half of dorsum of hand and palm, skin of palmar and dorsal surfaces of medial 1½ fingers
Medial root of median nerve (with lateral root) forms median nerve (C5, C6, C7, C8, T1)	Pronator teres, flexor carpi radialis, palmaris longus, flexor digitorum superficialis, abductor pollicis brevis, flexor policis brevis, opponens pollicis, first two lumbricals (by way of anterior interosseous branch), flexor pollicis longus, flexor digitorum profundus (lateral half), pronator quadratus; palmar cutaneous branch to lateral half of palm and digital branches to palmar surface of lateral 3½ fingers; articular branches to elbow, wrist, and carpal joints

Table 3–3 Summary of the Branches of the Lumbar and Sacral Plexuses and Their Distribution

Branches	Distribution
Femoral nerve (L2, L3, L4)	Iliacus, pectineus, sartorius, quadriceps femoris muscles; skin, medial cutaneous and intermediate cutaneous nerves of thigh, saphenous nerve to medial side of leg, medial side of foot as far as ball of big toe; articular branches to hip and knee joints
Obturator nerve (L2, L3, L4)	Pectineus, adductor longus, adductor brevis, adductor magnus (adductor portion), gracilis muscles; skin, medial side of thigh; articular branches to hip and knee joints
Sciatic nerve (L4, L5, S1, S2, S3)	
Common peroneal nerve	Biceps femoris muscle (short head); skin, lateral cutaneous nerve of calf, sural communicating branch to lateral side of leg, lateral side of foot and little toe
Superficial peroneal nerve	Peroneus longus and brevis muscles; skin, lower leg and dorsum of foot
Deep peroneal nerve	Tibialis anterior, extensor hallucis longus, extensor digitorum longus, peroneus tertius, extensor digitorum brevis muscles; skin, cleft between first and second toes; articular branches to tibiofibular, ankle, and foot joints
Tibial nerve	Semitendinosus, biceps femoris (long head), semimembranosus, adductor magnus (hamstring part), gastrocnemius, soleus, plantaris, popliteus, tibialis posterior, flexor digitorum longus, flexor hallucis longus muscles; skin, medial side of ankle; articular branches to hip, knee, and ankle joints
Medial plantar nerve	Abductor hallucis, flexor digitorum brevis, flexor hallucis brevis, first lumbrical muscles; skin, medial side of sole of foot; articular branches to foot joints
Lateral plantar nerve	Flexor accessorius, abductor digiti minimi, flexor digiti minimi brevis, second, third, and fourth lumbricals, adductor hallucis, all interossei muscles; skin of lateral side of sole of foot

REVIEW QUESTIONS

Directions: Each of the incomplete statements in this section is followed by completions of the statement. Select the ONE lettered completion that is BEST in each case.

1. Following complete transection of the ulnar nerve near the elbow joint the:
   (a) nerve fibers in the distal stump lose their blood supply
   (b) myelin in the distal stump remains intact
   (c) Schwann cells proliferate at the lesion and fill in the spaces between the endoneurial tubes in the stumps
   (d) proximal stump usually retracts
   (e) distal stump remains fixed in its anatomical position
2. The rate of regeneration in a peripheral nerve is:
   (a) 5–10 mm/day
   (b) 2–4 mm/day
   (c) 20 mm/day
   (d) 11–15 mm/day
   (e) 16–19 mm/day
3. Regeneration in a peripheral nerve can be limited by:
   (a) the length of segment of peripheral nerve destroyed
   (b) neuroma formation
   (c) infection of the wound
   (d) the presence of muscle between the cut ends
   (e) all of the above
4. From a practical standpoint, peripheral nerve regeneration can be enhanced by reuniting:
   (a) the axolemma
   (b) the endoneurium
   (c) the perineurium
   (d) the Schwann cell layer
   (e) the epineurium
5. The rate of regeneration in peripheral nerves is best correlated with:
   (a) nerve impulse velocity
   (b) slow axoplasmic flow
   (c) retrograde axoplasmic flow
   (d) fast axoplasmic flow
   (e) none of the above
6. Chromatolysis, which may be seen in an injured nerve cell, is due to the:
   (a) disappearance of the nucleolus
   (b) peripheral shift of the nucleus
   (c) deafferentation of the neuron surface
   (d) dispersal of the rough surfaced endoplasmic reticulum
   (e) swelling of the nerve cell body

Directions: Each of the numbered items in this section is followed by answers that are positively phrased. Select the ONE lettered answer that is an EXCEPTION.

7. The following statements concerning wallerian degeneration are correct **except:**
   (a) The axon breaks up into fragments
   (b) The Schwann cells multiply
   (c) In peripheral nerves the endoneurium disappears
   (d) In the central nervous system the debris is removed by the microglial cells
   (e) The myelin sheath breaks down into short segments and degenerate completely

8. The following statements concerning the failure of regeneration in the central nervous system may be correct **except:**
   (a) Sprouting filaments from the proximal end of the cut axon are absent
   (b) Endoneurial tubes are absent
   (c) Oligodendrocytes fail to form a band fiber
   (d) Scar tissue is formed by the astrocytes
   (e) Nerve growth inhibiting factors are present in the central nervous system
9. The partial return of function following injury to the central nervous system can be explained by the following factors **except:**
   (a) The damaged nerve fiber proximal to the lesion may form new synapses with neighboring normal neurons
   (b) Intense physiotherapy may enable the patient to use other muscles to compensate for the loss of paralyzed muscles
   (c) The presence of edema fluid increases the possibility of return of function of the damaged axon
   (d) Following a lesion of an afferent neuron, an increased number of receptor sites may develop on a postsynaptic membrane
   (e) Nonfunctioning neurons may take over the function of damaged neurons
10. The following statements concerning degeneration in the peripheral nervous system are correct **except:**
    (a) In a cut peripheral axon, degeneration extends proximally as far as the first node of Ranvier
    (b) In a damaged peripheral axon, the axonal and myelin debris is phagocytosed by Schwann cells and tissue macrophages
    (c) Following the death of a neuron, the space occupied by the cell body is left empty
    (d) Any small gap that exists between the proximal and distal stump of a sectioned peripheral nerve is filled with proliferating Schwann cells
    (e) A crushed peripheral nerve has a better functional recovery than a completely sectioned nerve
11. The following statements concerning the process of regeneration in the peripheral nervous system are correct **except:**
    (a) During regeneration, the new axon reaches about 80 per cent of the original diameter
    (b) The conduction velocity of a regenerated axon is identical to that of the original axon
    (c) Regeneration in a mixed peripheral nerve is less successful than in a pure sensory or motor nerve
    (d) A regenerated motor fiber on reaching a sensory ending does not assume the function of a sensory nerve
    (e) For practical purposes the overall regeneration rate in a peripheral nerve is 1.5 mm daily
12. The following statements concerning the central nervous system are correct **except:**
    (a) Following section of a motor nerve, the synaptic contacts with the nerve cell body may retract and lose contact
    (b) Following injury, chromatolysis is usually seen
    (c) The process of regeneration ceases after about 2 weeks
    (d) The absence of nerve growth factors in the central nervous system may inhibit the process of regeneration
    (e) When the proximal neuron in a functional pathway degenerates, the second neuron in many instances undergoes some transneuronal degeneration
13. The following statements concerning the central nervous system are correct **except:**
    (a) Regeneration is likely to be impeded by mechanical problems such as proliferation of astrocytes and hemorrhage
    (b) Regeneration may take the form of collateral sprouting, where an intact neuron sends out processes to denervated areas
    (c) In old age a person loses up to 20 per cent of the original number of neurons
    (d) Nonfunctioning neurons never take over the function of damaged neurons
    (e) Following a lesion of an afferent neuron, an increased number of receptor sites may develop on a postsynaptic membrane.

Directions: Read the following case history then answer the question.
A 38-year-old man was thrown from his horse while attempting to jump over a gate. He fell heavily on his head and was found unconscious. On recovering consciousness he was found to be paralyzed from the neck downward and had complete sensory loss below the neck. Radiological examination revealed a fracture dislocation of the sixth cervical vertebra. During the next few weeks there was some return of muscle function and some return of sensory appreciation.

14. This rapid recovery could be explained by which of the following fact or facts?
    (a) Some regeneration of the spinal axons had taken place.
    (b) The physiological function of some of the axons was returning as the edema subsided.
    (c) Traction applied to the vertebral column reduced pressure on the spinal cord from the displaced bony fragments of the fractured vertebra.
    (d) The great willpower exhibited by the patient was aided by the strong encouragement of the relatives and physiotherapists.

ANSWERS AND EXPLANATIONS

1. D. When a nerve is sectioned, especially near a joint, both the proximal and distal stumps retract for a variable distance. Surgical approximation of the stumps results in a more satisfactory restoration of nerve function.
2. B
3. E
4. E
5. E
6. D. The Nissl substance is formed of rough endoplasmic reticulum and in chromatolysis the Nissl substance is dispersed throughout the cell cytoplasm .
7. C. The endoneurium does not disappear and it plays a vital role in the regeneration process.
8. A. The proximal stump of an axon does send out large numbers of filaments, but the process ceases after about 2 weeks.
9. C
10. C. The space previously occupied by a nerve cell body in the peripheral nervous system is filled with new connective tissue laid down by local fibroblasts.
11. B. Because the diameter of the new axon is less than that of the original, the conduction velocity of the new axon is less than that of the original axon.
12. B. Following injury of a nerve cell in the central nervous system chromatolysis is rarely seen.
13. D. Nonfunctioning neurons may take over the function of damaged neurons.
14. B, C, and D

CHAPTER 4

Peripheral Nerves

CHAPTER OUTLINE

SUGGESTED PLAN FOR REVIEW OF CHAPTER 4

1. Clearly understand the structure of a peripheral nerve and know how peripheral nerve fibers can be classified. Do nerve fibers of different diameters have different physiological properties?
2. Learn the composition of the 12 cranial nerves. Which cranial nerves are purely motor, which are purely sensory, and which are mixed nerves?
3. Be able to define what a spinal nerve is. How does it arise from the spinal cord? What is an anterior nerve root, a posterior nerve root, an anterior ramus, and a posterior ramus?
4. Understand how the cauda equina is formed during development. Does it consist of anterior or posterior roots or both of these roots? Are the spinal nerves included in the definition of the cauda equina? Which segments of the spinal cord contribute to the cauda equina?
5. Learn the structure of a sensory ganglion of a spinal or a cranial nerve and be able to compare it with the structure of an autonomic ganglion.
6. Understand how a nerve plexus is formed and appreciate the advantages of having nerve plexuses in different parts of the body.

INTRODUCTION

The peripheral nerves are the cranial and spinal nerves. Each peripheral nerve trunk consists of parallel bundles of nerve fibers, which may be myelinated or nonmyelinated, surrounded by connective tissue sheaths. The afferent nerve fibers connect the receptors to the central nervous system, while the efferent fibers connect the central nervous system to the muscles, glands, and blood vessels. There are 12 pairs of cranial nerves and 31 pairs of spinal nerves.

STUCTURE OF PERIPHERAL NERVES

A nerve fiber is the name given to an axon (or dendrite) of a nerve cell. The structure of axons and dendrites is described on page ···. Each nerve trunk is surrounded by a dense connective tissue sheath called the **Epineurium** (Fig. 4-1). Within the sheath are bundles of nerve fibers, each of which is surrounded by a connective tissue sheath called the **Perineurium.** Between the individual nerve fibers is a loose, connective tissue referred to as the **Endoneurium.** The sheaths serve to support the nerve fibers and their blood vessels and lymph vessels.

CLASSIFICATION OF PERIPHERAL NERVE FIBERS

Peripheral nerve fibers can be classified into groups, depending on their speed of conduction and size. For details, see Table 4-1.

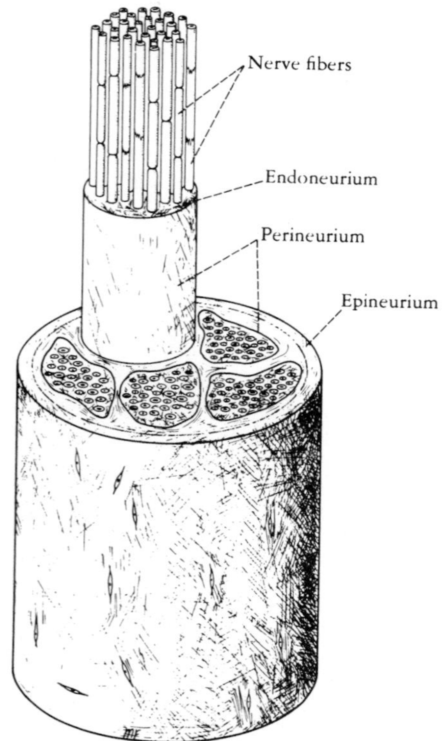

Figure 4–1 Structure of a peripheral nerve.

CRANIAL NERVES

There are 12 pairs of cranial nerves, which leave the brain and pass through foramina in the skull. Some of these nerves are composed entirely of afferent nerve fibers bringing sensations to the brain [olfactory (I), optic (II), vestibulocochlear (VIII)], others are composed entirely of efferent fibers [oculomotor (III), trochlear (IV), abducent (VI), accessory (XI), hypoglossal (XII)], while the remainder possess both afferent and efferent fibers [trigeminal (V), facial (VII), glossopharyngeal (IX), vagus (X)]. The cranial nerves are described in Chapters 18, 19, and 20.

SPINAL NERVES AND SPINAL NERVE ROOTS

There are 31 pairs of spinal nerves, which leave the spinal cord and pass through intervertebral foramina in the vertebral column. The spinal nerves are named according to the regions of the vertebral column with which they are associated: 8 cervical, 12 thoracic, 5 lumbar, 5 sacral, and 1 coccygeal. Note that there are 8 cervical nerves and only 7 cervical vertebrae and that there is 1 coccygeal nerve and there are 4 coccygeal vertebrae.

Two spinal roots, an anterior root and a posterior root, connect each spinal nerve to the spinal cord (Fig. 4-2). The **anterior root** consists of bundles of nerve fibers carrying nerve impulses away from the spinal cord; these nerve fibers are called efferent nerve fibers. The efferent fibers that pass to skeletal muscles and cause them to contract are called **motor fibers.** Their cells of origin lie in the anterior gray horn of the spinal cord. At certain levels the anterior roots also contain preganglionic nerve fibers of the autonomic system.

The **posterior root** consists of bundles of nerve fibers, called afferent fibers, that carry nervous impulses to the spinal cord. Since these fibers convey nerve impulses concerned with general sensations, they are called **sensory fibers.** The cell bodies of those nerve fibers are located in a swelling on the posterior root called the **posterior root ganglion** (Fig. 4-2).

The spinal nerve roots pass from the spinal cord to the level of their respective intervertebral foramina, where they unite to form a spinal nerve. Here the motor and sensory fibers mix so that a spinal nerve is made up of a mixture of motor and sensory fibers.

After emerging from the intervertebral foramen, each spinal nerve divides into a large **anterior ramus** and a smaller **posterior ramus,** each containing both motor and sensory fibers (Fig. 4-2). The posterior ramus runs posteriorly around the vertebral column to supply the muscles and skin of the back. The anterior ramus runs anteriorly to supply the muscles and skin over the anterolateral body wall and all the muscles and skin of the limbs.

CAUDA EQUINA

Because of the disproportionate growth in length of the vertebral column during fetal development, compared with

Table 4–1 Classification of Nerve Fibers by Speed of Conduction and Size

Fiber Type	Conduction Velocity (m/sec)	Fiber Diameter (μm)	Function	Myelination	Sensitivity to Local Anesthetics
A Fibers					
Alpha	70–120	12–20	Motor, skeletal muscle	Yes	Least
Beta	40–70	5–12	Sensory, touch, pressure vibration	Yes	
Gamma	10–50	3–6	Muscle spindle	Yes	
Delta	6–30	2–5	Pain (sharp, localized), temperature, touch	Yes	
B Fibers	3–15	<3	Preganglionic autonomic	Yes	
C Fibers	0.5–2.0	0.4–1.2	Pain (diffuse, deep), temperature, postganglionic autonomic	No	Most

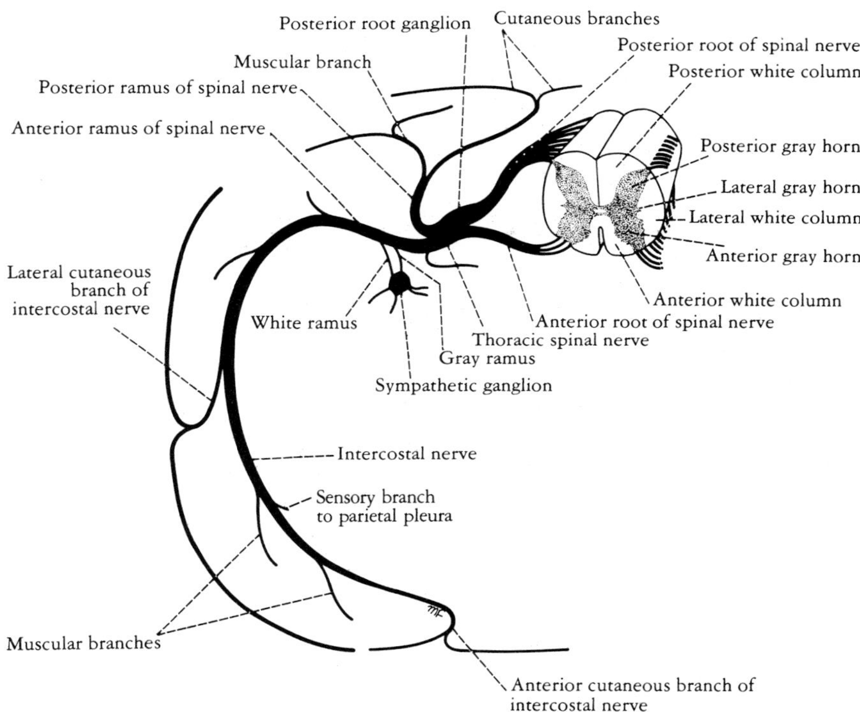

Figure 4–2 Cross section of the thoracic region of the spinal cord, showing roots, spinal nerve, and anterior and posterior rami and their branches. Note that an intercostal nerve is formed from the anterior rami of T1–11 spinal nerves.

that of the spinal cord, the length of the spinal nerve roots increases progressively from above downward (Fig. 4-3). In the upper cervical region the spinal nerve roots are short and run almost horizontally, but the roots of the lumbar and sacral nerves below the level of the termination of the cord (lower border of the first lumbar vertebra in the adult) form a vertical leash of nerves around the **filum terminale** (see p. 58). Together these lower nerve roots are called the **cauda equina** (Fig. 4-4).

POSTERIOR ROOT GANGLIA AND SENSORY GANGLIA OF CRANIAL NERVES

The sensory ganglia of the posterior spinal nerve roots (Fig. 4-2) and of the trunks of the trigeminal, facial, vestibulocochlear, glossopharyngeal, and vagal cranial nerves have the same structure. Each ganglion is covered by a layer of connective tissue that is continuous with the epineurium

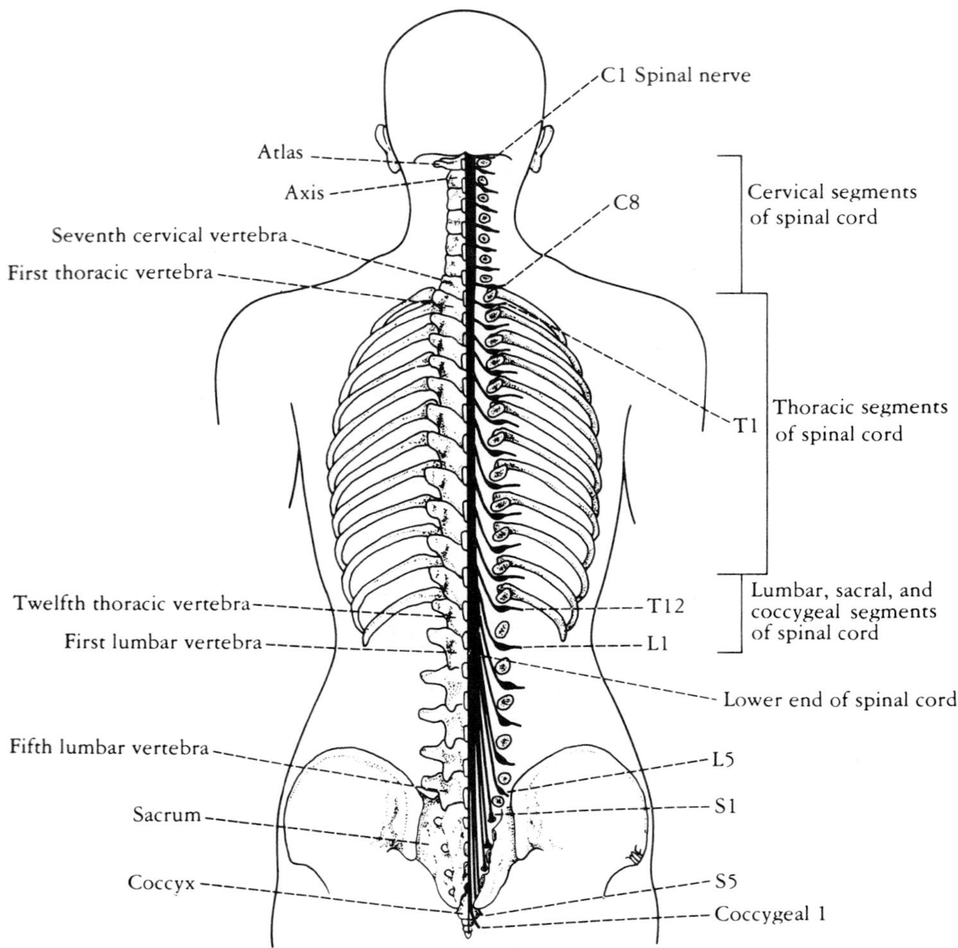

Figure 4–3 Posterior view of the spinal cord, showing the origins of the roots of the spinal nerves and their relationship to the different vertebrae. On the right, the laminae have been removed to expose the right half of the spinal cord and the nerve roots.

and perineurium of the peripheral nerve. The neurons are unipolar, possessing cell bodies that are rounded or oval. The sensory ganglia of the vestibulocochlear nerves differ in that the cells are bipolar. The peripheral axon terminates in a series of dendrites in a peripheral sensory ending, and the central axon enters the central nervous system.

Each nerve cell body is closely surrounded by a layer of flattened cells called **capsular cells** or **satellite cells.** The capsule cells are similar in structure to Schwann cells and are continuous with these cells as they envelop the peripheral and central processes of each neuron.

AUTONOMIC GANGLIA

The autonomic ganglia (sympathetic and parasympathetic ganglia) are situated at a distance from the brain and spinal cord (Fig. 4-2). They are located in the sympathetic trunks, in prevertebral plexuses (e.g., the celiac and mesenteric plexuses), and as ganglia in or close to viscera. Each ganglion is covered by a layer of connective tissue that is continuous with the epineurium and perineurium of the peripheral nerve. The neurons are multipolar and possess cell bodies that are irregular in shape. The dendrites of the neurons make synaptic connections with the myelinated axons of preganglionic neurons. The axons of the neurons are of small diameter (C fibers) and unmyelinated, and they pass to viscera, blood vessels, and sweat glands.

Each nerve cell body is closely surrounded by a layer of flattened cells called **capsular cells** or **satellite cells.** The capsular cells, like those of sensory ganglia, are similar in structure to Schwann cells and are continuous with them as they cover the peripheral and central processes of each neuron.

NERVE PLEXUSES

In many parts of the body peripheral nerves divide into branches that join neighboring peripheral nerves. If this should occur frequently, a network of nerves called a **nerve plexus** is formed. Since a peripheral nerve is composed of bundles of nerve fibers, a nerve plexus permits individual nerve fibers to pass from one peripheral nerve to another and in most instances branching of nerve fibers does not

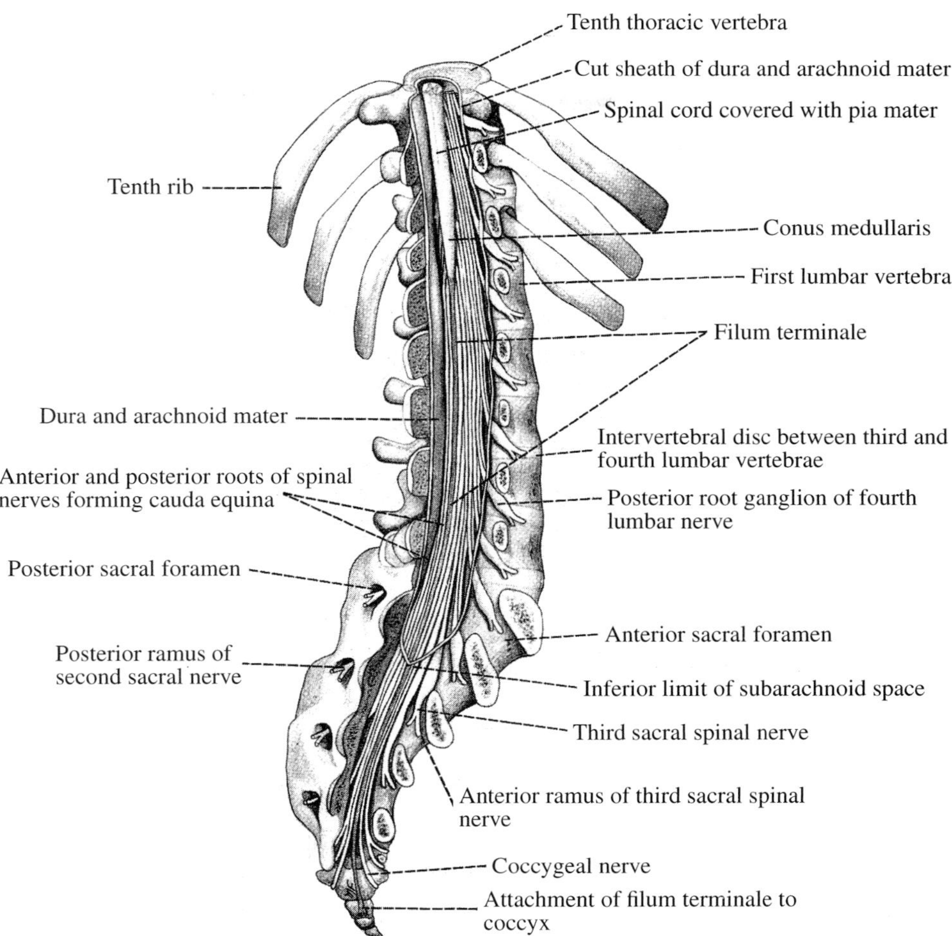

Figure 4–4 Oblique posterior view of the lower end of the spinal cord and the cauda equina. On the right, the laminae have been removed to expose the right half of the spinal cord and the nerve roots.

take place. A nerve plexus thus permits a redistribution of the nerve fibers within the different peripheral nerves.

At the root of the limbs the anterior rami of the spinal nerves form the following plexuses: cervical, brachial, lumbar, and sacral. This allows the nerve fibers derived from different segments of the spinal cord to be arranged and distributed efficiently in different nerve trunks to the various parts of the upper and lower limbs.

Cutaneous nerves, as they approach their final destination, commonly form fine plexuses, which again permit a rearrangement of nerve fibers before they reach their terminal sensory endings.

The autonomic nervous system also possesses numerous nerve plexuses, which consist of preganglionic and postganglionic nerve fibers and ganglia.

Segmental Innervation of Skin

The area of skin supplied by a single spinal nerve, and, therefore, a single segment of the spinal cord, is called a **dermatome.** On the trunk the dermatomes extend round the body from the posterior to the anterior median plane. Adjacent dermatomes overlap considerably, so that to produce a region of complete anesthesia at least three contiguous spinal nerves have to be sectioned. Dermatomal charts for the anterior and posterior surfaces of the body are shown in Figures 4-5 and 4-6.

In the limbs the arrangement of the dermatomes is more complicated, and the reason for this is the embryological rotation of the limbs as they grow out from the trunk.

In the face, the divisions of the trigeminal nerve supply a precise area of skin and there is little or no overlap to the cutaneous area of another division.

Segmental Innervation of Muscles

Skeletal muscle also receives a segmental innervation. Most of these muscles are innervated by more than one spinal nerve and, therefore, by the same number of segments of the spinal cord. Thus, to paralyze a muscle completely it would be necessary to section several spinal nerves or destroy several segments of the spinal cord.

To learn the segmental innervation of all the muscles of the body is an impossible task. Nevertheless, the segmental

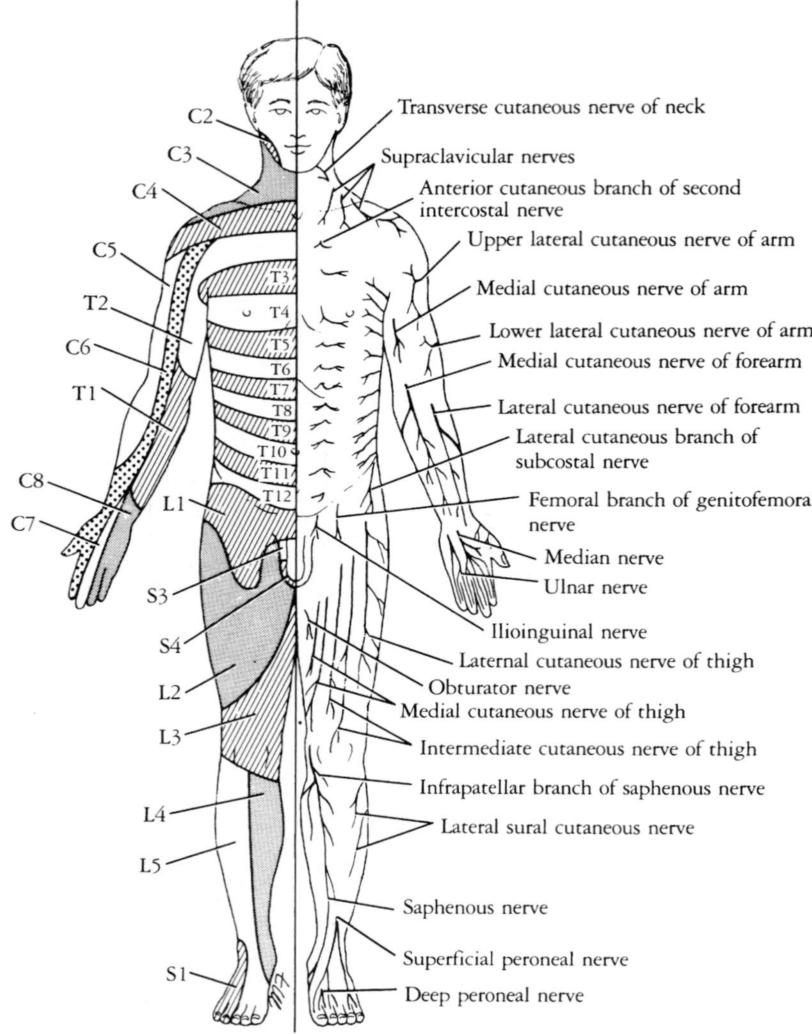

Figure 4–5 Anterior aspect of the body, showing the distribution of cutaneous nerves on the left side and dermatomes on the right side.

innervation of the following muscles should be known, because it is possible to test them by eliciting simple muscle reflexes in the patient:

Biceps brachii tendon reflex C5-**6** (flexion of the elbow joint by tapping the biceps tendon).

Triceps tendon reflex C6-**7,** and **8** (extension of the elbow joint by tapping the triceps tendon).

Brachioradialis tendon reflex C5-**6,** and 7 (supination of the radioulnar joints by tapping the insertion of the brachioradialis tendon).

Abdominal superficial reflexes (contraction of underlying abdominal muscles by stroking the skin). Upper abdominal skin T6-7; middle abdominal skin T8-9; lower abdominal skin T10-12.

Patellar tendon reflex (knee jerk) L2, **3,** and **4** (extension of knee joint on tapping the patellar tendon).

Achilles tendon reflex (ankle jerk) S**1** and 2 (plantar flexion of ankle joint on tapping the Achilles tendon—tendo calcaneus).

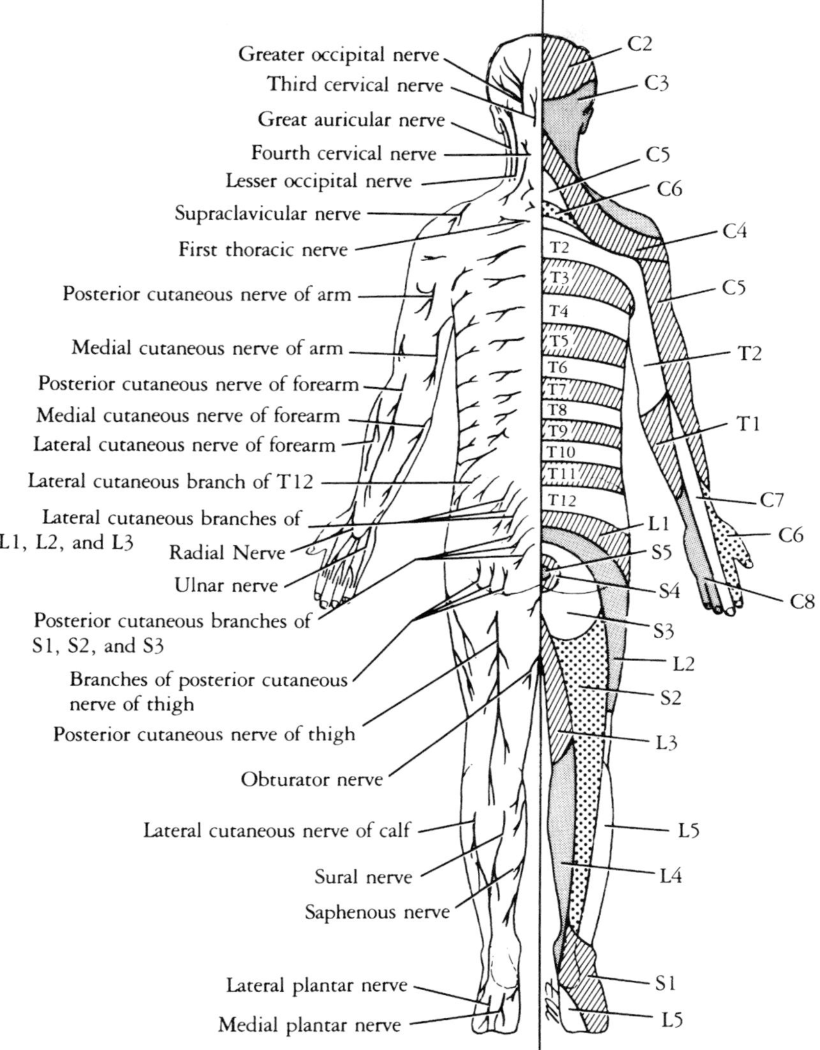

Figure 4–6 Posterior aspect of the body, showing the distribution of cutaneous nerves on the left side and dermatomes on the right side.

Clinical Notes

Some Basic Clinical Principles Underlying Peripheral Nerve Injuries

In open, dirty wounds, where there is a high risk of infection, the sectioned nerve should be ignored and the wound infection should be treated. Later, when the wound has healed satisfactorily, the nerve should be explored and the cut ends of the nerve sutured together.

For a patient with a healed wound and no evidence of nerve recovery, the treatment should be conservative. Sufficient time should be allowed to elapse to enable the regenerating nerve fibers to reach the proximal muscles. If recovery fails to occur, the nerve should be explored surgically.

In those cases in which connective tissue, bone fragments, or muscles come to lie between the cut ends of a severed nerve, the nerve should be explored and, if possible, the cut ends of the nerve should be brought together and sutured.

The nutrition of the paralyzed muscles must be maintained with adequate physiotherapy. Warm baths, massage, and warm clothing help to maintain adequate circulation.

The paralyzed muscles must not be allowed to be stretched by antagonist muscles or by gravity. Moreover, excessive shortening of the paralyzed muscles leads to contracture of these muscles.

Mobility must be preserved by daily passive movements of all joints in the affected area. Failure to do this results in the formation of adhesions and consequent limitation of movement.

Once voluntary movement returns in the most proximal muscles, the physiotherapist can assist the patient in performing active exercises. This not only aids in the return of a normal circulation to the affected part but also helps the patient to learn once again the complicated muscular performance of skilled movements.

Nerve Transplantation

Nerve grafts have been used with some success to restore muscle tone in facial nerve palsy. In mixed nerve injuries nerve grafts have succeeded only in restoring some sensory function and slight muscle activity. The presence of two suture lines and the increased possibility of mixing the nerve fibers is probably the reason for the lack of success with nerve grafts. In most nerve injuries, even when the gap between the proximal and distal ends is as great as 10 cm, it is usually possible to mobilize the nerve or alter its position in relation to joints so that the proximal and distal ends may be brought together without undue tension; the ends are then sutured together.

Tumors of Peripheral Nerves

A **benign fibroma** or a **malignant sarcoma** may arise in the connective tissue of the nerve and does not differ from similar tumors elsewhere. **Neurilemmomas** are believed to arise from Schwann cells. They arise from any nerve trunk, cranial or spinal, and in any part of its course. Primary tumors of the axons are very rare.

Herpes Zoster

Herpes zoster or shingles is caused by reactivation of the latent varicella-zoster virus in a patient who has had chickenpox. The infection involves the first sensory neuron in a cranial or spinal nerve. Inflammation and degeneration of the sensory neuron occur, causing pain and the formation of vesicles on the skin.

Polyneuropathy

Polyneuropathy is the simultaneous impairment of function of many peripheral nerves. There are many causes, including infection (endotoxin of diphtheria, Guillain-Barré syndrome), metabolic disorders (vitamin B_1 and B_2 deficiency, poisoning by heavy metals, drugs), and endocrine disorders (diabetes mellitus). Axon degeneration, involving both sensory and motor nerves, may take place and the neuron cell body may be affected.

REVIEW QUESTIONS

Directions: Each of the numbered items in this section is followed by answers that are positively phrased. Select the ONE lettered answer that is an **exception.**

1. The following statements concerning the cranial nerves are correct **except:**
   (a) There are 12 cranial nerves
   (b) They exit through the foramina in the skull
   (c) Many contain both motor and sensory axons
   (d) They exit from the brain only
   (e) They are paired
2. The following statements concerning the spinal nerves are correct **except:**
   (a) There are 31 spinal nerves
   (b) They leave the vertebral column through the intervertebral foramina
   (c) There are 7 in the cervical region
   (d) They are paired
   (e) There is 1 coccygeal nerve in the coccygeal region
3. The following statements concerning the spinal nerve roots are correct **except:**
   (a) The cells of origin of the voluntary motor fibers of the anterior root are located in the anterior gray column (horn) of the spinal cord
   (b) The posterior root contains sensory axons
   (c) The anterior root contains motor axons to skeletal muscle
   (d) The anterior root does not contain autonomic nerve fibers
   (e) The cells of origin of the posterior root nerve fibers are located in the posterior root ganglion
4. The following statements concerning a spinal nerve are correct **except:**
   (a) A spinal nerve is connected to the spinal cord by an anterior and a posterior ramus
   (b) The posterior ramus of a spinal nerve is smaller than the anterior ramus
   (c) The anterior ramus contains both sensory and motor axons
   (d) The spinal nerve is formed as it passes through an intervertebral foramen
   (e) The roots of a spinal nerve can be compressed by a prolapsed intervertebral disc
5. The following statements concerning nerve ganglia are correct **except:**
   (a) The nerve cells in a posterior root ganglion are unipolar
   (b) The nerve cells in the sensory ganglia of the vestibulocochlear nerve are bipolar
   (c) The nerve cells in the posterior root ganglion are devoid of capsular cells

(d) The nerve cells in an autonomic ganglion are of the multipolar type
(e) Autonomic ganglia are not situated close to the spinal cord

6. The following statements concerning the cauda equina are correct **except:**
(a) It is formed from the roots of the lumbar and sacral nerves below the level of the lower border of the first lumbar vertebra
(b) It is not bathed in cerebrospinal fluid
(c) It is made up of both anterior and posterior nerve roots
(d) The nerve roots form a leash of nerves around the filum terminale
(e) It lies below the lower end of the spinal cord

7. The following statements concerning large nerve plexuses are correct **except:**
(a) They do not contain sensory axons
(b) They permit nerve fibers to pass from one peripheral nerve to another
(c) They are commonly found at the root of a limb
(d) They permit nerve fibers from different segments of the spinal cord to enter a peripheral nerve
(e) In most instances individual nerve fibers do not branch at large nerve plexuses

8. The following statements concerning autonomic ganglia are correct **except:**
(a) They are present in both the sympathetic and parasympathetic parts of the autonomic nervous system
(b) They are covered with connective tissue that is continuous with the epineurium and perineurium of the nerves
(c) They are located, for example, in the celiac and mesenteric plexuses
(d) The dendrites of the nerve cells synapse with non-myelinated axons
(e) The axons of the neurons within the ganglia are type C fibers

9. The following statements concerning a peripheral nerve are correct **except:**
(a) The nerve is composed entirely of axons
(b) The endoneurium supports individual nerve fibers and plays a vital role in the regeneration of peripheral nerves
(c) Group A fibers serve as somatic afferent and efferent fibers
(d) Only myelinated nerve fibers are present in a peripheral nerve
(e) The connective tissue sheaths that surround a peripheral nerve contain blood vessels

Directions: Each of the incomplete statements in this section is followed by completions of the statement. Select the ONE lettered completion that is BEST in each case.

10. Group A alpha nerve fibers can have a:
(a) conduction velocity of 50-60 m/sec
(b) fiber diameter of 8-10 um
(c) motor skeletal muscle function
(d) lack of myelination
(e) great sensitivity to anesthetics

11. Group C nerve fibers have a:
(a) conduction velocity 0.5–2 m/sec
(b) fiber diameter of 12–20 um
(c) role in preganglionic nerve conduction
(d) myelin sheath
(e) low sensitivity to anesthetics

12. The epineurium is:
(a) formed of delicate connective tissue
(b) a sheath that surrounds bundles of nerve fibers within a nerve trunk
(c) devoid of lymph vessels
(d) not involved in the support of the nerve trunk
(e) formed of dense connective tissue which surrounds the entire nerve trunk

Directions: Read the case history and then answer the question. You will be required to select ONE BEST lettered answer.

A 45-year-old landscape gardener was seen in the neurology clinic. He complained of severe pain in the back that radiated down the back of the left leg along the distribution of the sciatic nerve. He also experienced numbness in the buttocks. He admitted to having lifted a large rock the previous day. The diagnosis was a central posterior protrusion of a prolapsed intervertebral disc between the fourth and fifth lumbar vertebrae with pressure on the cauda equina.

13. The following facts concerning this patient are correct **except:**
(a) Further protrusion of the disc could result in malfunctioning of the urinary bladder
(b) Provided that the pressure of the disc on the nerve fibers is removed in a timely manner, the axons in the cauda equina can then function normally and will result in cessation of pain and the return of normal sensation
(c) Continued pressure on the roots of the cauda equina could result in nerve degeneration and permanent damage to the axons
(d) Atrophy of the voluntary muscles of the lower limbs never occurs with pressure on the cauda equina

ANSWERS AND EXPLANATIONS

1. D. All the cranial nerves exit from the brain except the spinal part of the accessory nerve (XI), which exits from the upper five cervical segments of the spinal cord and joins the cranial part of the nerve within the skull; they then both exit through the jugular foramen.
2. C. There are 8 cervical spinal nerves in the cervical region.
3. D. The anterior root contains preganglionic autonomic nerve fibers (sympathetic T1–L2 and parasympathetic S2, S3, and S4).
4. A. A spinal nerve is connected to the spinal cord by anterior and posterior roots.
5. C. The nerve cells in a posterior root ganglion are surrounded with capsular or satellite cells.

6. B. The cauda equina is located in the subarachnoid space and is bathed with cerebrospinal fluid.
7. A. Large nerve plexuses often contain sensory axons.
8. D. The dendrites of the nerve cells synapse with myelinated preganglionic nerve fibers.
9. D. A peripheral nerve contains both myelinated motor and sensory fibers and nonmyelinated postganglionic autonomic fibers. In answer A, remember that the motor efferent fibers in a peripheral nerve are all axons; the sensory afferent fibers are also the axons of unipolar cells located in the posterior root ganglia or cranial nerve sensory ganglia.
10. C. See Table 4-1 for further information.
11. A. See Table 4-1 for further information.
12. E
13. D. Prolonged pressure of a prolapsed intervertebral disc on motor nerve fibers results in the atrophy of the muscles that they supply.

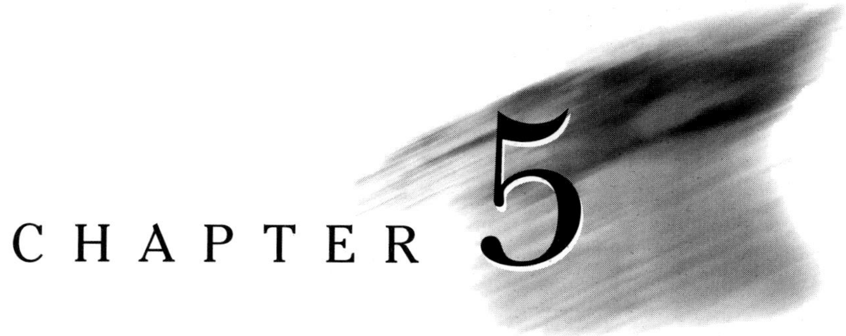

CHAPTER 5

Peripheral Nerve Endings

CHAPTER OUTLINE

SUGGESTED PLAN FOR REVIEW OF CHAPTER 5

1. Understand and be able to classify the different types of receptors.
2. Learn the detailed structure of hair follicle receptors, Meissner's corpuscles, and the pacinian corpuscles.
3. Understand the function of cutaneous receptors.
4. Learn what is meant by transduction of sensory stimuli into nerve impulses.
5. Learn the different types of joint receptors.
6. The structure and function of neuromuscular and neurotendinous spindles must be learned. These structures are basic to the understanding of skeletal muscle tone, muscle movements, and posture.

SUGGESTED PLAN FOR REVIEW OF CHAPTER 5 (*continued*)

7. Learn the anatomy and physiology of a stretch reflex. What is reciprocal inhibition?
8. Learn what gamma efferent nerve fibers are.
9. Be able to define a motor unit.
10. Learn in detail the structure and function of a neuromuscular junction in skeletal muscle.
11. Understand how nerves end on smooth muscle, cardiac muscle, and secretory cells.

INTRODUCTION

Special sensory nerve endings or **receptors** allow the individual to receive information from the environment and from within the body. **Exteroceptors** are those that respond to stimuli from the external environment and include those of the eye, ear, nose, and taste buds in the mouth. The skin receptors are sensitive to touch, pressure, and temperature changes. **Interoceptors** respond to stimuli from within the body and include **stretch receptors** within muscles, **visceroreceptors** in the walls of viscera, **chemoreceptors** such as the carotid and aortic bodies, and **baroreceptors** such as the carotid sinus.

CLASSIFICATION OF RECEPTORS

From a functional standpoint, sensory receptors can be classified into five basic types:

1. **Mechanoreceptors.** These respond to mechanical deformation.
2. **Thermoreceptors.** These respond to changes in temperature; some receptors respond to cold and others to heat.
3. **Nocioreceptors.** These respond to any stimuli that bring about damage to the tissue.
4. **Electromagnetic receptors.** The rods and cones of the eyes are sensitive to changes in light intensity and wavelength.
5. **Chemoreceptors.** These respond to chemical changes associated with taste and smell and oxygen and carbon dioxide concentrations in the blood.

Until more is known about the genesis of subjective sensations, the sensory receptors will be classified in this text, on a structural basis, into nonencapsulated and encapsulated receptors. Table 5-1 shows the classification and comparison of the receptor types. The eyes, ears, nose, and taste buds will be considered with the cranial nerves.

Nonencapsulated Receptors

FREE NERVE ENDINGS

Free nerve endings are found throughout the body, including the epithelia of the skin, cornea, and alimentary tract,

Table 5–1 Classification and Comparison of Receptor Types

Type of Receptor	Location	Stimulus	Sensory Modality	Adaptability	Nerve Fibers
Nonencapsulated receptors					
Free nerve endings	Epidermis, cornea, gut, dermis, ligaments, joint capsules, bone, dental pulp, etc.	Mechanoreceptor	Pain (fast), pain (slow), touch (crude), pressure, ? heat and cold	Rapid	A delta C
Merkel's discs	Hairless skin	Mechanoreceptor	Touch	Slow	A beta
Hair follicle receptors	Hairy skin	Mechanoreceptor	Touch	Rapid	A beta
Encapsulated receptors					
Meissner's corpuscles	Dermal papillae of skin of palm and sole of foot	Mechanoreceptor	Touch	Rapid	A beta
Pacinian corpuscles	Dermis, ligaments, joint capsules, peritoneum, exterior genitalia, etc.	Mechanoreceptor	Vibration	Rapid	A beta
Ruffini's corpuscles	Dermis of hairy skin	Mechanoreceptor	Stretch	Slow	A beta
Neuromuscular spindles	Skeletal muscle	Mechanoreceptor	Stretch—muscle length	Fast	A alpha A beta
Neurotendinous spindles	Tendons	Mechanoreceptor	Compression—muscle tension	Fast	A alpha

and in connective tissues, including the dermis, ligaments, joint capsules, tendons, perichondrium, periosteum, and dental pulp. The afferent nerve fibers from the free nerve endings are either myelinated or nonmyelinated. The terminal endings are devoid of a myelin sheath and there are no Schwann cells covering their tips.

The majority of these endings detect pain, while others detect crude touch, pressure, and tickle sensations, and possibly cold and heat.

MERKEL'S DISCS

Merkel's discs are found in hairless skin, for example, the fingertips, and also in hair follicles. The nerve fiber passes into the epidermis and terminates as a disc-shaped expansion that is applied closely to a dark-staining epithelial cell in the deeper part of the epidermis, called the **Merkel cell**. In hairy skin, clusters of Merkel's discs known as **tactile domes** are found in the epidermis between the hair follicles. They measure about 0.2 mm in diameter and are supplied by branches of a single myelinated axon. Merkel's discs are slowly adapting touch receptors that transmit information about the degree of pressure exerted on the skin, as, for example, when holding a pen.

HAIR FOLLICLE RECEPTORS

Nerve fibers wind around the follicle in its outer connective tissue sheath below the sebaceous gland (Fig. 5-1). Some branches surround the follicle while others run parallel to its long axis. Many naked axon filaments terminate among the cells of the outer root sheath. Bending of the hair stimulates the follicle receptor, which belongs to the rapidly adapting group of mechanoreceptors. While the hair remains bent, the receptor is silent, but when the hair is released, a further burst of nerve impulses is initiated.

Encapsulated Receptors

These receptors vary in size and shape, and the termination of the nerve is covered by a capsule.

MEISSNER'S CORPUSCLES

Meissner's corpuscles are located in the dermal papillae of the skin, especially the skin of the hand and the foot (Fig. 5-1). Each corpuscle is ovoid and consists of a stack of modified flattened Schwann cells arranged transversely across the long

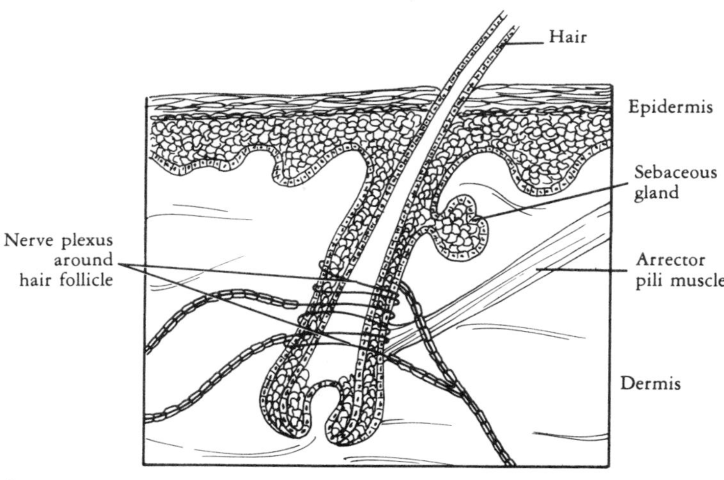

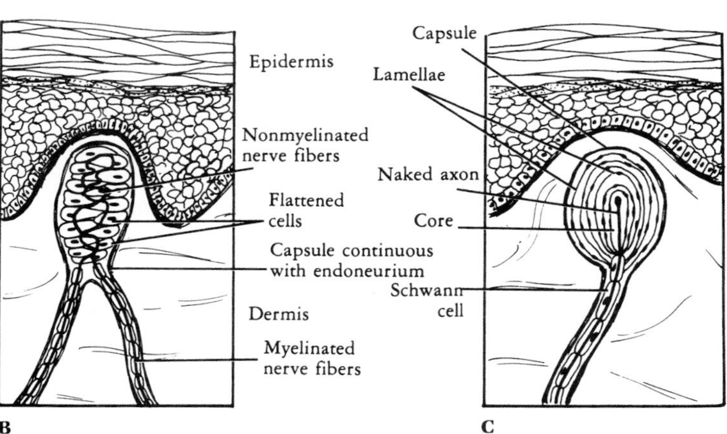

Figure 5–1 A. Nerve endings around a hair follicle. **B.** Meissner's corpuscle in skin. **C.** Pacinian corpuscle in skin.

axis of the corpuscle. The corpuscle is enclosed by a capsule of connective tissue that is continuous with the endoneurium of the nerves that enter it. A few myelinated nerve fibers enter the deep end of the corpuscle; myelinated and nonmyelinated branches decrease in size and ramify among the Schwann cells. There is a considerable reduction in the number of Meissner's corpuscles between birth and old age.

Meissner's corpuscles are extremely sensitive to touch and are rapidly adapting mechanoreceptors. They enable an individual to distinguish between two pointed structures when they are placed close together on the skin (two-point tactile discrimination).

PACINIAN CORPUSCLES

Pacinian corpuscles are widely distributed throughout the body and are present in large numbers in the dermis and subcutaneous tissue of the hands and feet (Fig. 5-1). Each corpuscle is ovoid, measuring about 2 mm long and about 100 to 500 mm across. It consists of a capsule and a central core containing the nerve ending. The capsule consists of numerous concentric lamellae of flattened cells.

A large myelinated nerve fiber enters the corpuscle and loses its myelin sheath and then its Schwann cell covering. The naked axon, surrounded by lamellae formed of flattened cells, passes through the center of the core and terminates in an expanded end.

Pacinian corpuscles are rapidly adapting mechanoreceptors and are particularly sensitive to vibration. They can respond to up to 600 stimuli per second.

RUFFINI'S CORPUSCLES

Ruffini's corpuscles are located in the dermis of hairy skin. Each corpuscle consists of several nonmyelinated nerve endings lying within a bundle of collagen fibers and surrounded by a cellular capsule. They are stretch receptors and respond when the skin is stretched. They are slowly adapting mechanoreceptors.

FUNCTIONS OF CUTANEOUS RECEPTORS

The main types of sensation that can be experienced by the skin are pain, temperature (heat and cold), touch, pressure, and vibration. Each receptor that has been described can be stimulated by a variety of stimuli such as mechanical deformation, application of chemicals, or change in the temperature. For a long time it was believed that the different histological types of receptors corresponded to specific sensations. However, it was soon pointed out that there are areas of the body that have only one or two histological types of receptors and yet they are sensitive to a variety of different stimuli. Moreover, in spite of the fact that we have these different receptors, all nerves only transmit nerve impulses. The type of sensation felt is determined by the specific area of the central nervous system to which the afferent nerve fiber passes. For example, if a pain nerve fiber is stimulated by heat, cold touch, or pressure, the individual will experience only pain.

TRANSDUCTION OF SENSORY STIMULI INTO NERVE IMPULSES

Transduction is the process by which one form of energy (the stimulus) is changed into another form of energy (electrochemical energy of the nerve impulse). The stimulus, when applied to the receptor, brings about a change in potential of the plasma membrane of the nerve ending. Since this process takes place in the receptor, it is referred to as the **receptor potential**. The receptor potential, if large enough, will generate an action potential at the first node of Ranvier. This sets in motion the saltatory conduction of an action potential that travels along the afferent nerve fiber to the central nervous system.

JOINT RECEPTORS

Four types of sensory endings can be located in the capsule and ligaments of synovial joints. Three of these endings are encapsulated and resemble pacinian, Ruffini's, and tendon stretch receptors. They provide the central nervous system with information regarding the position and movements of the joint. A fourth type of ending is nonencapsulated and is thought to be sensitive to excessive movements and to transmit pain sensations.

MUSCLE RECEPTORS

Neuromuscular Spindles

Neuromuscular spindles, or muscular spindles (Fig. 5-2), are found in skeletal muscles and are most numerous toward the tendinous attachment of the muscle. They provide sensory information that is used by the central nervous system in the control of muscle activity.

Each spindle is surrounded by a fusiform capsule of connective tissue. Within the capsule are slender **intrafusal muscle fibers**; the ordinary muscle fibers situated outside the spindles are referred to as **extrafusal fibers**. The intrafusal fibers of the spindles are of two types: the **nuclear bag** and **nuclear chain** fibers. The nuclear bag fibers have numerous nuclei in the equatorial region, which consequently is expanded; also, cross-striations are absent in this region. In the nuclear chain fibers, the nuclei form a single longitudinal row or chain in the center of each fiber at the equatorial region. The nuclear bag fibers extend beyond the capsule at each end to be attached to the endomysium of the extrafusal fibers.

Two types of sensory innervation of the muscle spindles exist, the annulospiral and the flower spray (Fig. 5-2). The **annulospiral endings** are located at the equator of the intrafusal fibers. The large myelinated nerve fiber pierces the capsule and loses its myelin sheath, and the naked axon winds spirally around the intrafusal fiber.

The **flower spray endings** are located chiefly on the nuclear chain fibers away from the equatorial region. A large myelinated nerve fiber pierces the capsule and loses its myelin sheath, and the naked axon breaks up into small branches with terminal expansions that resemble a spray of flowers.

Stretching (elongation) of the intrafusal muscle fibers causes stimulation of the annulospiral and flower spray endings and the passage of nerve impulses to the spinal cord in the afferent neurons.

Motor innervation of the intrafusal fibers is from small gamma efferent fibers (Fig. 5-2). The nerves terminate in small motor end-plates situated away from the equatorial region of the intrafusal fibers. Stimulation of the motor nerves causes both ends of the intrafusal fibers to contract and activates the sensory endings. The equatorial region, which is without cross-striations, is noncontractile.

The extrafusal muscle fibers receive their innervation from large alpha-sized axons.

FUNCTION OF THE NEUROMUSCULAR SPINDLE

Under resting conditions, the muscle spindles give rise to afferent nerve impulses all the time, and most of this information is not consciously perceived. When muscle activity occurs, either actively or passively, the intrafusal fibers are stretched and there is an increase in the rate of passage of nerve impulses to the spinal cord in the afferent neurons. Similarly, if the intrafusal fibers are now relaxed due to the cessation of muscle activity, the result is a decrease in the rate of passage of nerve impulses to the spinal cord. The neuromuscular spindle thus plays a very important role in keeping the central nervous system informed about muscle activity, thereby indirectly influencing the control of voluntary muscle.

STRETCH REFLEX

The neurons involved in the simple stretch reflex are as follows: Stretching a muscle results in the elongation of the intrafusal fibers and stimulation of the annulospiral and the flower spray endings. The nerve impulses reach the spinal cord in the afferent neurons and synapse with the large alpha motor neurons situated in the anterior gray horns of the spinal cord. Nerve impulses now pass via the efferent motor nerves and stimulate the extrafusal muscle fibers and the muscle contracts. This simple stretch reflex depends on a two-neuron arc, an afferent neuron and an efferent neuron. It is interesting to note that the muscle spindle afferent impulses inhibit the alpha motor neurons supplying the antagonist muscles. This effect is called **reciprocal inhibition**.

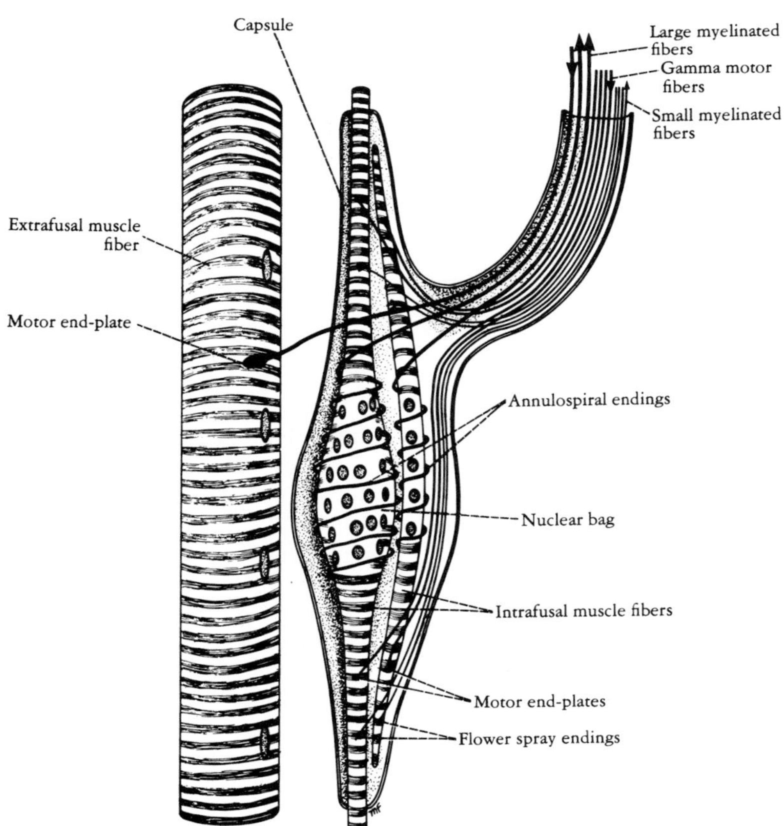

Figure 5–2 Neuromuscular spindle showing two types of intrafusal fibers: the nuclear bag and nuclear chain fibers.

Control of the Gamma Efferent Nerves

In the brain and spinal cord there are centers that give rise to tracts that synapse with gamma motor neurons in the spinal cord. Included in these centers are the reticular formation, the basal nuclei (basal ganglia), and the cerebellum. By this means these centers can greatly influence voluntary muscle activity. The gamma efferent motor fibers cause shortening of the intrafusal fibers, stretching of the equatorial regions, and stimulation of the annulospiral and flower spray endings. This in turn will initiate the reflex contraction of the extrafusal fibers described previously. It is estimated that about one-third of all the motor fibers passing to a muscle are gamma efferents; the remaining two-thirds are the large alpha motor fibers. It is believed that the nuclear bag fibers are concerned with dynamic responses and are associated more with position and velocity of contraction, whereas the nuclear chain fibers are associated with slow static contractions of voluntary muscle.

Neurotendinous Spindles (Golgi Tendon Organs)

Neurotendinous spindles are present in tendons near the junctions of tendons with muscles. Each spindle consists of a fibrous capsule that surrounds a small bundle of tendon fibers. One or more myelinated sensory nerve fibers pierce the capsule, lose their myelin sheath, branch, and terminate in expanded endings. The nerve endings are activated by being squeezed when tension develops in the tendon. Unlike the neuromuscular spindle, which is sensitive to changes in muscle length, the neurotendinous organ detects changes in muscle tension.

FUNCTION OF THE NEUROTENDINOUS SPINDLES

Increased muscle tension stimulates the neurotendinous spindles and an increased number of nerve impulses reaches the spinal cord through the afferent nerve fibers. These fibers synapse with the large alpha motor neurons situated in the anterior gray horns of the spinal cord. Unlike the muscle spindle reflex, this reflex is inhibitory and inhibits muscle contraction. In this manner the tendon reflex prevents the development of too much tension in the muscle. Although this tendon reflex is probably important in protecting the muscle from developing too much tension and thus tearing or being avulsed from its bony attachments, its main function is to provide the central nervous system with information that can influence voluntary muscle activity.

EFFECTOR ENDINGS

Innervation of Skeletal Muscle

Skeletal muscle is innervated by one or more nerves. In the limbs and head and neck the innervation is usually single, but in the large muscles of the abdominal wall the innervation is multiple, the latter muscles having retained their embryonic segmental nerve supply.

The nerve supply to a muscle contains motor and sensory fibers. The motor fibers are of three types: (1) large alpha myelinated fibers, (2) small gamma myelinated fibers, and (3) fine nonmyelinated C fibers. The large myelinated axons of the alpha anterior horn cells supply the extrafusal fibers that form the main mass of the muscle. The small gamma myelinated fibers supply the intrafusal fibers of the neuromuscular spindles. The fine nonmyelinated fibers are postganglionic autonomic efferents that supply the smooth muscle in the walls of blood vessels.

The sensory fibers are of three main types: (1) the myelinated fibers that originate in the annulospiral and flower spray endings of the neuromuscular spindles; (2) the myelinated fibers that originate in the neurotendinous spindles; and (3) the myelinated and nonmyelinated fibers that originate from a variety of sensory endings in the connective tissue of the muscle.

MOTOR UNIT

The motor unit can be defined as the single alpha motor neuron and the muscle fibers that it innervates. The muscle fibers of a single motor unit are widely scattered throughout the muscle. Where fine, precise muscle control is required, such as in the extraocular muscles or the small muscles of the hand, the motor units possess only a few muscle fibers. However, in a large limb muscle, such as the gluteus maximus, where precise control is not necessary, a single motor nerve may innervate many hundreds of muscle fibers.

NEUROMUSCULAR JUNCTIONS IN SKELETAL MUSCLE

As each large alpha myelinated fiber enters a skeletal muscle, it branches many times. A single branch then terminates on a muscle fiber at a site referred to as a **neuromuscular junction** or **motor end-plate** (Fig. 5-3). The great majority of muscle fibers are innervated by just one motor end-plate. On reaching the muscle fiber, the nerve loses its myelin sheath and breaks up into a number of fine branches. Each branch ends as a naked axon and forms the **neural element** of the motor end-plate (Fig. 5-3). The axon contains numerous mitochondria and vesicles. At the site of the motor end-plate the surface of the muscle fiber is elevated slightly to form the **muscular element** of the plate, often referred to as the **sole plate**.

The naked axon lies in a groove on the surface of the muscle fiber. Each groove is formed by the infolding of the sarcolemma. The groove may branch many times, each branch containing a division of the axon. It is important to realize that the axons are truly naked; the Schwann cells merely serve as a cap or roof to the groove and never project into it. The floor of the groove is formed of sarcolemma, which is thrown into numerous folds, called **junctional folds**; these serve to increase the surface area of the sarcolemma that lies close to the naked axon (Fig. 5-3). The plasma membrane of the axon (the axolemma or presynaptic membrane) is separated, by a space about 30 to 50 nm wide, from the plasma membrane of the muscle fiber (the sarcolemma or postsynaptic membrane). This space constitutes the **synaptic cleft**.

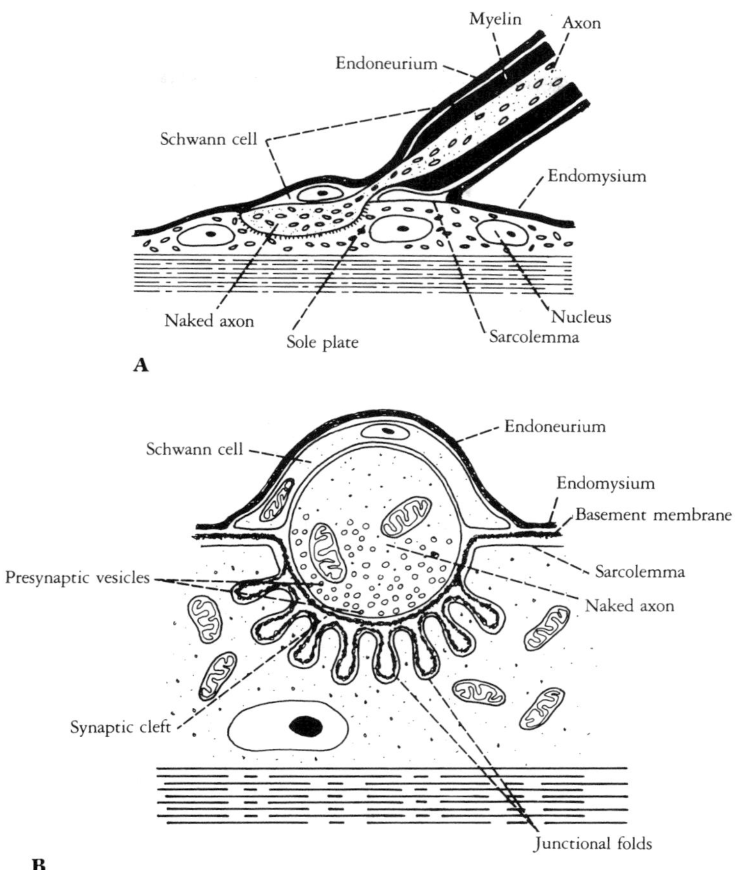

Figure 5–3 **A.** Skeletal neuromuscular junction. **B.** Enlarged view of a muscle fiber showing a terminal naked axon lying in the surface groove of a muscle fiber.

A nerve impulse (action potential), on reaching the presynaptic membrane of the motor end-plate, causes the opening of voltage-gated Ca^{2+} channels that allow Ca^{2+} ions to enter the axon. This stimulates the fusion of some of the synaptic vesicles with the presynaptic membrane and causes the release of acetylcholine into the synaptic cleft. The acetylcholine is thus discharged into the cleft by a process of **exocytosis** and diffuses rapidly across the cleft to reach the nicotinic type of Ach receptors on the postsynaptic membrane of the junctional folds. The postsynaptic membrane possesses large numbers of Ach-gated channels.

Once the Ach-gated channels are opened, the postsynaptic membrane becomes more permeable to Na^+ ions which flow into the muscle cell and a local potential called the **end-plate potential** is created. (The Ach-gated channels are also permeable to K^+ ions, which flow out of the cell, but to a lesser extent). If the end-plate potential is large enough, the voltage-gated channels for Na^+ ions are opened and an action potential will be initiated and will spread along the surface of the sarcolemma. The wave of depolarization is carried into the muscle fiber to the contractile myofibrils through the system of T tubules. This leads to the release of Ca^+ ions from the sarcoplasmic reticulum that in turn causes the muscle to contract.

The amount of acetylcholine released at the motor end-plate will depend on the number of nerve impulses arriving at the nerve terminal. Once the acetylcholine crosses the synaptic cleft and triggers the ionic channels on the postsynaptic membrane, it immediately undergoes hydrolysis due to the presence of the enzyme **acetylcholinesterase (AChE).** The enzyme is adherent to the collagen fibrils of the basement membranes in the cleft; some of the acetylcholine also diffuses away from the cleft. The acetylcholine remains for about 1 msec in contact with the postsynaptic membrane, and it is rapidly destroyed to prevent reexcitation of the muscle fiber. After the fall in concentration of Ach in the cleft, the ionic channels close and remain closed until the arrival of more Ach.

Skeletal muscle fiber contraction is thus controlled by the frequency of the nerve impulses that arrive at the motor nerve terminal. A resting muscle fiber shows small occasional depolarizations (end-plate potentials) at the motor end-plate, which are insufficient to cause an action potential and make the fiber contract. These are believed to be due to the sporadic release of acetylcholine into the synaptic cleft from a single presynaptic vesicle.

The sequence of events that takes place at a motor end-plate upon stimulation of a motor nerve can be summarized as follows:

ACh -> Nicotinic Type of ACh Receptor, Ach-gated channels opened ⟶ Na^+ influx ⟶ End-plate potential created.

End-plate potential (if large enough) -> Na^+ gated channels opened ⟶ Na^+ influx-> Action potential created.

Action potential -> Increased release of Ca^{2+} -> muscle fiber contraction.

Immediate hydrolysis of acetylcholine by AChE -> Ach-gated channels closed -> muscle fiber repolarization

NEUROMUSCULAR JUNCTIONS IN SMOOTH MUSCLE

In smooth muscle, where the action is slow and widespread, such as within the wall of the intestine, the autonomic nerve fibers branch extensively, so that a single neuron exerts control over a large number of muscle fibers. In some areas, for example, the longitudinal layer of smooth muscle in the intestine, only a few muscle fibers are associated with autonomic endings, the wave of contraction passing from one muscle cell to another by means of gap junctions.

In smooth muscle, in which the action is fast and precision is required, such as in the iris, the branching of the nerve fibers is less extensive, so that a single neuron exerts control over only a few muscle fibers.

The autonomic nerve fibers, which are postganglionic, are nonmyelinated and terminate as a series of varicosed branches. At the site where transmission is to occur, the Schwann cell is retracted so that the axon lies within a shallow groove on its surface. Part of the axon thus is naked, permitting free diffusion of the transmitter substance from the axon to the muscle cell. Here the axoplasm contains numerous vesicles similar to those seen at the motor end-plate of skeletal muscle.

Smooth muscle is innervated by sympathetic and parasympathetic parts of the autonomic system. Those nerves that are cholinergic liberate acetylcholine at their endings by a process of exocytosis, the acetylcholine being present in the vesicles at the nerve ending. Those nerves that are noradrenergic liberate **norepinephrine** at their endings by a process of exocytosis, the norepinephrine being present in dark-cored vesicles at the nerve endings. Both acetylcholine and norepinephrine bring about depolarization of the muscle fibers innervated, which thereupon contract. The fate of these neurotransmitter substances differs. The acetylcholine is hydrolyzed in the presence of AChE in the sarcolemma of the muscle fiber and the norepinephrine is taken up by the nerve endings. It is important to note that in some areas of the body (e.g., bronchial muscle) the norepinephrine liberated from postganglionic sympathetic fibers causes smooth muscle to relax and not contract.

NEUROMUSCULAR JUNCTIONS IN CARDIAC MUSCLE

Cardiac muscle is innervated by nonmyelinated postganglionic sympathetic and parasympathetic nerve fibers. At the site where transmission takes place, the axon becomes naked because of the retraction of the Schwann cell. This permits free diffusion of the neurotransmitter substance from the axon to the muscle cell. Because of the presence of gap junctions between adjacent muscle cells, excitation and contraction rapidly spread from fiber to fiber.

NERVE ENDINGS ON SECRETORY CELLS OF GLANDS

Nonmyelinated postganglionic sympathetic and parasympathetic nerves run close to the secretory cells. The nerve fibers entering some glands innervate only the blood vessels.

CLINICAL NOTES

NEUROMUSCULAR BLOCKING AGENTS

d-Tubocurarine produces flaccid paralysis of skeletal muscle, first affecting the extrinsic muscles of the eyes and then those of the face, the extremities, and finally the diaphragm. **Dimethyltubocurarine, gallamine,** and **benzoquinonium** have similar effects.

These drugs combine with the receptor sites at the postsynaptic membrane normally used by acetylcholine, and thus block the neurotransmitter action of acetylcholine. They are therefore referred to as competitive blocking agents, since they are competing for the same receptor site as does acetylcholine. As these drugs are slowly metabolized, the paralysis passes off.

Decamethonium and **succinylcholine** also paralyze skeletal muscle, but their action differs from that of competitive blocking agents because they produce their effect by causing depolarization of the motor end-plate. Acting like acetylcholine, they produce depolarization of the postsynaptic membrane and the muscle contracts once. This is followed by a flaccid paralysis and a blockage of neuromuscular activity. Although the blocking action endures for some time, the drugs are metabolized and the paralysis passes off. The actual paralysis is produced by the continued depolarization of the postsynaptic membrane. It must be remembered that continuous depolarization does not produce continuous skeletal muscle contraction. Repolarization has to take place before further depolarization can occur.

Neuromuscular blocking agents are commonly used with general anesthetics to produce the desired degree of muscle relaxation without using larger doses of general anesthetics. Because the respiratory muscles are paralyzed, facilities for artificial respiration are essential.

ANTICHOLINESTERASES

Physostigmine and **neostigmine** have the capacity to combine with acetylcholinesterase and prevent the esterase from inactivating acetylcholine. In addition, neostigmine has a direct stimulating action on skeletal muscle. The actions of both drugs are reversible and they have been used with success in the treatment of myasthenia gravis.

BACTERIAL TOXINS

Clostridium botulinum, the causative organism in certain cases of food poisoning, produces a toxin that inhibits the release of acetylcholine at the neuromuscular junction. Death results from paralysis of the respiratory muscles. The course of the disease can be improved by the administration of calcium gluconate or guanidine which promote the release of Ach from the nerve terminals.

Myasthenia Gravis

Myasthenia gravis is a disease characterized by drooping of the upper eyelids (ptosis), double vision (diplopia), difficulty in swallowing (dysphagia), difficulty in talking (dysarthria), and general muscle weakness and fatigue. Initially, the disease most commonly involves the muscles of the eye and the pharynx, and the symptoms can be relieved with rest. In the progressive form of the disease, the weakness becomes steadily worse and ultimately death occurs.

The condition is an autoimmune disorder in which antibodies are produced against the acetylcholine receptors on the postsynaptic membrane. This results in a reduced amplitude in end-plate potentials. The condition can be temporarily relieved by anticholinesterase drugs such as neostigmine, which potentiates the action of acetylcholine.

REVIEW QUESTIONS

Directions: Each of the incomplete statements in this section is followed by completions of the statement. Select ONE lettered completion that is BEST in each case.

1. One characteristic of a Meissner's corpuscle is that it:
   (a) increases in number with age
   (b) is present in small numbers in the skin of the palm of the hand
   (c) is a mechanoreceptor
   (d) is composed of a stack of endoneurial cells
   (e) is supplied by C nerve fibers
2. One characteristic of a Pacinian corpuscle is that it:
   (a) is flat in shape
   (b) contains a core of connective tissue devoid of nerve fibers
   (c) slow in adapting
   (d) has a large myelinated nerve fiber that enters the capsule
   (e) responds to stretch
3. One characteristic of Merkel's discs is that it:
   (a) is not present in hairless skin
   (b) is a mechanoreceptor
   (c) responds to vibration
   (d) is innervated by A delta nerve fibers
   (e) is fast adapting
4. The neurotendinous spindles are:
   (a) present in the tendon at only one end of a skeletal muscle
   (b) devoid of a fibrous capsule
   (c) innervated by nonmyelinated nerve fibers
   (d) used to detect changes in muscle tension
   (e) activated by being elongated

Directions: Each of the numbered items in this section is followed by answers that are positively phrased. Select the ONE lettered answer that is an **exception.**

5. The following statements concerning the pacinian corpuscle are correct **except:**
   (a) It is present in large numbers in the dermis and subcutaneous tissues
   (b) It measures about 2 mm long
   (c) The expanded end of the axon is covered by Schwann cells
   (d) It is particularly sensitive to vibration
   (e) The capsule consists of numerous concentric lamellae of flattened cells
6. The following statements concerning the neuromuscular spindles correct **except:**
   (a) They are most numerous toward the tendinous attachment of skeletal muscle
   (b) If the intrafusal fibers are relaxed, there is an increase in the rate of passage of nerve impulses to the spinal cord
   (c) The intrafusal fibers receive their motor innervation from gamma nerve fibers
   (d) Flower spray endings are located on the nuclear chain fibers away from the equatorial region
   (e) The extrafusal fibers receive their nerve supply from alpha-sized axons

7. The following statements concerning the innervation of skeletal muscle are correct **except:**
   (a) Each muscle of the anterior abdominal wall receives multiple innervations
   (b) The motor nerve supply to a muscle contains motor and sensory fibers
   (c) The motor fibers consist of alpha myelinated fibers and gamma myelinated fibers
   (d) A motor unit is composed of a single muscle fiber and its nerve supply
   (e) The arterial supply to a muscle receives fine nonmyelinated nerve fibers
8. The following statements concerning a neuromuscular junction in skeletal muscle are correct **except:**
   (a) The motor nerve loses its myelin sheath on reaching the muscle fiber
   (b) The terminal axon is surrounded by Schwann cell cytoplasm
   (c) The terminal axon breaks up into a number of branches
   (d) The terminal axon lies in a groove on the surface of the muscle fiber
   (e) The terminal axon contains mitochondria and vesicles in its cytoplasm
9. The following statements concerning the muscular element of the motor end-plate are correct **except:**
   (a) The endomysium lines the grooves on the surface of the muscle fibers
   (b) The surface area of the sarcolemma is increased by the presence of junctional folds
   (c) The width of the space between the presynaptic membrane and the postsynaptic membrane measures about 20 to 50 nm
   (d) The neurotransmitter is acetylcholine
   (e) The receptor on the postsynaptic membrane is nicotinic
10. The following statements concerning the events that take place at a motor end-plate are correct **except:**
   (a) The neurotransmitter is released from the presynaptic vesicles
   (b) The end-plate potential is created by the acetylcholine reaching the receptors on the postsynaptic membrane, resulting in an increased permeability to Na^+ ions
   (c) Acetylcholinesterase limits the action of acetylcholine by the process of hydrolysis, which takes place inside the sarcoplasmic reticulum
   (d) The T tubules serve to conduct the wave of depolarization to the myofibrils
   (e) The wave of depolarization carried to the myofibrils causes the release of Ca^+ ions from the sarcoplasmic reticulum, which in turn causes the muscle to contract
11. The following statements concerning the innervation of smooth muscle are correct **except:**
   (a) The wave of contraction of smooth muscle travels from one muscle fiber to another by means of gap junctions
   (b) The presynaptic membrane of the autonomic nerve fiber that innervates the muscle fiber is naked and not covered by a Schwann cell
   (c) Smooth muscle is innervated by sympathetic and parasympathetic parts of the autonomic nervous system
   (d) Each smooth muscle fiber is innervated by several autonomic neurons
   (e) The autonomic innervation is from postganglionic neurons
12. The following statements concerning neuromuscular junctions in cardiac muscle are correct **except:**
   (a) The nerves run in the connective tissue between the cardiac muscle fibers
   (b) The nerve fibers are myelinated
   (c) The terminal axon is naked and devoid of Schwann cells
   (d) Gap junctions on the cardiac muscle fibers permit the excitation and contraction to spread rapidly from fiber to fiber
   (e) Both sympathetic and parasympathetic nerves innervate cardiac muscle

Directions: Read the case history then answer the question. You will be required to select ONE BEST lettered answer. Study the following case history and select the best answer to the question following it.

A 10-year-old girl was walking along a dusty road when suddenly the wind blew a foreign particle into her right eye, causing her to cry out with pain. Because the pain persisted, she was taken to the emergency department of a local hospital.

13. The following facts concerning this patient are correct **except:**
   (a) The cornea is extremely sensitive and a foreign object causes considerable discomfort that often remains for several hours following the removal of the object
   (b) The cornea is not sensitive to stimuli other than pain
   (c) The only sensory receptors present in the cornea are free nerve endings
   (d) The free nerve endings are located between the epithelial cells on the surface of the cornea
   (e) The sensory receptors of the cornea exhibit rapid adaptability

ANSWERS AND EXPLANATIONS

1. C. See Table 5-1.
2. D. See Table 5-1.
3. B. See Table 5-1.
4. D
5. C. The expanded end of the axon is naked.
6. B. If the intrafusal fibers are relaxed, there is a decrease in the rate of passage of nerve impulses to the spinal cord.
7. D. A motor unit is a single motor nerve cell and all the muscle fibers that it supplies.
8. B. The terminal axon is truly naked; the Schwann cell merely serves as a cap or roof to the groove in the sarcolemma.
9. A. The endomysium does not line the grooves in the sarcolemma at the motor end-plate.
10. C. Acetylcholinesterase is located in the basement membranes of the synaptic cleft and on the postsynaptic membrane.
11. D. Each smooth muscle fiber is innervated by a single autonomic neuron.
12. B. The postganglionic nerve fibers are nonmyelinated.
13. B. The cornea is mainly sensitive to pain, although touch and temperature and possibly pressure can be felt. The discomfort in the eye remains for several hours after a foreign object has been removed, even though the free nerve endings have rapid adaptability. This can be explained by the fact that the surface of the cornea has been damaged by the foreign object and this damage remains after the object has been removed.

CHAPTER 6

Spinal Cord

CHAPTER OUTLINE

SUGGESTED PLAN FOR REVIEW OF CHAPTER 6

1. Spend a long time absorbing the contents of this chapter. The information is repeatedly used in describing the various nerve pathways as they ascend and descend in the spinal cord.
2. Understand the general shape and arrangement of the spinal cord. Know the vertebral level of the lower end of the spinal cord in the adult and young child. What is a spinal segment?
3. Learn the arrangement of the gray and white matter at different segmental levels of the spinal cord. Be able to draw a representative cross section taken from the cervical, thoracic, lumbar, and sacral levels of the cord.
4. Be able to define the phrenic nucleus and the accessory nucleus.
5. Learn the location and function of the substantia gelatinosa, the nucleus proprius, the nucleus dorsalis (Clark's column), the visceral nucleus, and the lateral gray column cells.
6. Define the gray commissure and the central canal.

SUGGESTED PLAN FOR REVIEW OF CHAPTER 6 (*continued*)

7. Learn the approximate position of the nerve fiber tracts in the white matter. You will need this knowledge when you learn about the various pathways in the central nervous system. Be able to draw a cross section of the spinal cord with the different tracts in position.
8. Understand the three meninges and learn the extent of the subarachnoid space with its cerebrospinal fluid (CSF), especially its lower extent in the vertebral column.
9. Know the main blood supply to the spinal cord. Appreciate the seriousness of the situation should the blood supply be compromised.

INTRODUCTION

The spinal cord is an elongated cylindrical part of the central nervous system (Fig. 6-1). It is situated in the upper two-thirds of the vertebral column and is continuous above with the brain. Like the vertebral column, the spinal cord is segmented, though the segments are not visible externally. Left and right spinal nerves, one pair per segment, connect the spinal cord to the tissues of the trunk, appendages, and the viscera.

The spinal cord contains large numbers of ascending and descending pathways, which serve as conduits for nervous information passing to and from different parts of the body to the brain. The spinal cord is also an important center for reflex activity, which is closely supervised by the brain.

ORGANIZATION OF SPINAL CORD

The spinal cord begins superiorly at the foramen magnum in the skull, where it is continuous with the medulla oblongata of the brain. It terminates inferiorly in the adult at the level of the **lower border of the first lumbar vertebra**. In the young child it is relatively longer and ends at the upper border of the third lumbar vertebra. The spinal cord is situated within the vertebral canal of the vertebral column and is surrounded by three meninges, the **dura mater**, the **arachnoid mater**, and the **pia mater** (Fig. 6-1). Further protection is provided by the cerebrospinal fluid, which surrounds the spinal cord in the subarachnoid space.

The spinal cord is roughly cylindrical (Fig. 6-1). However, in the cervical region, where it gives origin to the brachial plexus, and in the lower thoracic and lumbar regions, where it gives origin to the lumbosacral plexus, there are fusiform enlargements, called the **cervical and lumbar enlargements** (Fig. 6-2). Inferiorly, the spinal cord tapers off into the **conus medullaris**, from the apex of which a prolongation of the pia mater, the **filum terminale**, descends to be attached to the back of the coccyx (Fig. 6-1).

Along the entire length of the spinal cord are attached 31 pairs of spinal nerves by the **anterior or motor roots** and the **posterior or sensory roots** (Fig. 6-1). Each root is attached to the cord by a series of rootlets, which extend the whole length of the corresponding segment of the cord. Each posterior nerve root possesses a **posterior root ganglion**, the cells of which give rise to peripheral and central nerve fibers.

STRUCTURE OF SPINAL CORD

The spinal cord is composed of an inner core of **gray matter**, which is surrounded by an outer covering of **white matter** (Fig. 6-1). For a comparison of the structural details in different regions of the spinal cord, see Table 6-1.

Gray Matter

The gray matter, on cross section, is seen as an H-shaped pillar with **anterior and posterior gray columns, or horns**, united by a thin **gray commissure** containing the small **central canal** (Fig. 6-3). A **small lateral gray column or horn** is present in the thoracic and upper lumbar segments of the cord.

STRUCTURE OF GRAY MATTER

As in other regions of the central nervous system, the gray matter of the spinal cord consists of a mixture of nerve cells and their processes, neuroglia, and blood vessels.

Nerve Cell Groups in the Anterior Gray Columns

The majority of the nerve cells are large and multipolar and their axons pass out in the anterior roots of the spinal nerves as **alpha efferents**, which innervate skeletal muscles.
The smaller nerve cells are also multipolar and the axons of many of these pass out in the anterior roots of the spinal nerves as **gamma efferents**, which innervate the intrafusal muscle fibers of neuromuscular spindles.

The nerve cells of the anterior gray column can be divided into three basic groups: medial, central, and lateral.

The medial group is responsible for innervating the skeletal muscles of the neck and trunk (Fig. 6-3). The central group is present in some cervical and lumbosacral segments. In the cervical part of the cord some of these nerve

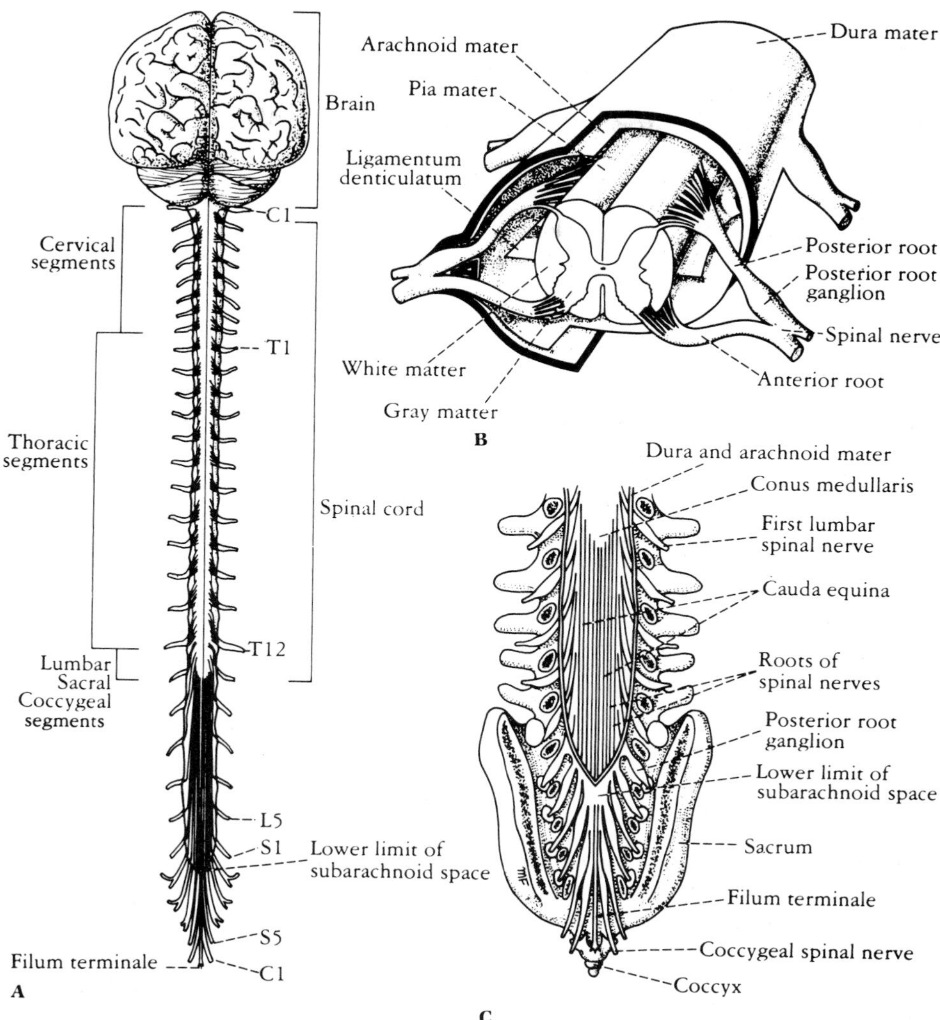

Figure 6–1 A. Brain and spinal cord posterior view. B. Transverse section of the spinal cord in the thoracic region, showing anterior and posterior roots of a spinal nerve and the meninges. C. Posterior view of the lower end of the spinal cord and the cauda equina.

cells (segments C3, C4, and C5) specifically innervate the diaphragm and are collectively referred to as the **phrenic nucleus**. In the upper five or six cervical segments, some of the nerve cells innervate the sternocleidomastoid and trapezius muscles and are referred to as the **accessory nucleus**. The axons of these cells form the spinal part of the accessory nerve. The **lumbosacral nucleus** present in the second lumbar down to the first sacral segments of the cord has an unknown distribution. The lateral group is present in the cervical and lumbosacral segments of the cord and is responsible for innervating the skeletal muscles of the limbs.

Nerve Cell Groups in the Posterior Gray Columns

There are four nerve cell groups of the posterior gray column.

The **substantia gelatinosa group** is situated at the apex of the posterior gray column throughout the length of the spinal cord (Fig. 6-3). It receives afferent fibers concerned with pain, temperature, and touch from the posterior root.

The **nucleus proprius** is situated anterior to the substantia gelatinosa throughout the spinal cord (Fig. 6-3). This nucleus receives fibers from the posterior white column that are associated with the senses of position and movement (proprioception), two-point discrimination, and vibration.

The **nucleus dorsalis (Clark's column)** is situated at the base of the posterior gray column and extends from the eighth cervical segment caudally to the third or fourth lumbar segment (Fig. 6-3). The cells are associated with proprioceptive endings (neuromuscular spindles and tendon spindles).

The **visceral afferent nucleus** is situated lateral to the nucleus dorsalis; it extends from the first thoracic to the third lumbar segment of the spinal cord and is associated with receiving visceral afferent information.

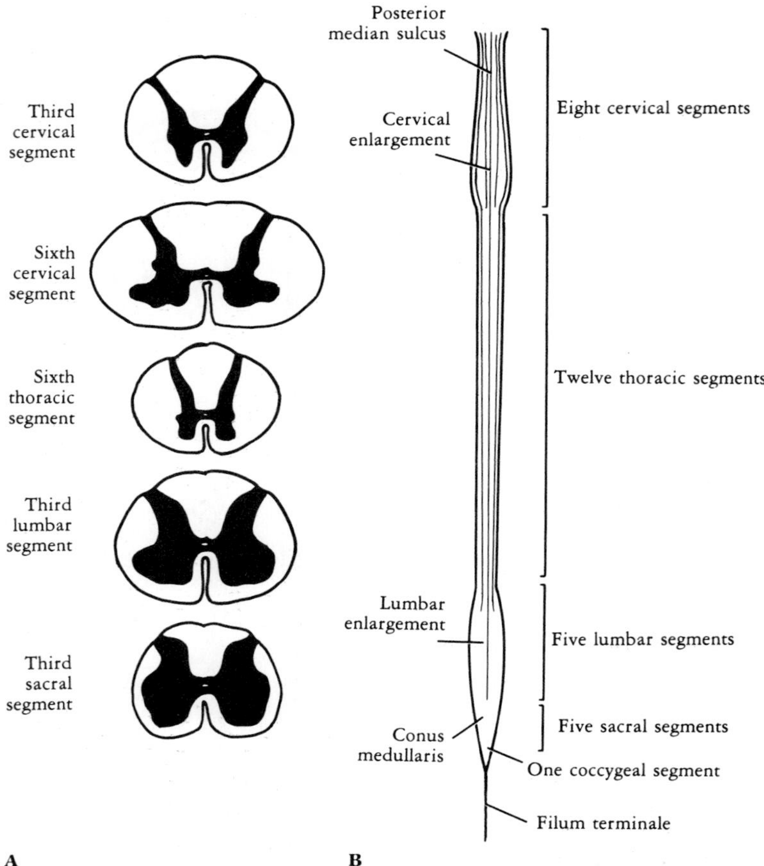

Figure 6–2 A. Transverse sections of the spinal cord at different levels. **B**. Posterior view of the spinal cord, showing cervical and lumbar enlargements.

Nerve Cell Groups in the Lateral Gray Columns

These cells extend from the first thoracic to the second or third lumbar segment of the spinal cord (Fig. 6-3) and give rise to preganglionic sympathetic fibers.

A similar group of cells found in the second, third, and fourth sacral segments of the spinal cord give rise to preganglionic parasympathetic fibers.

THE GRAY COMMISSURE AND CENTRAL CANAL

In transverse sections of the spinal cord, the anterior and posterior gray columns on each side are seen to be connected by a transverse **gray commissure**, so that the gray matter resembles the letter H (Fig. 6-3). In the center of the gray commissure is situated the **central canal**.

In most individuals, the central canal is present throughout the spinal cord (Fig. 6-2). Superiorly, it is continuous with the central canal of the caudal half of the medulla oblongata, and above this it opens into the cavity of the fourth ventricle. Inferiorly in the conus medullaris, it expands into the **terminal ventricle**. It is filled with cerebrospinal fluid and is lined with ciliated columnar epithelium, the **ependyma**.

White Matter

The white matter, for purposes of description, can be divided into **anterior, lateral, and posterior white columns**. The anterior column on each side lies between the midline and the point of emergence of the anterior nerve roots; the lateral column lies between the emergence of the anterior nerve roots and the entry of the posterior nerve roots; the posterior column lies between the entry of the posterior nerve roots and the midline.

STRUCTURE OF WHITE MATTER

As in other regions of the central nervous system, the white matter of the spinal cord consists of a mixture of nerve fibers, neuroglia, and blood vessels. It surrounds the gray matter and its white color is due to the high proportion of myelinated nerve fibers.

Table 6–1 Comparison of Structural Details in Different Regions of the Spinal Cord

Region	Shape	White Matter	Gray Matter: Anterior Gray Column	Gray Matter: Posterior Gray Column	Gray Matter: Lateral Gray Column
Cervical	Oval	Fasciculus cuneatus present, fasciculus gracilis present	Medial group of cells for neck muscles, central group of cells for accessory nucleus (C1–5) and phrenic nucleus (C3, C4, and C5), lateral group of cells for upper limb muscles	Substantia gelatinosa present, continuous with spinal nucleus of fifth cranial nerve at level C2, nucleus proprius present, nucleus dorsalis (Clark's column) absent	Absent
Thoracic	Round	Fasciculus cuneatus present (T1–6), fasciculus gracilis present	Medial group of cells for trunk muscles	Substantia gelatinosa present, nucleus proprius present, nucleus dorsalis (Clark's column) present, visceral afferent nucleus present	Present, gives rise to preganglionic sympathetic fibers
Lumbar	Round to oval	Fasciculus cuneatus absent, fasciculus gracilis present	Medial group of cells for lower limb muscles, central group of cells for lumbosacral nerve	Substantia gelatinosa present, nucleus proprius present, nucleus dorsalis (Clark's column) L1–4, visceral afferent nucleus present	Present at (L1, L2[3]), gives rise to preganglionic sympathetic fibers
Sacral	Round	Small amount; fasciculus cuneatus absent; fasciculus gracilis present	Medial group of cells for lower limb and perineal muscles	Substantia gelatinosa present, nucleus proprius present	Absent, group of cells present at S2, S3, S4, for parasympathetic outflow

Note: The information in this table is useful for identifying the specific level of the spinal cord from which a section has been taken.

ARRANGEMENT OF NERVE FIBER TRACTS

The spinal tracts are divided into ascending, descending, and intersegmental tracts, and their relative positions in the white matter are shown in Figure 6-3. The connections and functions of the various tracts are given in Chapter 7.

MENINGES OF THE SPINAL CORD

The spinal cord, like the brain, is surrounded by three meninges: the dura mater, the arachnoid mater, and the pia mater.

Dura Mater

The dura mater is a dense, fibrous membrane that encloses the spinal cord and cauda equina (Fig. 6-1). It is continuous above through the foramen magnum with the meningeal layer of dura covering the brain. Inferiorly, it ends on the filum terminale at the level of the lower border of the second sacral vertebra. The dural sheath lies loosely in the vertebral canal and is separated from the walls of the canal by the **extradural space**. This contains loose areolar tissue and the **internal vertebral venous plexus**. The dura mater extends along each nerve root and becomes continuous with the epineurium of each spinal nerve. The inner surface of the dura mater is in contact with the arachnoid mater.

Arachnoid Mater

The arachnoid mater is a delicate impermeable membrane that covers the spinal cord and lies between the pia mater internally and the dura mater externally (Fig. 6-1). It is separated from the pia mater by a wide space, the **subarachnoid space**, which is filled with **cerebrospinal fluid**. The arachnoid mater is continuous above through the foramen magnum with the arachnoid covering the brain. Inferiorly, it ends on the filum terminale at the level of the lower border of the second sacral vertebra (Fig. 6-1). The arachnoid mater continues along the spinal nerve roots, forming small lateral extensions of the subarachnoid space.

Pia Mater

The pia mater, a vascular membrane that closely covers the spinal cord, is thickened on either side between the nerve roots to form the **ligamentum denticulatum**, which passes laterally to adhere to the arachnoid and dura (Fig. 6-1). It is by this means that the spinal cord is suspended in the middle of the dural sheath. The pia mater extends along each

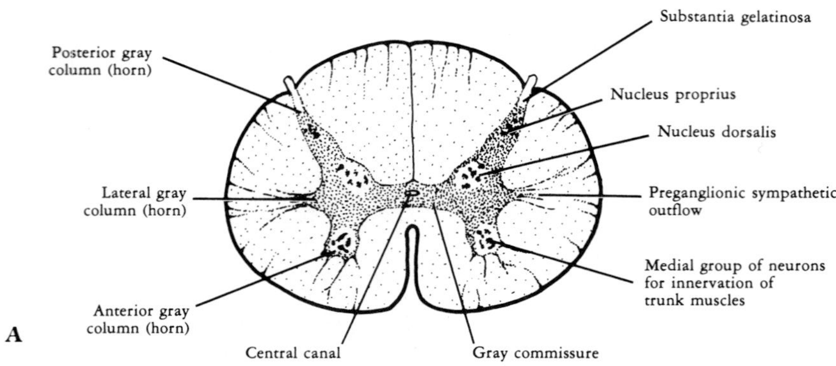

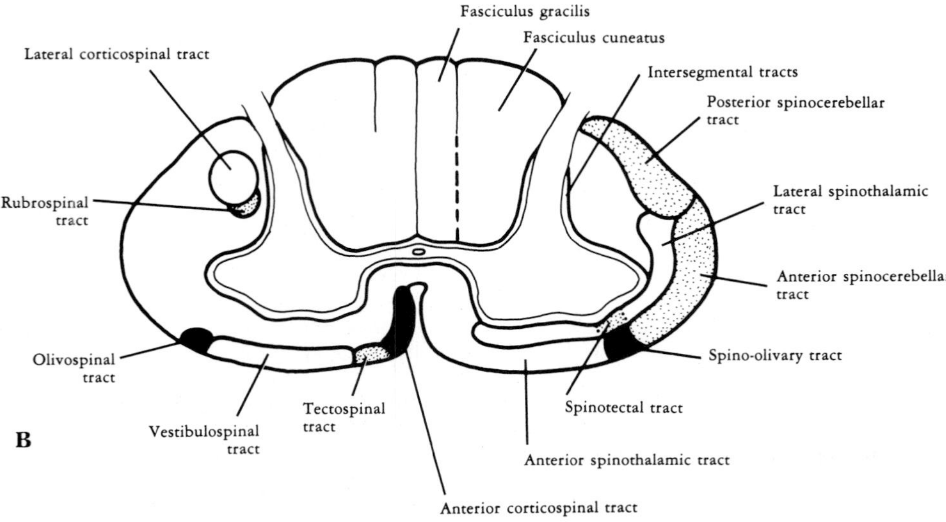

Figure 6–3 **A**. Transverse section of the sixth thoracic segment of the spinal cord showing the arrangement of the gray matter. **B**. Transverse section of the spinal cord at the midcervical level, showing the general arrangement of the ascending tracts on the right and the descending tracts on the left.

nerve root and becomes continuous with the epineurium of each spinal nerve.

CEREBROSPINAL FLUID

The cerebrospinal fluid (CSF) is present in the subarachnoid space and in the central canal of the spinal cord. It is produced by the **choroid plexuses** within the lateral, third, and fourth ventricles of the brain. The spinal part of the subarachnoid space extends down as far as the lower border of the second sacral vertebra.

In addition to removing waste products associated with neuronal activity, the CSF, together with the bony and ligamentous walls of the vertebral canal, effectively protects the spinal cord from trauma. For further details on the cerebrospinal fluid.

BLOOD SUPPLY OF THE SPINAL CORD

The **posterior spinal arteries**, which arise either directly or indirectly from the vertebral arteries, run inferiorly along the side of the spinal cord, close to the attachments of the posterior spinal nerve roots (Fig. 6-4). The **anterior spinal arteries**, which arise from the vertebral arteries, unite to form a single artery, which runs down within the anterior median fissure of the spinal cord. Both the posterior and anterior spinal arteries are small and are not sufficient to supply the entire length of the spinal cord.

The posterior and anterior spinal arteries are reinforced by **radicular arteries** (Fig. 6-4), which are branches of local arteries (deep cervical, intercostal, and lumbar arteries). Radicular arteries enter the vertebral canal through the in-

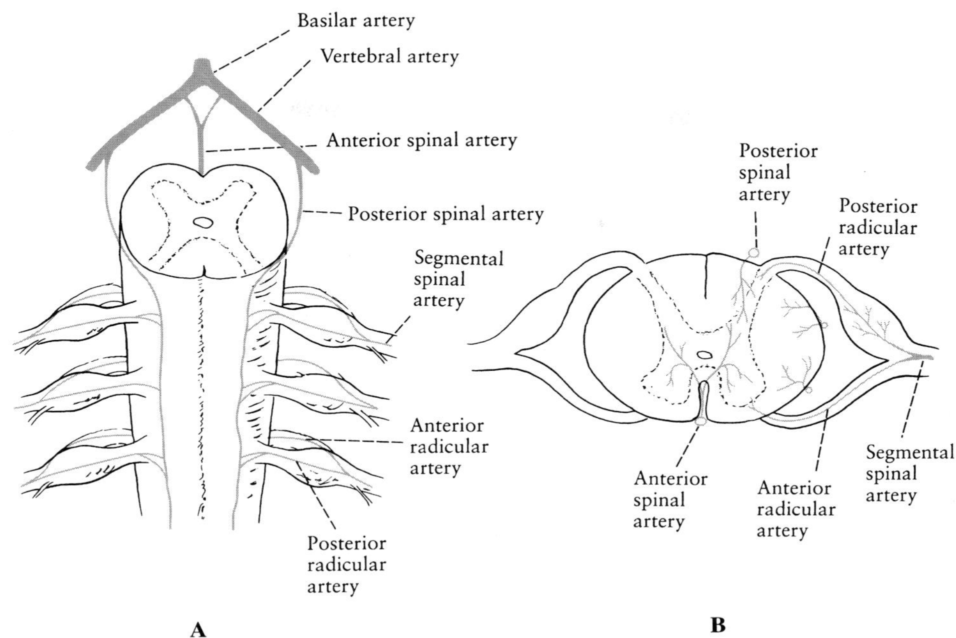

Figure 6–4 Spinal cord showing the arterial supply. **A.** Formation of one anterior and two posterior spinal arteries. **B.** Transverse section of the spinal cord showing the segmental spinal arteries and the radicular arteries.

tervertebral foramina. Commonly, one of the anterior radicular arteries is larger than the remainder and is referred to as the **arteria radicularis magna** (artery of Adamkiewicz). It usually arises from an intersegmental branch of the descending aorta in the lower thoracic or upper lumbar vertebral levels. Usually it arises on the left-hand side. The importance of this artery lies in the fact that it may be the major source of blood to the lower two-thirds of the spinal cord.

The branches of the anterior spinal artery supply approximately the anterior two-thirds of the spinal cord, while the remaining posterior third is supplied by branches from the posterior spinal arteries. A small area on the periphery of the spinal cord is supplied by small arteries from a plexus in the pia mater.

The veins of the spinal cord drain into six tortuous longitudinal channels that communicate superiorly within the skull with the veins of the brain and the venous sinuses. They drain mainly into the internal vertebral venous plexus.

Clinical Notes

Relationship of Spinal Cord Segments to Vertebral Numbers

Because the spinal cord is shorter than the vertebral column, the spinal cord segments do not correspond numerically with the vertebrae that lie at the same level (see Fig.4-3). Table 6-2 shows which spinal segment is related to a given vertebral body.

Table 6–2 Relationship of Spinal Cord Segments to Vertebral Numbers

Vertebrae	Spinal Segment
Cervical vertebrae	Add 1
Upper thoracic vertebrae	Add 2
Lower thoracic vertebrae (7–9)	Add 3
Tenth thoracic vertebra	L1 and 2 cord segments
Eleventh thoracic vertebra	L3 and 4 cord segments
Twelfth thoracic vertebra	L5 cord segment
First lumbar vertebra	Sacral and coccygeal cord segments

Spinal Cord Injuries

In the cervical region, dislocation or fracture dislocation is common, but the large size of the vertebral canal often prevents severe injury to the spinal cord. In fracture dislocations of the thoracic region, displacement of the bony fragments is often considerable and because of the small size of the vertebral canal, severe injury to this region of the spinal cord results. In fracture dislocations of the lumbar region, the spinal cord may escape injury since the cord only extends down as far as the level of the lower border of the first lumbar vertebra (Fig. 4-4). The large size of the vertebral foramen in this region gives the roots of the cauda equina ample room, so that nerve injury may be minimal.

Spinal Nerve Injuries

Disease and the Intervertebral Foramina

At the intervertebral foramen, the spinal nerve may be pressed upon by disease of the surrounding structures. Herniations of the intervertebral disc, fractures of the vertebral bodies, and osteoarthritis involving the joints of the articular processes or the joints between the vertebral bodies may result in pressure on the emerging spinal nerve.

Cervical Disc Herniations

The discs most susceptible to this condition are those between the fifth and sixth and the sixth and seventh cervical vertebrae. Each spinal nerve emerges above the corresponding vertebra; thus, the lateral protrusion of the disc between the fifth and sixth cervical vertebrae may compress the C6 spinal nerve or its roots. Central protrusions may press on the spinal cord.

Lumbar Disc Herniations

These are more common than cervical disc herniations. The discs between the fourth and fifth lumbar vertebrae and between the fifth lumbar vertebra and the sacrum are commonly affected. It should be remembered that in the thoracic and lumbar regions the nerve roots emerge **below** the vertebra of the corresponding number. Thus, the L5 nerve root exits between the L5 and S1 vertebrae. A lateral herniation may press on one or two roots and a central protrusion may press on the whole cauda equina.

Ischemia of the Spinal Cord

This can easily follow minor damage to the arterial supply, as the result of nerve block procedures, aortic surgery or surgery on the vertebral column, or any operation in which severe hypotension occurs.

REVIEW QUESTIONS

Directions: Each of the numbered items in this section is followed by answers that are positively phrased. Select the ONE lettered answer that is an EXCEPTION.

1. The following statements concerning the spinal cord are correct **except:**
   (a) The spinal cord is segmented though the segments are not visible on the surface
   (b) Each segment of the spinal cord has a pair of spinal nerves
   (c) The spinal cord is an important reflex center
   (d) The spinal cord in the young child terminates inferiorly at the level of the twelfth thoracic vertebra
   (e) The spinal cord in the adult terminates inferiorly at the level of the lower border of the first lumbar vertebra
2. The following statements concerning the protection of the spinal cord from external injury are correct **except:**
   (a) The spinal cord is located within the vertebral canal of the vertebral column
   (b) The spinal cord is covered by the ligamentum denticulatum
   (c) The spinal cord is floating in the cerebrospinal fluid
   (d) The spinal cord is surrounded by the pia mater, arachnoid mater, and dura mater
   (e) The spinal cord is protected by fatty areolar tissue in the vertebral canal
3. The following statements concerning the shape of the spinal cord are correct **except:**
   (a) The sacral enlargement is caused by the terminal ventricle
   (b) The cervical enlargement is caused by the presence of the brachial plexus
   (c) The lumbar enlargement is caused by the presence of the lumbosacral plexus
   (d) The conus medullaris is located at the lower end of the spinal cord
   (e) The spinal cord is roughly cylindrical throughout its length
4. The following statements concerning the gray matter of the spinal cord are correct **except:**
   (a) The central canal contains cerebrospinal fluid
   (b) The lateral gray columns (horns) are present in the thoracic region
   (c) The anterior and posterior gray columns (horns) are present throughout the length of the spinal cord
   (d) The gray commissure connects the tips of the posterior gray columns (horns)
   (e) The gray matter is surrounded by an outer covering of white matter
5. The following statements concerning the gray matter of the spinal cord are correct **except:**
   (a) The phrenic nucleus is present in the third, fourth, and fifth cervical segments
   (b) The accessory nucleus lies at the level of the fifth and sixth cervical segments
   (c) The substantia gelatinosa occupies the tip of the

posterior gray column throughout the length of the spinal cord
(d) The nucleus dorsalis (Clark's column) extends from the eighth cervical segment caudally to the third or fourth lumbar segment of the cord
(e) The nucleus proprius extends throughout the length of the spinal cord

6. The following statements concerning the efferent outflows of the autonomic system in the spinal cord are correct **except:**
(a) The sympathetic outflow occurs at segmental levels T1–L2
(b) The sympathetic outflow occupies the lateral gray column (horn)
(c) The parasympathetic outflow occupies the posterior gray column (horn)
(d) The parasympathetic outflow occurs at segmental levels S2, S3, and S4
(e) The cells of origin give rise to axons that are called preganglionic nerve fibers

7. The following statements concerning the meninges are correct **except:**
(a) The dura mater covering the spinal cord is continuous above through the foramen magnum with the meningeal layer of dura of the brain
(b) The dura mater of the spinal cord ends below at the level of the second sacral vertebra
(c) The arachnoid mater covering the spinal cord ends below at the level of the second sacral vertebra
(d) The subarachnoid space is filled with cerebrospinal fluid
(e) The pia mater surrounds the spinal cord but does not extend along the spinal nerve roots

8. The following statements concerning the spinal cord are correct **except:**
(a) The ligamentum denticulatum attaches the pia mater covering the spinal cord to the dura between the nerve roots
(b) The posterior spinal arteries supply the posterior third of the spinal cord
(c) The radicular arteries reinforce only the anterior spinal artery
(d) Each spinal nerve is attached to the spinal cord by an anterior and a posterior nerve root
(e) Each root of the spinal nerve is attached to the spinal cord by a series of rootlets that extend the whole length of each segment of the spinal cord

Directions: Each of the incomplete statements in this section is followed by completions of the statement. Select the ONE lettered completion that is BEST in each case.

For questions 9-12, study Figure 6-5, showing a transverse section of a thoracic segment of the spinal cord.

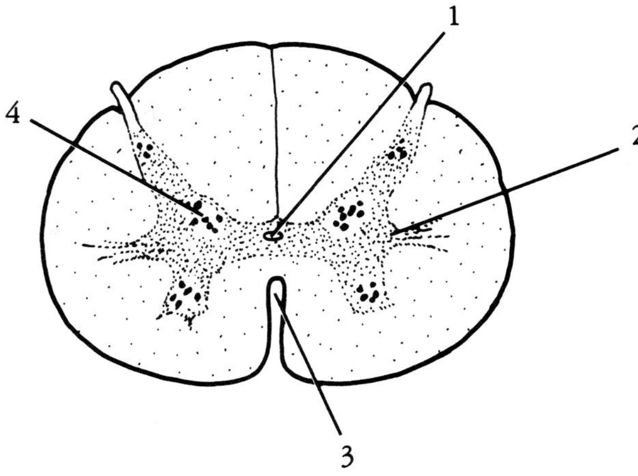

Figure 6–5 Transverse section of a thoracic segment of the spinal cord.

9. Identify structure number 1.
(a) Nucleus dorsalis
(b) Central canal
(c) Anterior median fissure
(d) Posterior median septum
(e) Posterior gray horn

10. Identify structure number 2.
(a) Anterior gray horn
(b) Posterior gray horn
(c) Lateral gray horn
(d) Lateral white column
(e) Ligamentum denticulatum

11. Identify structure number 3.
(a) Posterior median fissure
(b) Anterior median fissure
(c) Preparation artefact
(d) Anterior white column
(e) Arachnoid mater

12. Identify structure number 4.
(a) Nucleus dorsalis
(b) Nucleus proprius
(c) Substantia gelatinosa
(d) Phrenic nucleus
(e) Accessory nucleus

For questions 13-16 study Figure 6-6, showing a transverse section of a cervical segment of the spinal cord

13. Identify structure number 1.
(a) Posterior spinocerebellar tract
(b) Lateral corticospinal tract
(c) Fasciculus cuneatus
(d) Rubrospinal tract
(e) Anterior spinocerebellar tract

14. Identify structure number 2.
(a) Vestibulospinal tract
(b) Olivospinal tract
(c) Rubrospinal tract
(d) Lateral corticospinal tract
(e) Anterior corticospinal tract

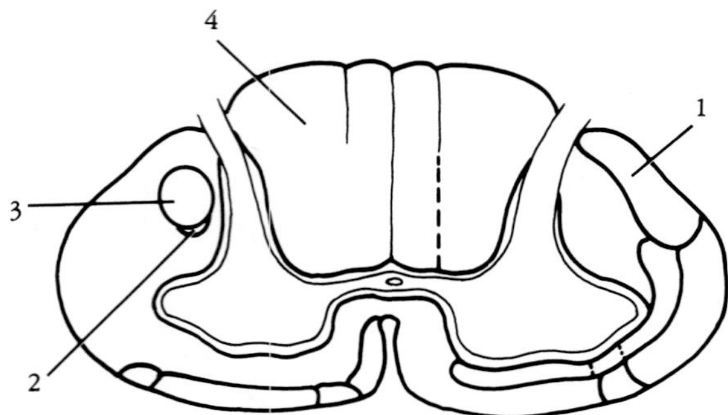

Figure 6–6 Transverse section of a cervical segment of the spinal cord.

15. Identify structure number 3.
    (a) Rubrospinal tract
    (b) Anterior corticospinal tract
    (c) Lateral spinothalamic tract
    (d) Lateral corticospinal tract
    (e) Anterior spinothalamic tract
16. Identify structure number 4.
    (a) Fasciculus gracilis
    (b) Posterior spinocerebellar tract
    (c) Fasciculus cuneatus
    (d) Intersegmental tracts
    (e) Lateral corticospinal tract

For questions 17-21, study Figure 6-7, showing a sagittal MRI of the vertebral column.

17. Identify structure number 1.
    (a) Margin of the foramen magnum
    (b) Medulla oblongata
    (c) Occipital condyle
    (d) Spinal cord
    (e) Body of the second cervical vertebra
18. Identify structure number 2.
    (a) Intervertebral disc C4-5
    (b) Body of the fourth cervical vertebra
    (c) Intervertebral disc C3-4
    (d) Prolapsed intervertebral disc C5-6
    (e) Body of the third cervical vertebra
19. Identify structure number 3.
    (a) Body of the fourth cervical vertebral
    (b) Body of the second cervical vertebra
    (c) Body of the third cervical vertebra
    (d) Pedicle of the third cervical vertebra
    (e) Intervertebral disc C5-6
20. Identify structure number 4.
    (a) Spinal cord
    (b) Normal intervertebral disc C5-6
    (c) Prolapsed intervertebral disc C5-6
    (d) Internal vertebral vein
    (e) Body of the fourth cervical vertebra
21. Identify structure number 5.
    (a) Medulla oblongata
    (b) Thoracic region of spinal cord

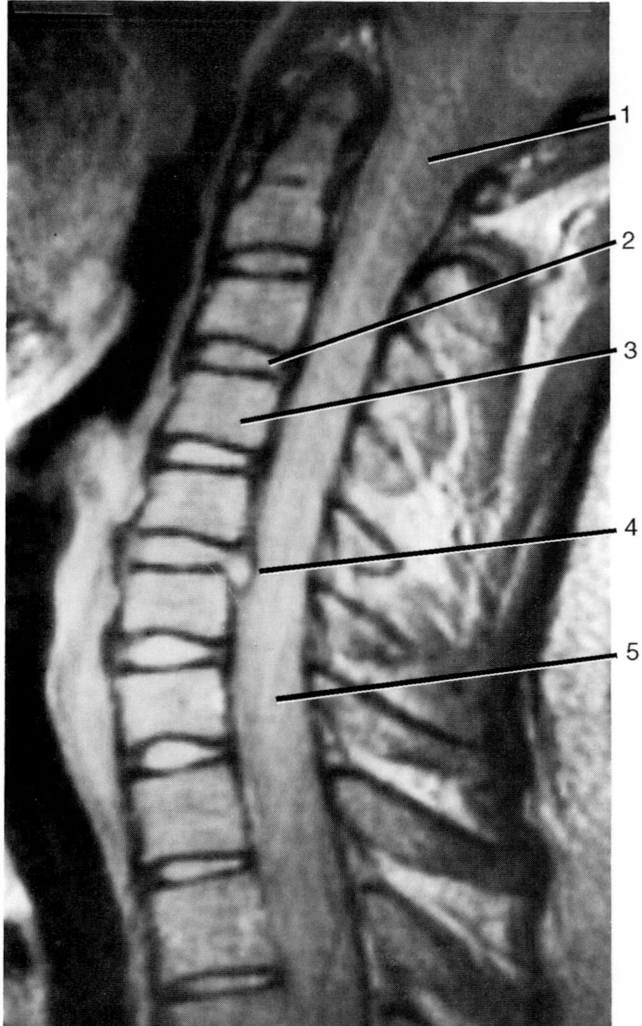

Figure 6–7 Sagittal MRI of the vertebral column.

    (c) Cervical region of spinal cord
    (d) Posterior longitudinal ligament
    (e) Ligamentum flavum

Directions: Read the case history then answer the question. You will be required to select ONE BEST lettered answer. Study the following case history and select the best answer to the question following it.

A 38-year-old man was examined by a neurologist because of a complaint of severe burning pain over the left shoulder and upper part of the left arm that had started 3 weeks previously. The pain was accentuated by moving his neck and by coughing. After a full clinical examination followed by an MRI, a diagnosis of prolapse of the intervertebral disc between the fifth and sixth cervical vertebrae was made. There was no evidence of muscle weakness.

22. The following anatomical facts concerning this case are correct **except:**
    (a) The posterior root of the sixth cervical nerve was being pressed on by the prolapsed disc.
    (b) When an intervertebral disc prolapses, the nucleus pulposus moves anteriorly.
    (c) The common site for a disc to press on a nerve root is in the intervertebral foramen.
    (d) In the cervical region the spinal nerves emerge above the vertebra of the same number.
    (e) In the cervical region there are eight cervical nerves but only seven cervical vertebrae.

ANSWERS AND EXPLANATIONS

1. D. In the young child the spinal cord is relatively long and ends below at the level of the upper border of the third lumbar vertebra.
2. B. The ligamentum denticulatum is formed of pia mater and extends laterally to be attached to the arachnoid mater and dura mater; it serves to suspend the spinal cord in the middle of the dural sheath.
3. A. There is no enlargement of the spinal cord in the sacral region.
4. D. The gray commissure connects the anterior and posterior gray columns on each side so that the gray matter resembles the letter H.
5. B. The accessory nucleus occupies the upper five cervical segments of the spinal cord.
6. C. The parasympathetic outflow at levels S2, S3, and S4 does not occupy the posterior gray column (horn) and the nerve cells do not form a separate lateral gray column.
7. E. The pia mater extends laterally around each nerve root as far as the beginning of the spinal nerve.
8. C. The radicular arteries reinforce both the anterior and the posterior spinal arteries.
9. B
10. C
11. B
12. A
13. A
14. C
15. D
16. C
17. B
18. C
19. A
20. C
21. C
22. B. When herniation of an intervertebral disc occurs, the posterior part of the anulus fibrosus of the disc ruptures and the nucleus pulposus is forced out posteriorly, like toothpaste out of a tube. This herniation can occur in the midline or posterolaterally close to the intervertebral foramen, as in this patient.

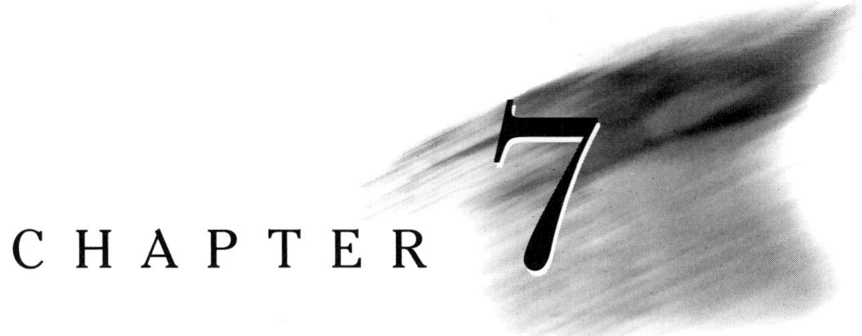

CHAPTER 7

Ascending and Descending Tracts and Reflex Activity

CHAPTER OUTLINE

SUGGESTED PLAN FOR REVIEW OF CHAPTER 7

1. Each of the ascending and descending tracts listed in this chapter must be memorized. The function of each pathway must be committed to memory.
2. Distinguish between light touch and discriminative touch.
3. Understand the analgesia system and the gating theory.
4. Know what enkephalins and endorphins are.
5. Be able to define a reflex arc. Know what is meant by the law of reciprocal innervation and the crossed extensor reflex.
6. Know what a Renshaw cell is.

By the time you have finished this chapter, it should be possible for you to make simple line drawings of each of the ascending and descending pathways showing their cells of origin, their course through the central nervous system, and their destination. Particular attention should be paid to whether a particular tract crosses the midline to the opposite side of the central nervous system or remains on the same side. If the tract does cross the midline, the level of crossover is important.

INTRODUCTION

The ascending and descending tracts of the spinal cord are situated in the white matter. They are the axons of nerve cells that carry nerve impulses up to the brain and down from the brain to the different segments of the spinal cord.

The position of the tracts has been determined by clinical and pathological studies and by animal experimentation. It must be emphasized that the positions of the tracts are only approximate and considerable overlap and mixing occur. Nevertheless, from a practical standpoint, the arrangement of the tracts outlined below can be of considerable clinical value in making neurological diagnoses.

ASCENDING TRACTS

On entering the spinal cord, the sensory nerve fibers of different functions are sorted out and segregated into bundles of nerves or tracts (Fig. 7-1). Some of the nerve fibers serve to link different segments of the spinal cord, while others ascend from the spinal cord to higher centers and thus connect the spinal cord with the brain. The bundles of the ascending fibers are referred to as the **ascending tracts**.

In its simplest form, the ascending pathway to consciousness consists of three neurons. The first neuron, the **first-order neuron**, has its cell body in the **posterior root ganglion** of the spinal nerve. A peripheral process connects with a sensory receptor ending, whereas a central process enters the spinal cord through the posterior root to synapse on the **second-order neuron**. The second-order neuron gives rise to an axon that crosses to the opposite side and ascends to a higher level of the central nervous system, where it synapses with the **third-order neuron**. The third-order neuron is usually in the thalamus and gives rise to a projection fiber that passes to a sensory region of the cerebral cortex. The three-neuron chain described is the most common arrangement, but some afferent pathways use more or fewer neurons. Many of the neurons branch and participate in reflex activity.

Functions of the Ascending Tracts

Painful and thermal sensations ascend in the lateral spinothalamic tract; light (crude) touch and pressure ascend in the anterior spinothalamic tract. Discriminative touch—that is, the ability to localize accurately the area of the body touched and also to be aware that two points are touched simultaneously, even though they are close together (two-point discrimination)—ascends in the posterior white columns. Also ascending in the posterior white columns is information from muscles and joints pertaining to movement and position of different parts of the body. In addition, vibratory sensations ascend in the posterior white column. Unconscious information from muscles, joints, the skin, and subcutaneous tissue reaches the cerebellum by way of the anterior and posterior spinocerebellar tracts and by the cuneocerebellar tract. Pain, thermal, and tactile information is passed to the superior colliculus of the midbrain through the spinotectal tract for the purpose of spinovisual reflexes. The spinoreticular tract provides a pathway from the muscles, joints, and skin to the reticular formation, while the spino-olivary tract provides an indirect pathway for further afferent information to reach the cerebellum.

Pain and Temperature Pathways

LATERAL SPINOTHALAMIC TRACT

The pain and thermal receptors in the skin and other tissues are free nerve endings. The pain impulses are transmitted to the spinal cord in fast-conducting delta A type fibers and slow-conducting C type fibers. The fast-conducting fibers alert the individual to the initial sharp pain and the slow-conducting fibers are responsible for the prolonged burning, aching pain. The sensations of heat and cold also travel by delta A and C fibers.

The axons entering the spinal cord from the posterior root ganglion proceed to the tip of the posterior gray column and divide into ascending and descending branches (Fig. 7-2). These branches travel for a distance of one or two segments

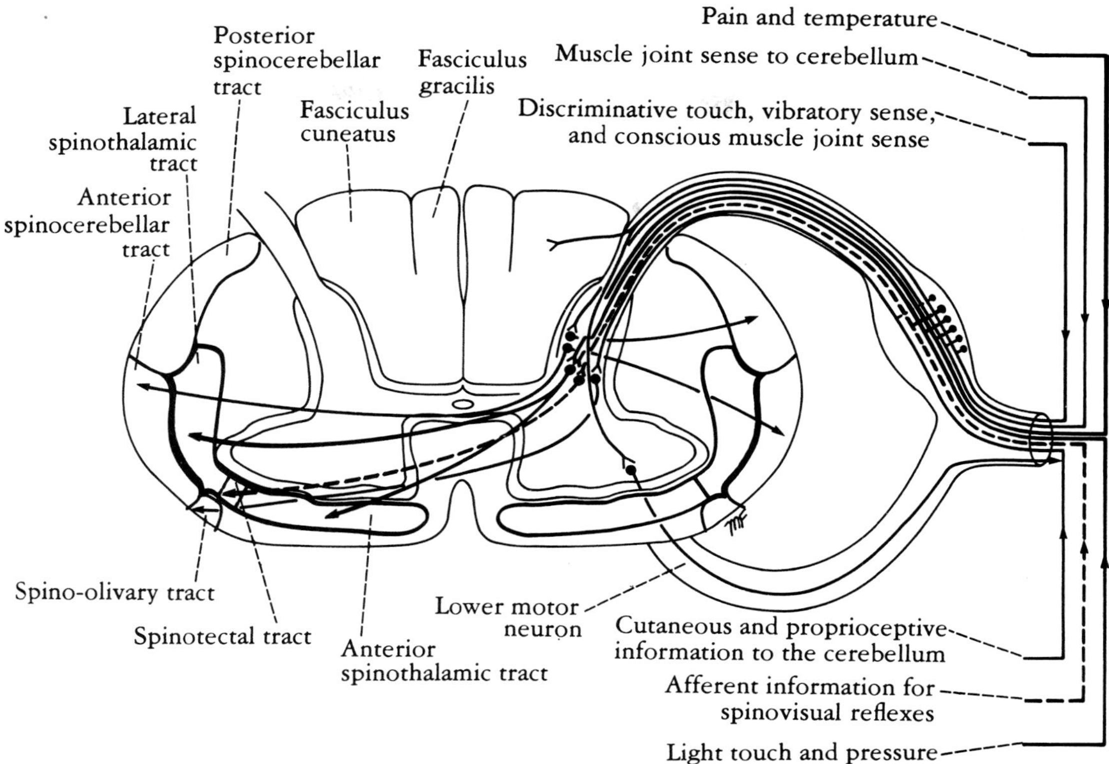

Figure 7–1 Transverse section of the spinal cord showing the organization of the main ascending tracts.

of the spinal cord and form the **posterolateral tract of Lissauer**. These fibers of the first-order neuron terminate by synapsing with cells in the posterior gray column, including cells in the substantia gelatinosa. Substance P, a peptide, is thought to be the neurotransmitter at these synapses.

The axons of the second-order neurons now **cross obliquely to the opposite side in the anterior gray and white commissures within one spinal segment of the cord** and ascend in the contralateral white column as the lateral spinothalamic tract (Fig. 7-2). As the lateral spinothalamic tract ascends through the spinal cord, new fibers are added to the anteromedial aspect of the tract, so that in the upper cervical segments of the cord the sacral fibers are lateral and the cervical segments are medial.

As the lateral spinothalamic tract ascends through the medulla oblongata, it is accompanied by the anterior spinothalamic tract and the spinotectal tract, which all together form the **spinal lemniscus** (Fig. 7-2).

The spinal lemniscus continues to ascend through the posterior part of the pons (Fig. 7-2). In the midbrain it lies in the tegmentum lateral to the medial lemniscus. Many of the fibers of the lateral spinothalamic tract end by synapsing with the third-order neuron in the ventral posterolateral nucleus of the thalamus (Fig. 7-2). It is believed that here crude pain and temperature sensations are appreciated and emotional reactions are initiated.

The axons of the third-order neurons in the ventral posterolateral nucleus of the thalamus now pass through the posterior limb of the internal capsule and the corona radiata to reach the somesthetic area in the postcentral gyrus of the cerebral cortex (Fig. 7-2). The contralateral half of the body is represented as inverted, with the hand and mouth situated inferiorly and the leg situated superiorly, and with the foot and anogenital region on the medial surface of the hemisphere. The role of the cerebral cortex is the interpretation of the sensory information at the level of consciousness.

Other Terminations of the Lateral Spinothalamic Tract

Pain impulses ascending through the lateral spinothalamic tract travel in two pathways

The initial sharp, pricking pain terminates in the ventral posterolateral nucleus of the thalamus and is then relayed to the cerebral cortex.

The burning pain terminates in the reticular formation, which then activates the entire nervous system. These impulses alert the individual to an injury, and although the site of the injury is poorly localized, nevertheless they arouse the nervous system and create a sense of urgency.

THE ANALGESIA SYSTEM

Experimental stimulation of certain areas of the brainstem can reduce or block sensations of pain. These areas include the periventricular area of the diencephalon, the periaqueductal gray matter of the midbrain, and midline nuclei of

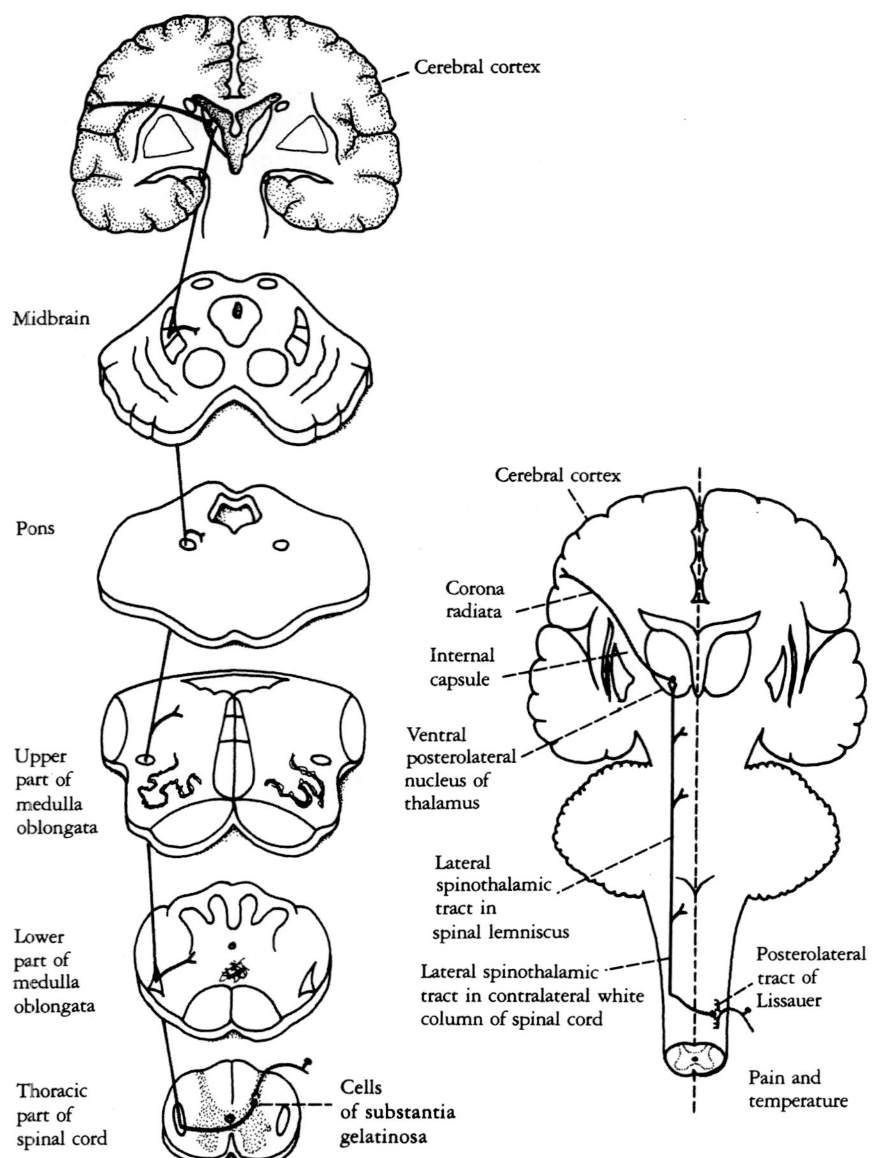

Figure 7–2 Pain and temperature pathways—lateral spinothalamic tract.

the brainstem. It is believed that fibers of the reticulospinal tract pass down to the spinal cord and synapse on cells concerned with pain sensation in the posterior gray column. The analgesic system can suppress both sharp pricking pain and burning pain sensations.

Recently two compounds with morphine-like actions, called the **enkephalins** and the **endorphins**, have been isolated in the central nervous system. It has been suggested that these compounds and serotonin serve as neurotransmitter substances in the analgesic system of the brain and that they may inhibit the release of substance P in the posterior gray column.

THE GATING THEORY

Massage and the application of liniments to painful areas of the body can be very effective in relieving pain. Although the precise mechanism for these phenomena is not understood, the gating theory was proposed some years ago. It was suggested that at the site where the pain fiber enters the central nervous system, inhibition could occur by means of connector neurons excited by large, myelinated afferent fibers carrying nonpainful information of touch and pressure. The excess tactile stimulation, produced by massage, for example, "closed the gate" for pain. Once the nonpainful tactile stimulation ceased, however, "the gate was opened" and the painful stimuli ascended the lateral spinothalamic tract. While the gate theory may partially explain the phenomena, it is probable that the analgesia system, noted above, is also involved with the liberation of enkephalins and endorphins in the posterior gray columns.

Light (Crude) Touch and Pressure Pathways

ANTERIOR SPINOTHALAMIC TRACT

The axons enter the spinal cord from the posterior root ganglion and proceed to the tip of the posterior gray column, where they divide into ascending and descending branches (Fig. 7-3). These branches travel for a distance of one or two segments of the spinal cord, contributing to the **posterolateral tract of Lissauer**. It is believed that these fibers of the first-order neuron terminate by synapsing with cells in the substantia gelatinosa group in the posterior gray column.

The axons of the second-order neuron now **cross very obliquely to the opposite side in the anterior gray and white commissures** and ascend in the opposite anterolateral white column as the anterior spinothalamic tract (Fig. 7-3). As the anterior spinothalamic tract ascends through the spinal cord, new fibers are added to the medial aspect of the tract, so that in the upper cervical segments of the cord the sacral fibers are mostly lateral and the cervical segments are mostly medial.

As the anterior spinothalamic tract ascends through the medulla oblongata, it accompanies the lateral spinothalamic tract and the spinotectal tract, all of which form the **spinal lemniscus** (Fig. 7-3).

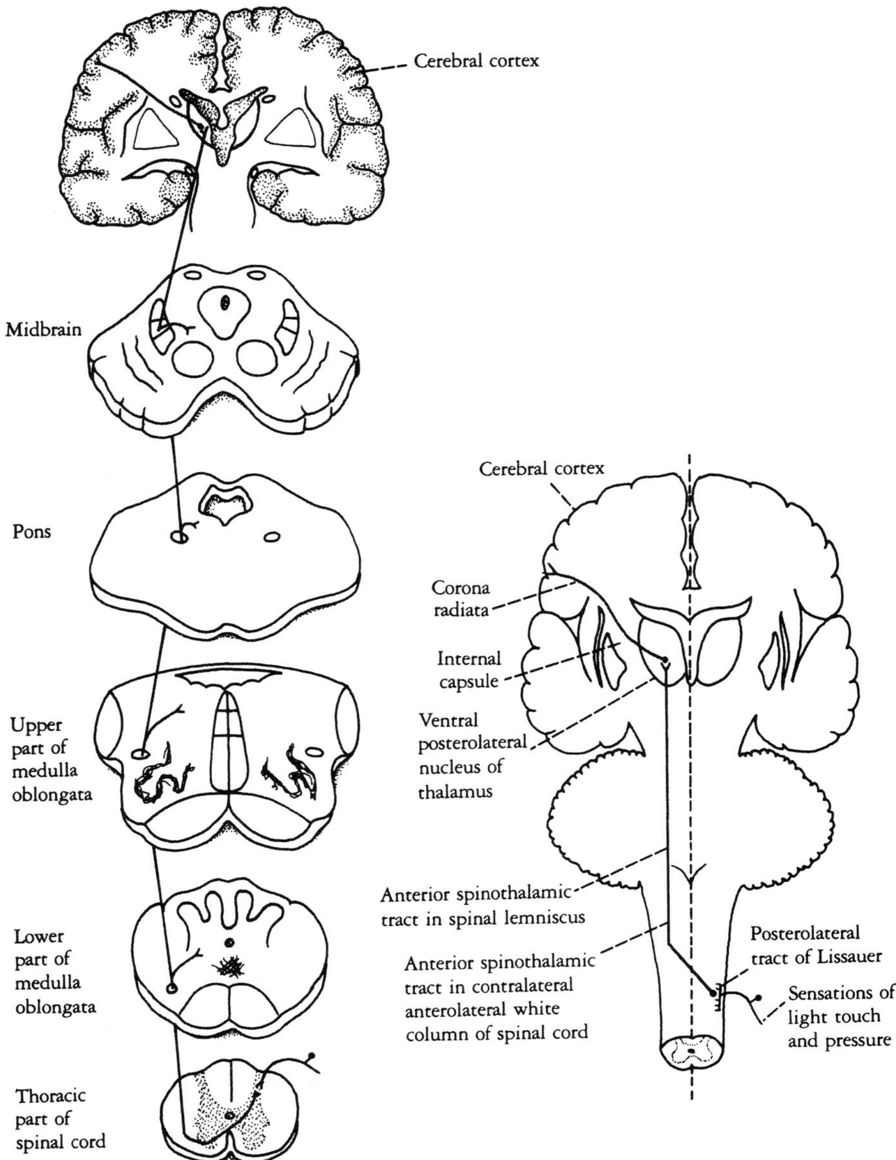

Figure 7–3 Light touch and pressure pathways—anterior spinothalamic tract.

The spinal lemniscus continues to ascend through the posterior part of the pons, and the tegmentum of the midbrain and the fibers of the anterior spinothalamic tract terminate by synapsing with the third-order neuron in the ventral posterolateral nucleus of the thalamus (Fig. 7-3). Crude awareness of touch and pressure is believed to be appreciated here.

The axons of the third-order neurons in the ventral posterolateral nucleus of the thalamus pass through the posterior limb of the **internal capsule** and the **corona radiata** to reach the somesthetic area in the postcentral gyrus of the cerebral cortex. The contralateral half of the body is represented inverted, with the hand and mouth situated inferiorly. The conscious appreciation of touch and pressure depends on the activity of the cerebral cortex. The sensations can only be crudely localized and very little discrimination of intensity is possible.

Discriminative Touch, Vibratory Sense, and Conscious Muscle Joint Sense

POSTERIOR WHITE COLUMN: FASCICULUS GRACILIS AND FASCICULUS CUNEATUS

The axons enter the spinal cord from the posterior root ganglion and pass directly to the posterior white column of the **same side** (Fig. 7-4). Here the fibers divide into long ascending and short descending branches. The descending

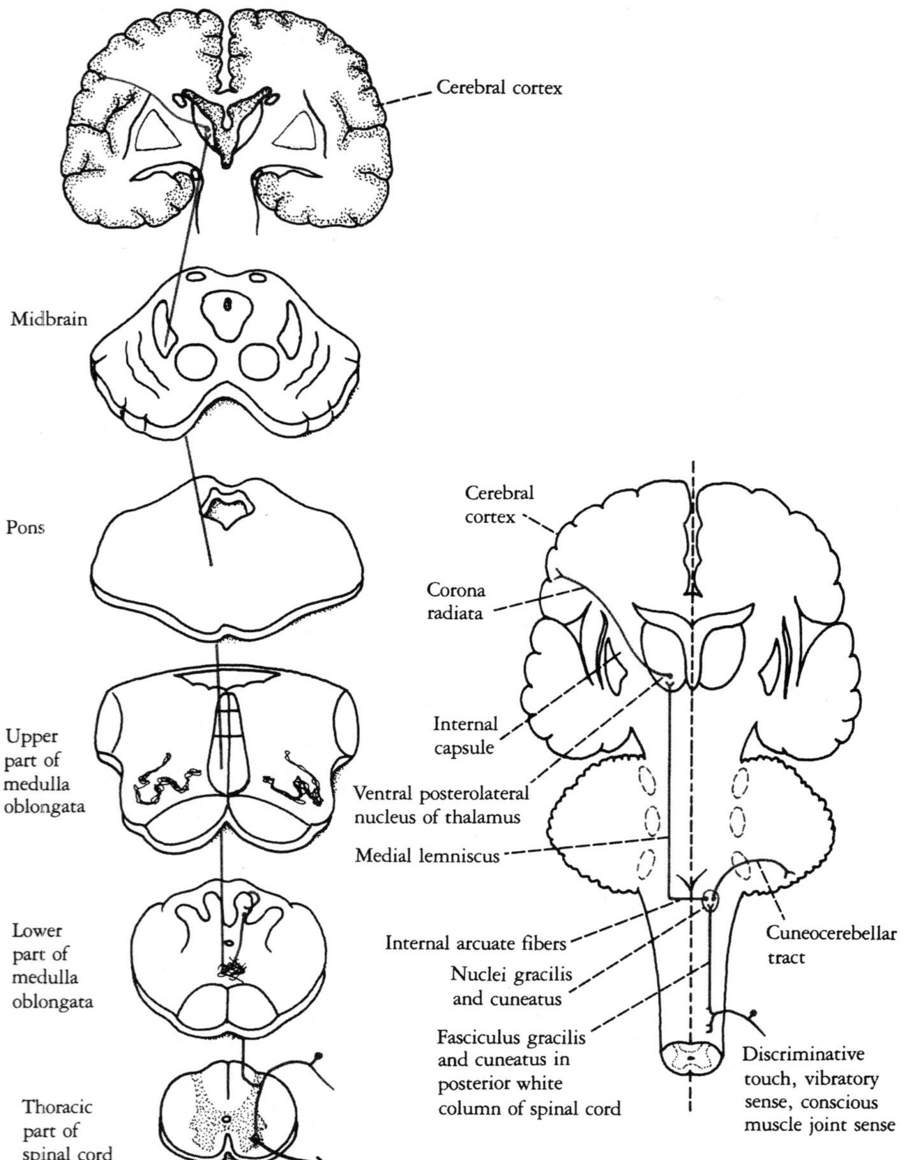

Figure 7–4 Discriminative touch, vibratory sense, and conscious muscle joint sense pathways—fasciculus gracilis and cuneatus.

branches pass down a variable number of segments, giving off collateral branches that synapse with cells in the posterior gray horn, with internuncial neurons, and with anterior horn cells. It is clear that these short descending fibers are involved with intersegmental reflexes.

The long ascending fibers may also end by synapsing with cells in the posterior gray horn, with internuncial neurons, and with anterior horn cells. This distribution may extend over many segments of the spinal cord. As in the case of the short descending fibers, they are involved with intersegmental reflexes.

Many of the long ascending fibers travel upward in the posterior white column as the **fasciculus gracilis and fasciculus cuneatus** (Fig. 7-4). The fasciculus gracilis is present throughout the length of the spinal cord and contains the long ascending fibers from the sacral, lumbar, and lower six thoracic spinal nerves. The fasciculus cuneatus is situated laterally in the upper thoracic and cervical segments of the spinal cord and is separated from the fasciculus gracilis by a septum. The fasciculus cuneatus contains the long ascending fibers from the upper six thoracic and all the cervical spinal nerves.

The fibers of the fasciculus gracilis and cuneatus ascend ipsilaterally and terminate by synapsing on the second-order neurons in the **nuclei gracilis and cuneatus** of the medulla oblongata (Fig. 7-4). The axons of the second-order neurons, called the **internal arcuate fibers**, sweep anteromedially around the central gray matter and cross the median plane, decussating with the corresponding fibers of the opposite side in the **sensory decussation** (Fig. 7-4). The fibers then ascend as a single compact bundle, the **medial lemniscus**, through the medulla oblongata, the pons, and the midbrain (Fig. 7-4). The fibers terminate by synapsing on the third-order neurons in the ventral posterolateral nucleus of the thalamus.

The axons of the third-order neuron leave and pass through the posterior limb of the **internal capsule and corona radiata** to reach the somesthetic area in the postcentral gyrus of the cerebral cortex. The contralateral half of the body is represented inverted, with the hand and mouth situated inferiorly. In this manner, the impressions of touch with fine gradations of intensity, exact localization, and two-point discrimination can be appreciated. Vibratory sense and the position of the different parts of the body can be consciously recognized.

A number of fibers in the fasciculus cuneatus from the cervical and upper thoracic segments, having terminated on the second-order neuron of the nucleus cuneatus, are relayed and travel as the axons of the second-order neurons to enter the cerebellum through the inferior cerebellar peduncle of the same side (Fig.7-4). The pathway is referred to as the **cuneocerebellar tract** and the fibers are known as the **posterior external arcuate fibers**. The function of these fibers is to convey information of muscle joint sense to the cerebellum.

The main somatosensory pathways are summarized in Table 7-1.

Muscle Joint Sense Pathways to the Cerebellum

POSTERIOR SPINOCEREBELLAR TRACT

The axons entering the spinal cord from the posterior root ganglion (Fig. 7-5) enter the posterior gray column and terminate by synapsing on the second-order neurons in the **nucleus dorsalis (Clark's column).** The axons of the second-order neurons enter the posterolateral part of the lateral white column on the **same side** and ascend as the posterior spinocerebellar tract to the medulla oblongata. Here the tract joins the inferior cerebellar peduncle and terminates in the cerebellar cortex (Fig. 7-5). Note that it does not ascend to the cerebral cortex. Since the nucleus dorsalis (Clark's

Table 7–1 Summary of the Main Somatosensory Pathways to Consciousness

Sensation	Receptor	First-Order Neuron	Second-Order Neuron	Third-Order Neuron	Pathways	Destination
Pain and temperature	Free nerve endings	Posterior root ganglion	Substantia gelatinosa	Posterior lateral nucleus of thalamus	Lateral spinothalamic, spinal lemniscus	Postcentral gyrus
Light touch, pressure	Free nerve endings	Posterior root ganglion	Substantia gelatinosa	Posterior lateral nucleus of thalamus	Anterior spinothalamic, spinal lemniscus	Postcentral gyrus
Discriminative touch, vibratory sense, conscious muscle joint sense	Meissner's corpuscle, pacinian corpuscle, muscle spindle, tendon organ	Posterior root ganglion	Nuclei gracilis and cuneatus	Posterior lateral nucleus of thalamus	Fasciculus gracilis and cuneatus, medial lemniscus	Postcentral gyrus

Note that all ascending pathways send branches to the reticular activating system.

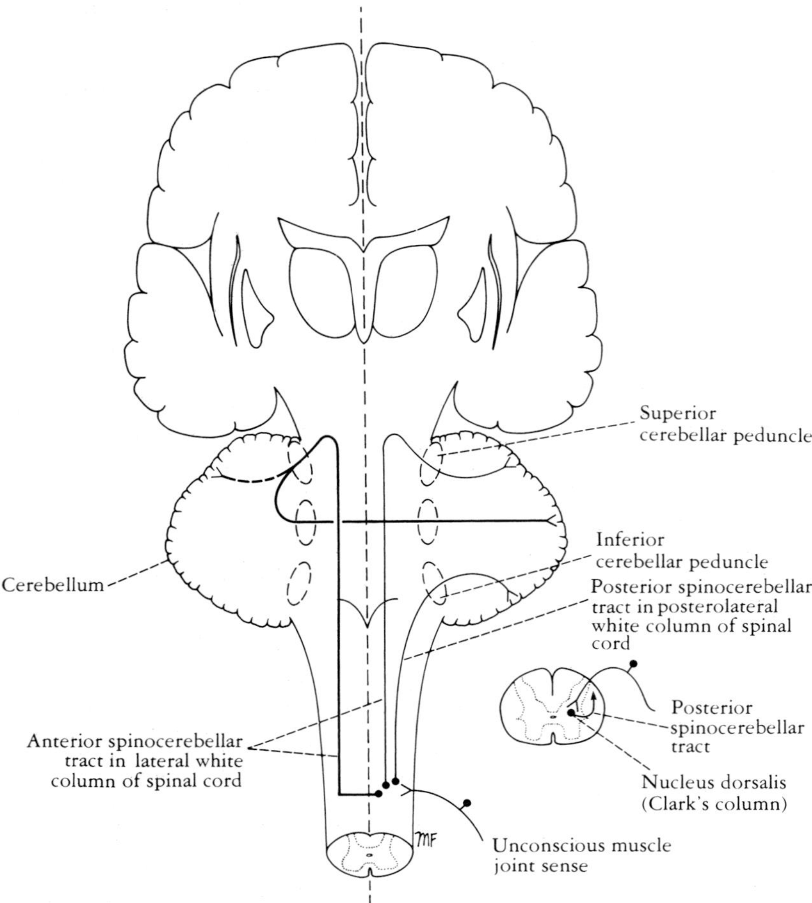

Figure 7–5 Muscle joint sense pathways to the cerebellum—anterior and posterior spinocerebellar tracts.

column) extends only from the eighth cervical segment caudally to the third or fourth lumbar segment, axons entering the spinal cord from the posterior roots of the lower lumbar and sacral segments ascend in the posterior white column until they reach the third or fourth lumbar segment, where they enter the nucleus dorsalis.

The posterior spinocerebellar fibers receive muscle joint information from the muscle spindles, tendon organs, and joint receptors of the trunk and lower limbs. This information concerning tension of muscle tendons and the movements of muscles and joints is used by the cerebellum in the coordination of limb movements and the maintenance of posture.

ANTERIOR SPINOCEREBELLAR TRACT

The axons entering the spinal cord from the posterior root ganglion terminate in the posterior gray column by synapsing with the second-order neurons in the nucleus dorsalis (Fig. 7-5). The majority of the axons of the second-order neurons **cross** to the opposite side and ascend as the anterior spinocerebellar tract in the contralateral white column; the minority of the axons ascend as the anterior spinocerebellar tract in the lateral white column of the **same side** (Fig. 7-5). The fibers, having ascended through the medulla oblongata and pons, enter the cerebellum through the superior cerebellar peduncle and terminate in the cerebellar cortex. It is believed that those fibers that crossed over to the opposite side in the spinal cord **cross back** within the cerebellum (Fig. 7-5). The anterior spinocerebellar tract conveys muscle joint information from the muscle spindles, tendon organs, and joint receptors of the trunk and the upper and lower limbs. It is also believed that the cerebellum receives information from the skin and superficial fascia by this tract.

The muscle joint sense pathways to the cerebellum are summarized in Table 7-2.

CUNEOCEREBELLAR TRACT

These fibers have already been described on page 75. They originate in the nucleus cuneatus and enter the cerebellum through the inferior cerebellar peduncle of the same side (Fig. 7-4). The fibers are known as the **posterior external arcuate fibers** and their function is to convey information of muscle joint sense to the cerebellum.

Other Ascending Pathways

SPINOTECTAL TRACT

The axons enter the spinal cord from the posterior root ganglion and travel to the gray matter where they synapse on unknown second-order neurons (Fig. 7-6). The axons of the second-order neurons **cross** the median plane and ascend as the spinotectal tract in the anterolateral white column lying close to the lateral spinothalamic tract. After they pass through the medulla oblongata and pons, they terminate by synapsing with neurons in the superior colliculus of the midbrain (Fig. 7-6). This pathway provides afferent information for spinovisual reflexes and brings about movements of the eyes and head toward the source of the stimulation.

Spionoreticular Tract

The axons enter the spinal cord from the posterior root ganglion and terminate on unknown second-order neurons in

Table 7–2 Summary of Muscle Joint Sense Pathways to the Cerebellum

Sensation	Receptor	First-Order Neuron	Second-Order Neuron	Pathways	Destination
Unconscious muscle joint sense	Muscle spindles, tendon organs, joint receptors	Posterior root ganglion	Nucleus dorsalis	Anterior and posterior spinocerebellar tract	Cerebellar cortex

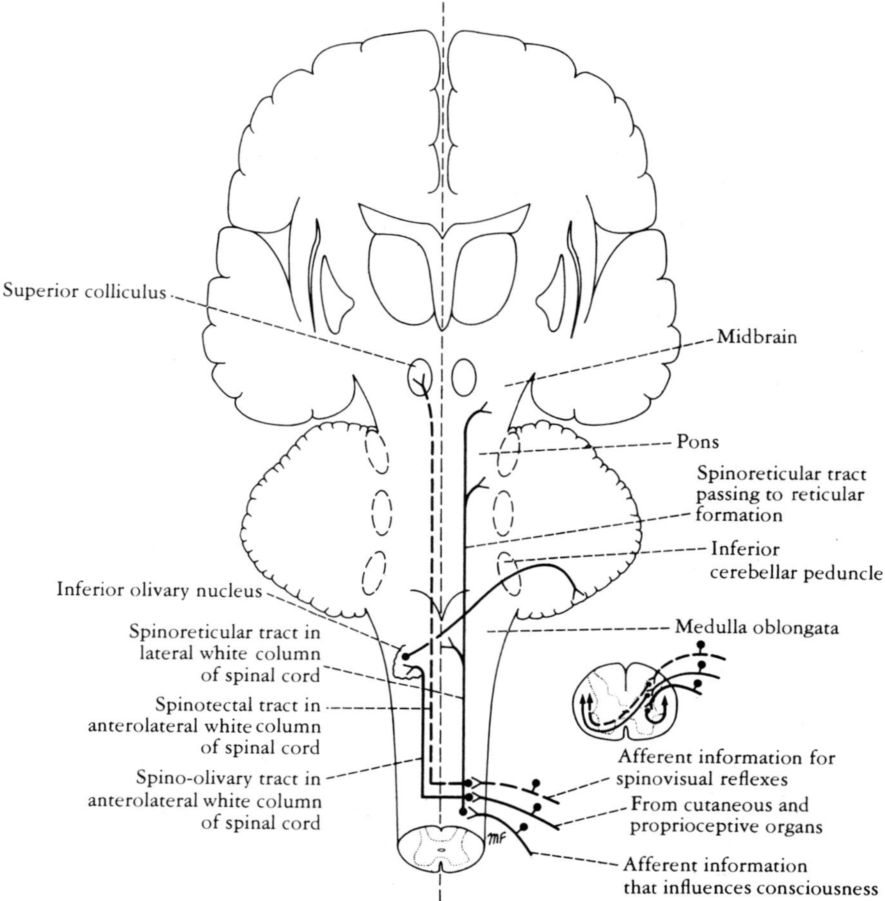

Figure 7–6 Spinotectal, spinoreticular, and spino-olivary tracts.

the gray matter (Fig. 7-6). The axons from these second-order neurons ascend the spinal cord as the spinoreticular tract in the lateral white column mixed with the lateral spinothalamic tract. The majority of the fibers are **uncrossed** and terminate by synapsing with neurons of the reticular formation in the medulla oblongata, pons, and midbrain (Fig. 7-6). The spinoreticular tract provides an afferent pathway for the reticular formation, which plays an important role in influencing levels of consciousness. (For details, see p. 123.)

Spino-Olivary Tract

The axons enter the spinal cord from the posterior root ganglion and terminate on unknown second-order neurons in the posterior gray column (Fig. 7-6). The axons from the second-order neurons **cross** the midline and ascend as the spino-olivary tract in the white matter at the junction of the anterior and lateral columns. The axons end by synapsing on third-order neurons in the inferior olivary nuclei in the medulla oblongata (Fig. 7-6). The axons of the third-order neurons cross the midline and enter the cerebellum through the inferior cerebellar peduncle. The spino-olivary tract conveys information to the cerebellum from cutaneous and proprioceptive organs.

Visceral Sensory Tracts

Sensations that arise in viscera located in the thorax and abdomen enter the spinal cord through the posterior roots. The cell bodies of the first-order neuron are situated in the posterior root ganglia. The peripheral processes of these cells receive nerve impulses from pain* and stretch receptor endings in the viscera. The central processes, having entered the spinal cord, synapse with second-order neurons in the gray matter, probably in the posterior or lateral gray columns.

The axons of the second-order neurons are believed to join the spinothalamic tracts and ascend and terminate on the third-order neurons in the ventral posterolateral nucleus of the thalamus. The final destination of the axons of the third-order neurons has not been established, but it may well be in the postcentral gyrus of the cerebral cortex.

Sensations from a full rectum and a full urinary bladder experienced before defecation and micturition are carried by ascending tracts located in the posterior white columns of the spinal cord.

Many of the visceral afferent fibers that enter the spinal cord branch and participate in reflex activity.

DESCENDING TRACTS

The motor neurons situated in the anterior gray columns (horns) of the spinal cord send axons to innervate skeletal muscle through the anterior roots of the spinal nerves. These motor neurons are sometimes referred to as the **lower motor neurons**.

The lower motor neurons are constantly bombarded by nervous impulses that descend from the medulla, pons, midbrain, and cerebral cortex, as well as those that enter along sensory fibers from the posterior roots. The nerve fibers that descend in the white matter from different supraspinal nerve centers are segregated into nerve bundles called the **descending tracts.** These supraspinal neurons and their tracts are sometimes referred to as the **upper motor neurons** and they provide numerous separate pathways that can influence motor activity.

The descending pathway from the cerebral cortex is often made up of three neurons. The first neuron, the **first-order neuron,** has its cell body in the cerebral cortex. Its axon descends to synapse on the **second-order neuron**, an internuncial neuron, situated in the anterior gray column of the spinal cord. The axon of the second-order neuron is short and synapses with the **third-order neuron**, the lower motor neuron, in the anterior gray column. The axon of the third-order neuron innervates the skeletal muscle through the anterior root and spinal nerve. In some instances, the axon of the first-order neuron terminates directly on the third-order neuron (as in reflex arcs).

Functions of the Descending Tracts

The **corticospinal tracts** (Fig. 7-7A) are the pathways concerned with voluntary, discrete, skilled movements, especially those of the distal parts of the limbs. The **reticulospinal tracts** (Fig. 7-7A) may facilitate or inhibit the activity of the alpha and gamma motor neurons in the anterior gray columns and may therefore facilitate or inhibit voluntary movement or reflex activity. The **tectospinal tract** (Fig. 7-7A) is concerned with reflex postural movements in response to visual stimuli. Those fibers that are associated with the sympathetic neurons in the lateral gray column are concerned with the pupillodilation reflex in response to darkness. The **rubrospinal tract** (Fig. 7-7A) acts on both the alpha and gamma motor neurons in the anterior gray columns and facilitates the activity of flexor muscles and inhibits the activity of extensor or antigravity muscles. The **vestibulospinal tract** (Fig. 7-7A), by acting on the motor neurons in the anterior gray columns, facilitates the activity of the extensor muscles, inhibits the activity of the flexor muscles, and is concerned with the postural activity associated with balance. The **olivospinal tract** (Fig. 7-7A) may play a role in muscular activity, but its precise function is unknown. The **descending autonomic fibers** are concerned with the control of visceral activity.

Corticospinal Tracts

Fibers of the corticospinal tract arise as axons of pyramidal cells situated in the fifth layer of the cerebral cortex (Fig. 7-8). About one-third of the fibers originate from the primary motor cortex (area 4), one-third from the secondary motor cortex (area 6), and one-third from the parietal lobe (are as 3, 1, and 2); thus, two-thirds of the fibers arise from the

*The causes of visceral pain include ischemia, chemical damage, spasm of smooth muscle, and distention.

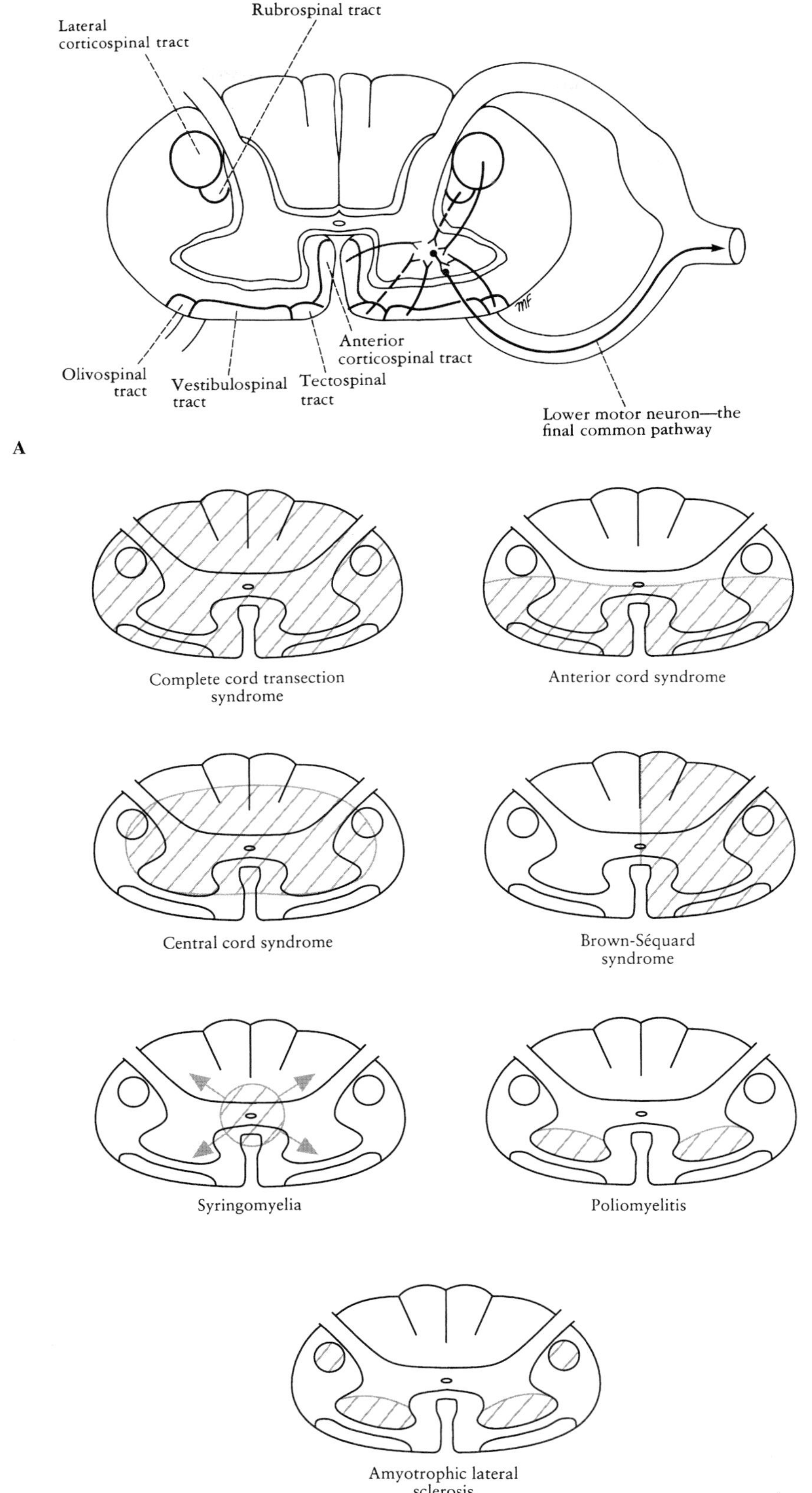

Figure 7–7 **A**. Transverse section of the spinal cord, showing termination of the descending motor tracts. **B**. Spinal cord syndromes.

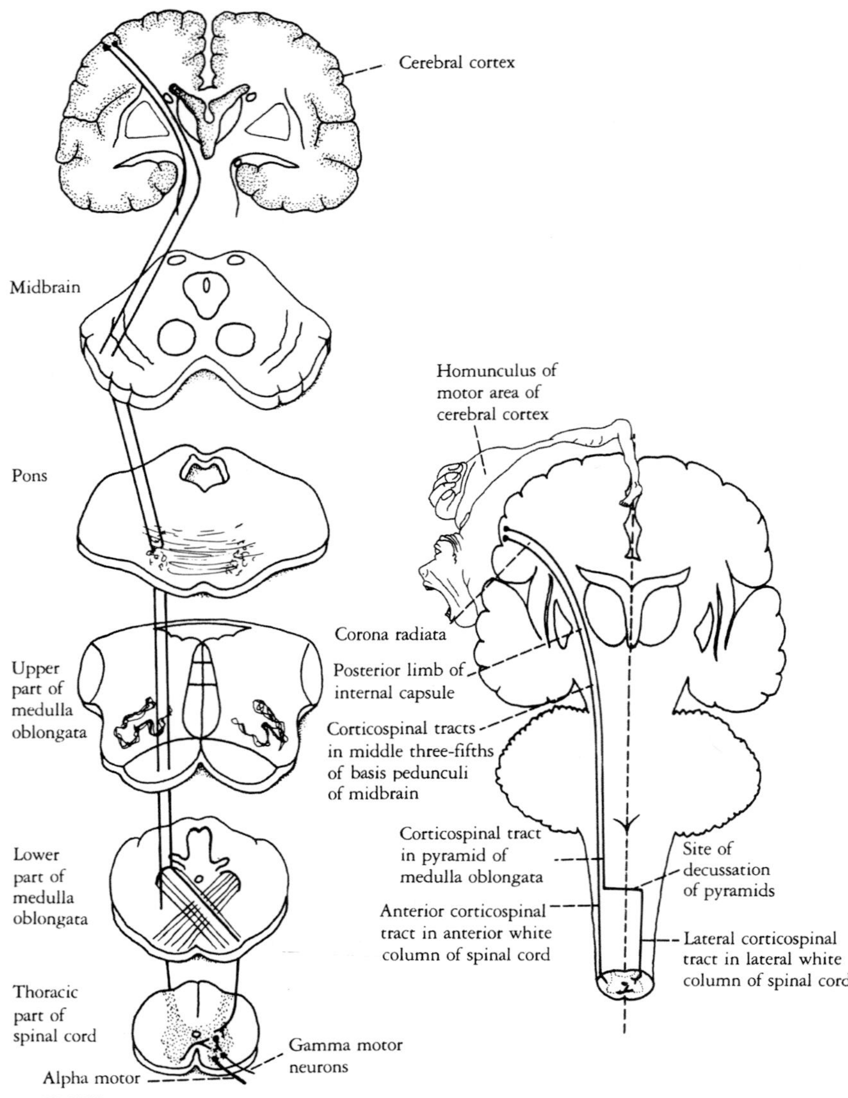

Figure 7–8 Corticospinal tracts.

precentral gyrus and one-third from the postcentral gyrus.* Since electrical stimulation of different parts of the precentral gyrus produces movements of different parts of the opposite side of the body, we can represent the parts of the body in this area of the cortex. Such a homunculus is shown in Figure 7-8. Note that the region controlling the face is situated inferiorly and the lower limb is situated superiorly and on the medial surface of the hemisphere. The homunculus is a distorted picture of the body, with the various parts having a size proportional to the area of the cerebral cortex devoted to their control. It is interesting to find that the majority of the corticospinal fibers are myelinated and are relatively slow-conducting, small fibers.

*These fibers do not control motor activity but influence sensory input to the nervous system.

The descending fibers converge in the **corona radiata** and then pass through the posterior limb of the **internal capsule** (Fig. 7-8). Here the fibers are organized so that those closest to the genu are concerned with cervical portions of the body, while those situated more posteriorly are concerned with the lower extremity. The tract then continues through the middle three-fifths of the **basis pedunculi of the midbrain** (Fig. 7-8). Here, the fibers concerned with cervical portions of the body are situated medially, while those concerned with the leg are placed laterally.

On entering the pons, the tract is broken into many bundles by the **transverse pontocerebellar fibers**. In the medulla oblongata, the bundles become grouped together along the anterior border to form a swelling known as the **pyramid** (hence the alternative name, **pyramidal tract**; see Fig. 8-1). At the junction of the medulla oblongata and the spinal cord, the majority of the fibers cross the midline at the **decussation of the pyramids** (Fig. 7-8) and enter the lateral white column of the spinal cord to form **the lateral corticospinal tract**. The remaining fibers **do not cross** in the decussation but descend in the anterior white column of the spinal cord as the **anterior corticospinal tract** (Fig. 7-8). These fibers eventually **cross** the midline and terminate in the anterior gray column of the spinal cord segments in the cervical and upper thoracic regions.

The lateral corticospinal tract descends the length of the spinal cord and its fibers terminate in the anterior gray column of all the spinal cord segments.

The majority of the corticospinal fibers synapse with internuncial neurons, which in turn synapse with alpha motor neurons and some gamma motor neurons. Only the largest corticospinal fibers synapse directly with the motor neurons.

The corticospinal tracts form the pathway that confers speed and agility to voluntary movements and are thus used in performing rapid skilled movements. Many of the simple, basic voluntary movements are believed to be mediated by other descending tracts.

BRANCHES OF CORTICOSPINAL TRACTS

1. Branches are given off early in their descent and return to the cerebral cortex to inhibit activity in adjacent regions of the cortex.
2. Branches pass to the caudate and lentiform nuclei, the red nuclei, and the olivary nuclei and the reticular formation. These branches keep the subcortical regions informed about the cortical motor activity. Once alerted, the subcortical regions may react and send their own nervous impulses to the alpha and gamma motor neurons by other descending pathways.

Reticulospinal Tracts

Throughout the midbrain, pons, and medulla oblongata, groups of scattered nerve cells and nerve fibers exist and are collectively known as the **reticular formation** (see p. 121). From the pons, these neurons send axons, which are mostly uncrossed, down into the spinal cord and form the **pontine reticulospinal tract** (Fig. 7-9). From the medulla, similar

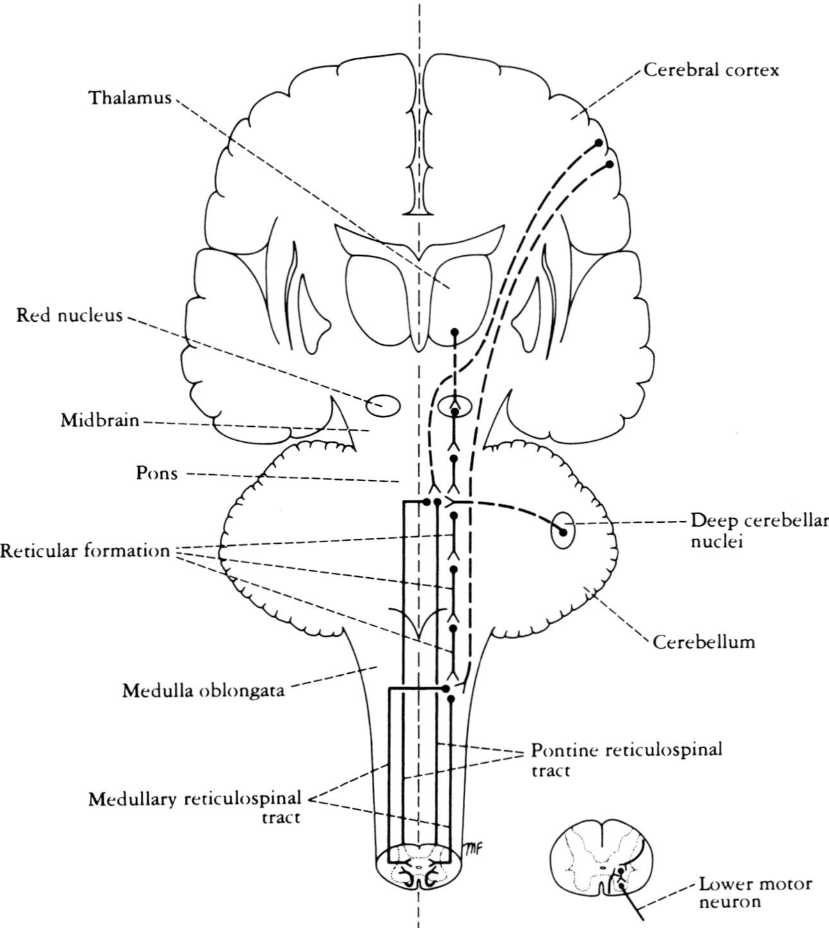

Figure 7–9 Reticulospinal tracts.

neurons send axons, which are **crossed** and **uncrossed**, to the spinal cord and form the **medullary reticulospinal tract**.

The reticulospinal fibers from the pons descend through the anterior white column, while those from the medulla oblongata descend in the lateral white column (Fig. 7-9). Both sets of fibers enter the anterior gray columns of the spinal cord and may facilitate or inhibit the activity of the alpha and gamma motor neurons. By this means the reticulospinal tracts influence voluntary movements and reflex activity. The reticulospinal fibers are also now thought to include the descending autonomic fibers. The reticulospinal tracts thus provide a pathway by which the hypothalamus can control the sympathetic outflow and the sacral parasympathetic outflow.

Tectospinal Tract

Fibers of this tract arise from nerve cells in the **superior colliculus** of the midbrain (Fig. 7-10). The majority of the fibers **cross** the midline soon after their origin and descend through the brainstem close to the **medial longitudinal fasciculus**. The tectospinal tract descends through the anterior white column of the spinal cord. The majority of the fibers terminate in the anterior gray column in the upper cervical segments of the spinal cord by synapsing with internuncial neurons. These fibers are believed to be concerned with reflex postural movements in response to visual stimuli.

Rubrospinal Tract

The **red nucleus** is situated in the tegmentum of the midbrain at the level of the superior colliculus (Fig. 7-11). The axons of neurons in this nucleus **cross** the midline at the level of the nucleus and descend as the rubrospinal tract through the pons and medulla oblongata to enter the lateral white column of the spinal cord. The fibers terminate by synapsing with internuncial neurons in the anterior gray column of the cord.

The neurons of the red nucleus receive afferent impulses through connections with the cerebral cortex and the cerebellum. This is believed to be an important indirect pathway by which the cerebral cortex and the cerebellum can influence the activity of the alpha and gamma motor neu-

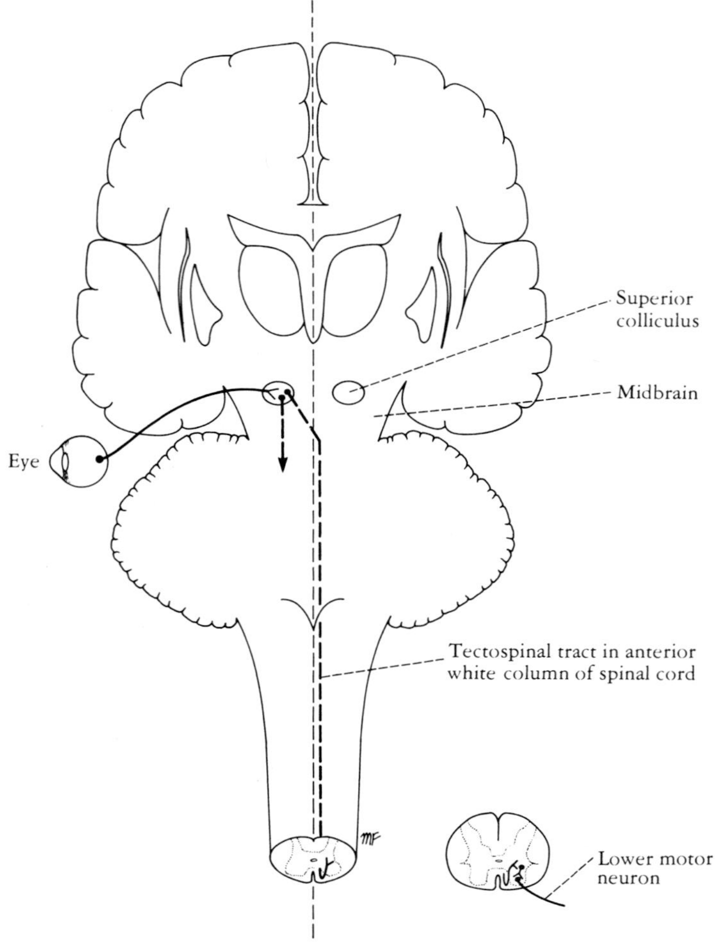

Figure 7–10 Tectospinal tract.

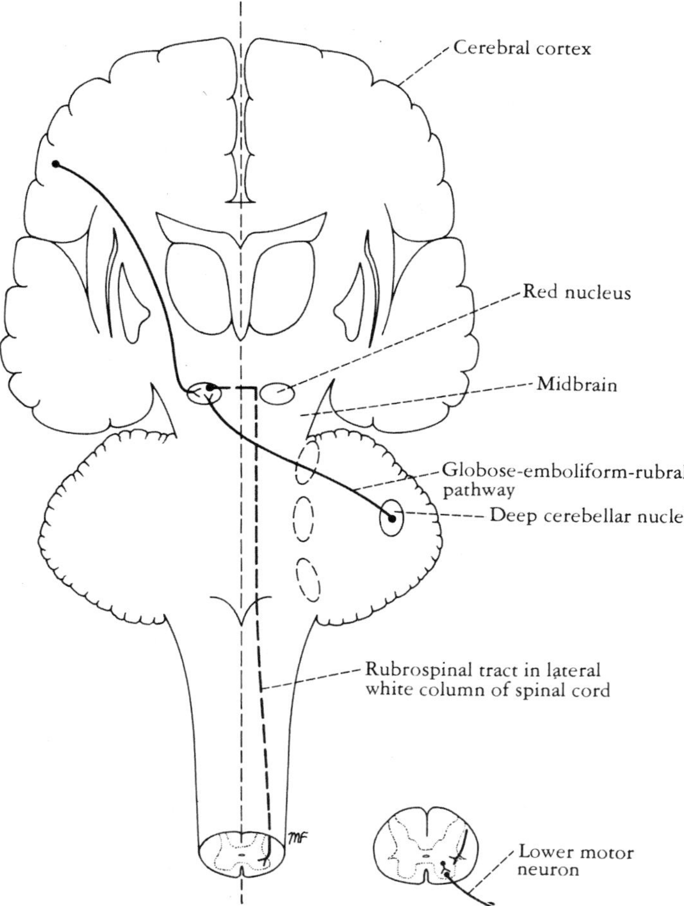

Figure 7–11 Rubrospinal tract.

rons of the spinal cord. The tract facilitates the activity of the flexor muscles and inhibits the activity of the extensor or antigravity muscles.

Vestibulospinal Tract

The **vestibular nuclei** are situated in the pons and medulla oblongata beneath the floor of the fourth ventricle (Fig. 7-12). The vestibular nuclei receive afferent fibers from the inner ear through the vestibular nerve and from the cerebellum. The neurons of the lateral vestibular nucleus give rise to the axons that form the vestibulospinal tract. The tract descends **uncrossed** through the medulla and through the length of the spinal cord in the anterior white column. The fibers terminate by synapsing with internuncial neurons of the anterior gray column of the spinal cord.

The inner ear and the cerebellum, by means of this tract, facilitate the activity of the extensor muscles and inhibit the activity of the flexor muscles in association with the maintenance of balance.

Olivospinal Tract

The olivospinal tract was thought to arise from the inferior olivary nucleus and to descend in the lateral white column of the spinal cord to influence the activity of the motor neurons in the anterior gray column. There is now considerable doubt that it exists.

Descending Autonomic Fibers

The higher centers of the central nervous system associated with the control of autonomic activity are situated in the cerebral cortex, hypothalamus, amygdaloid complex, and reticular formation. Although distinct tracts have not been recognized, it is known, as the result of study of spinal cord lesions, that descending autonomic tracts do exist and probably form part of the reticulospinal tract.

The fibers arise from neurons in the higher centers and **cross** the midline in the brainstem. They are believed to descend in the lateral white column of the spinal cord and to terminate by synapsing on the autonomic motor cells in the

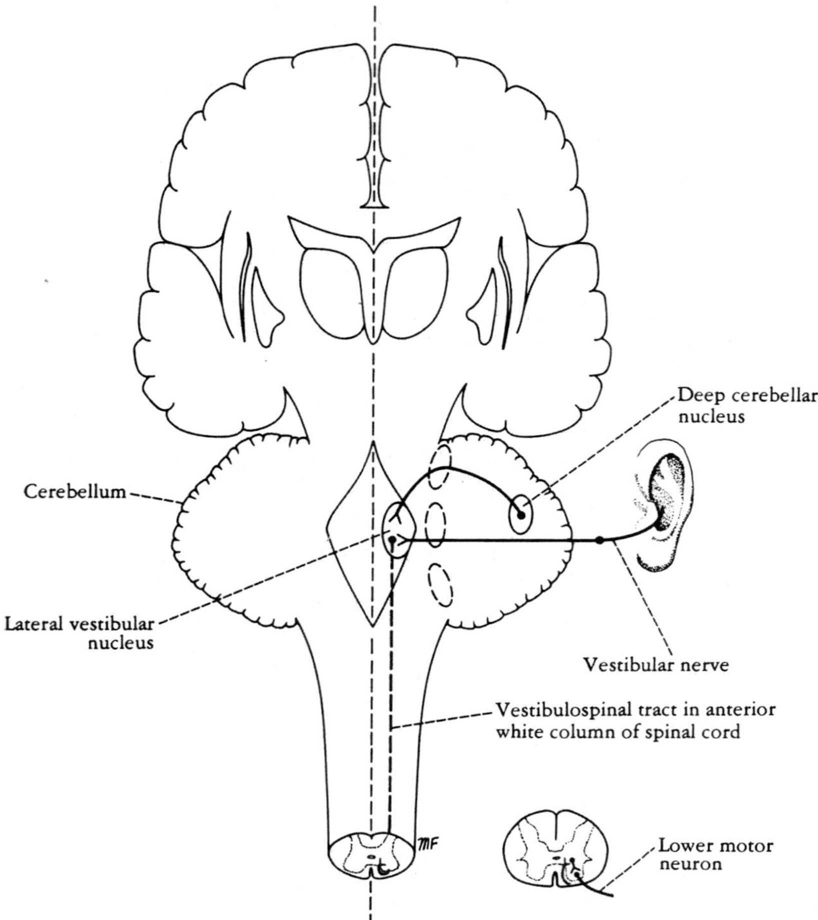

Figure 7–12 Vestibulospinal tract.

lateral gray columns in the thoracic and upper lumbar (sympathetic outflow) and midsacral (parasympathetic) levels of the spinal cord.

A summary of the main descending pathways to the spinal cord is shown in Table 7-3.

INTERSEGMENTAL TRACTS

Short ascending and descending tracts, which originate and end within the spinal cord, exist in the anterior, lateral, and posterior white columns. The function of these pathways is to interconnect the neurons of different segmental levels, and they are particularly important in intersegmental spinal reflexes.

REFLEX ARC

A **reflex** can be defined as an involuntary response to a stimulus. It depends on the integrity of the reflex arc (Fig. 7-13). In its simplest form, a reflex arc consists of the following anatomical structures: (1) a receptor organ, (2) an afferent neuron, (3) an effector neuron, and (4) an effector organ. Such a reflex arc involving only one synapse is referred to as a **monosynaptic reflex arc**. Interruption of the reflex arc at any point along its course would abolish the response.

In the spinal cord, reflex arcs play an important role in maintaining muscle tone, which is the basis for body posture. The receptor organ is situated in the skin, muscle, or tendon. The cell body of the afferent neuron is located in the posterior root ganglion, and the central axon of this first-order neuron terminates by synapsing on the effector neuron. Since the afferent fibers are of large diameter and are rapidly conducting, and because of the presence of only one synapse, a very quick response is possible.

Law of Reciprocal Innervation

In considering reflex skeletal muscle activity, it is important to understand the law of reciprocal innervation (Fig. 7-14). Simply stated, it means that the flexor and extensor reflexes

Table 7–3 Summary of the Main Descending Pathways to the Spinal Cord

Pathway	Function	Origin	Site of Crossover	Destination	Branches to
Corticospinal tracts	Rapid, skilled, voluntary movements, especially distal ends of limbs	Primary motor cortex (area 4), secondary motor cortex (area 6), parietal lobe (areas 3, 1, 2)	Most cross at decussation of pyramids and descend as lateral corticospinal tracts; some continue as anterior corticospinal tracts and cross over at level of destination	Internuncial neurons or alpha motor neurons	Cerebral cortex, basal nuclei, red nuclei, olivary nuclei, reticular formation
Reticulospinal tracts	Inhibit or facilitate voluntary movement; hypothalamus controls sympathetic, parasympathetic outflows	Reticular formation	Some cross at various levels	Alpha and gamma motor neurons	Multiple areas of central nervous system as they descend
Tectospinal tracts	Reflex postural movements for sight	Superior colliculus	Soon after origin	Alpha and gamma motor neurons	?
Rubrospinal tracts	Facilitate activity of flexor muscles and inhibit activity of extensor muscles	Red nucleus	Immediately	Alpha and gamma motor neurons	?
Vestibulospinal tracts	Facilitate activity of extensor muscles and inhibit flexor muscles	Vestibular nuclei	Uncrossed	Alpha and gamma motor neurons	?
Olivospinal tracts	?	Inferior olivary nucleus		? Alpha and gamma motor neurons	
Descending autonomic fibers	Control sympathetic and parasympathetic systems	Cerebral cortex, hypothalamus, amygdaloid complex, reticular formation	Cross in brainstem	Sympathetic and parasympathetic outflows	

Note that the corticospinal tracts are believed to control the prime mover muscles (especially the highly skilled movements), whereas the other descending tracts are important in controlling the simple basic movements.
For simplicity the internuncial neurons are omitted from this table.

of the same limb cannot be made to contract simultaneously. For this law to work, the afferent nerve fibers responsible for flexor reflex muscle action must have branches that synapse with the extensor motor neurons of the same limb, causing them to be inhibited.

Crossed Extensor Reflex

The evocation of a reflex on one side of the body causes opposite effects on the limb of the other side of the body. This crossed extensor reflex (Fig. 7-14) can be demonstrated as follows: Afferent stimulation of the reflex arc that causes the ipsilateral limb to flex results in the contralateral limb being extended.

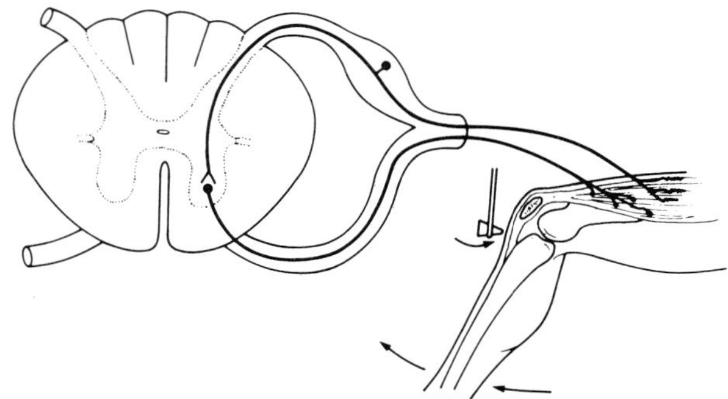

Figure 7–13 Monosynaptic reflex arc.

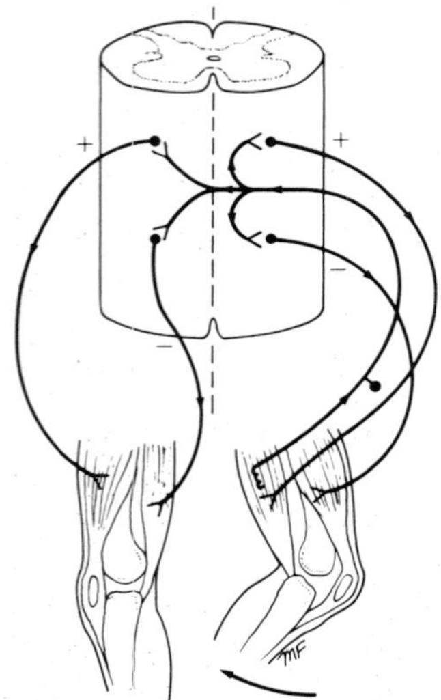

Figure 7–14 Law of reciprocal innervation and the crossed extensor reflex.

HIGHER NEURONAL CENTERS AND THE ACTIVITIES OF THE SPINAL REFLEXES

The spinal segmental reflex arc involving motor activity is greatly influenced by higher centers in the brain. These influences are mediated through the corticospinal, reticulospinal, tectospinal, rubrospinal, and vestibulospinal tracts. In the clinical condition known as spinal shock, which follows the sudden removal of these influences by severance of the spinal cord, the segmental spinal reflexes are depressed. When the so-called spinal shock disappears in a few weeks, the segmental spinal reflexes return and the muscle tone is increased. This so-called **decerebrate rigidity** is due to the overactivity of the gamma efferent nerve fibers to the muscle spindles, which results from the release of these neurons from the higher centers. The next stage may be **paraplegia in extension** with domination of the increased tone of the extensor muscles over the flexor muscles. Some neurologists believe that this condition is due to incomplete severance of all the descending tracts with persistence of the vestibulospinal tract. Should all the descending tracts be severed, the condition of **paraplegia in flexion** occurs. In this condition, the reflex responses are flexor in nature and the tone of the extensor muscles is diminished.

RENSHAW CELLS AND LOWER MOTOR NEURON INHIBITION

Lower motor neuron axons give off collateral branches as they pass through the white matter to reach the anterior roots of the spinal nerve. These collaterals synapse on neurons described by Renshaw, which in turn synapse on the lower motor neurons. These internuncial neurons are believed to provide feedback on the lower motor neurons, inhibiting their activity.

CLINICAL NOTES

SPINAL SHOCK SYNDROME

Spinal shock syndrome is a clinical condition that follows severe damage to the spinal cord. All cord functions below the level of the lesion become depressed or lost, and sensory impairment and a flaccid paralysis occur. The shock can last less than 24 hours or persist for as long as 1 to 4 weeks.

COMPLETE CORD TRANSECTION SYNDROME

This syndrome results in (1) complete loss of all sensibility below the level of the lesion and (2) complete loss of all voluntary movement below the level of the lesion (Fig. 7-7B).

ANTERIOR CORD SYNDROME

Anterior cord syndrome results in (1) bilateral lower motor neuron paralysis in the segment of the lesion, (2) bilateral spastic paralysis below the level of the lesion, and (3) bilateral loss of pain, temperature, and light touch below the level of the lesion. Tactile discrimination and vibratory and proprioceptive sensations are preserved because the posterior white columns on both sides are undamaged (Fig. 7-7B).

CENTRAL CORD SYNDROME

This syndrome results in (1) bilateral lower motor neuron paralysis in the segment of the lesion, (2) bilateral spastic paralysis below the level of the lesion with characteristic sacral "sparing," and (3) bilateral loss of pain, temperature, and light touch and pressure sensations below the level of the lesion with characteristic sacral "sparing" (Fig. 7-7B).

BROWN-SÉQUARD SYNDROME OR HEMISECTION OF THE SPINAL CORD

This condition results in (1) ipsilateral lower motor neuron paralysis in the segment of the lesion, (2) ipsilateral spastic paralysis below the level of the lesion, (3) ipsilateral band of cutaneous anesthesia in the segment of the lesion, (4) ipsilateral loss of tactile discrimination and of vibratory and proprioceptive senses below the level of the lesion, (5) contralateral loss of pain and temperature sense below the level of the lesion, and (6) contralateral but not complete loss of tactile sense below the level of the lesion (Fig. 7-7B).

POLIOMYELITIS

Poliomyelitis is an acute viral infection of the anterior horn cells of the spinal cord and the motor nuclei of the cranial nerves with consequent muscle paralysis (Fig. 7-7B). Following death of the anterior horn cells there is paralysis and wasting of the muscles. The muscles of the lower limb are more often affected than are those of the upper limb. In severe poliomyelitis, respiration may be threatened due to the paralysis spreading to the intercostal muscles and diaphragm.

MULTIPLE SCLEROSIS

Multiple sclerosis (MS) is a common disease confined to the central nervous system and causing widespread demyelination of the ascending and descending tracts in the brain and spinal cord. The loss of the myelin sheath results in the breakdown of the insulation around the axons and the velocity of the action potentials is reduced and ultimately becomes blocked. Weakness of the limbs is the most common sign of the disease and ataxia due to involvement of the tracts of the cerebellum may also be present. The cause of MS is not known although there is evidence that autoantigens to myelin may develop and be responsible in some cases.

AMYOTROPHIC LATERAL SCLEROSIS (LOU GEHRIG'S DISEASE)

Amyotrophic lateral sclerosis (ALS) is a chronic progressive disease of unknown origin. It results in the destruction of the motor neurons of the anterior gray horns and the corticospinal tracts of the spinal cord (Fig.7-7B). The lower motor neuron signs of progressive muscular atrophy, paresis, and fasciculations are superimposed on the signs and symptoms of upper motor neuron disease with paresis, spasticity, and the Babinski response. The motor nuclei of some cranial nerves may also be involved.

SYRINGOMYELIA

This disease is a developmental abnormality resulting in the formation of a cavity in the cervical segments of the spinal cord and brainstem (Fig. 7-7B). The condition interrupts the lateral and anterior spinothalamic tracts as they cross the spinal cord in the commissures. The patient has segmental losses of pain and thermal sensibility, which are often bilateral, and some impairment of touch sensation. These result in skin burns, especially to the fingers. Atrophy of the anterior horn cells leads to wasting and weakness of the muscles of the upper limb. A Horner's syndrome may be present. This is caused by the interruption of the descending autonomic fibers in the lateral white column by the expanding lesion.

REVIEW QUESTIONS

Directions: Each of the incomplete statements in this section is followed by completions of the statement. Select the one lettered completion that is BEST in each case.

1. The lateral spinothalamic tract originates from neurons located in the:
   (a) posterior root ganglion
   (b) substantia gelatinosa
   (c) nucleus proprius
   (d) phrenic nucleus
   (e) anterior horn
2. The fasciculus gracilis originates from neurons located in the:
   (a) dentate nucleus
   (b) olive
   (c) posterior root ganglion
   (d) pyramid
   (e) nucleus proprius
3. The anterior spinothalamic tract originates from neurons located in the:
   (a) thalamus
   (b) hypothalamus
   (c) lateral gray horn
   (d) substantia gelatinosa
   (e) accessory nucleus
4. The posterior spinocerebellar tract originates from neurons located in the:
   (a) cerebellum
   (b) nucleus dorsalis (Clark's column)
   (c) phrenic nucleus
   (d) lumbosacral nucleus
   (e) anterior gray horn
5. The anterior spinothalamic tract:
   (a) crosses the midline of the spinal cord
   (b) crosses the midline of the medulla oblongata
   (c) crosses the midline of the midbrain
   (d) is uncrossed in the spinal cord
   (e) is uncrossed in the medulla oblongata
6. The lateral corticospinal tract:
   (a) crosses the midline of the spinal cord
   (b) crosses the midline of the medulla oblongata
   (c) crosses the midline of the midbrain
   (d) crosses the midline in the pons
   (e) is uncrossed in the medulla oblongata
7. The anterior corticospinal tract:
   (a) crosses the midline of the spinal cord
   (b) crosses the midline of the medulla oblongata
   (c) crosses the midline of the pons
   (d) crosses the midline of the midbrain
   (e) is uncrossed in the spinal cord

8. The fasciculus gracilis:
   (a) crosses the midline of the spinal cord
   (b) crosses the midline of the medulla oblongata
   (c) crosses the midline of the midbrain
   (d) crosses the midline of the pons
   (e) remains uncrossed in the brain and spinal cord
9. The nucleus dorsalis is located in the spinal cord at the segmental levels:
   (a) T1-L3
   (b) C8-L3 or L4
   (c) S2,3,4
   (d) L4,5,S1,2,3
   (e) L2,3,4
10. The parasympathetic outflow is located in the spinal cord at the segmental levels:
    (a) L2,3,4
    (b) T1-L2
    (c) S2,3,4
    (d) L4,5
    (e) C3-6
11. The lateral corticospinal tract terminates at the:
    (a) substantia gelatinosa
    (b) ventroposterolateral nucleus of the thalamus
    (c) Clark's column
    (d) ventroposteromedial nucleus of the thalamus
    (e) motor anterior gray column (horn) cells of the spinal cord
12. The lateral spinothalamic tract terminates at the:
    (a) nerve cells in the lateral gray horn of the spinal cord
    (b) ventroposterolateral nucleus of the thalamus
    (c) caudate nucleus
    (d) lentiform nucleus
    (e) olivary nucleus
13. The fasciculus cuneatus terminates at the:
    (a) Clark's column
    (b) dentate nucleus
    (c) second order neuron in the nucleus cuneatus
    (d) nerve cells in the lateral gray horn of the spinal cord
    (e) olivary nucleus

Directions: Each of the numbered items in this section is followed by answers that are positively phrased. Select the ONE lettered answer that is an EXCEPTION.

14. Normal muscle tone is dependent on the integrity of the following **except:**
    (a) Posterior root of the spinal nerve
    (b) Afferent fibers from facial and other muscles of the head
    (c) Hyperactive reflexes
    (d) Spinal nerves
    (e) Lower motor neurons in anterior roots of the spinal nerves
15. Following section of a motor nerve, an atonic muscle has the following characteristics **except:**
    (a) It is soft and flabby
    (b) The muscle atrophies
    (c) There is a loss of tendon reflexes
    (d) The muscle ceases to respond to faradic stimulation after 4 to 7 days
    (e) The muscle fibers are not replaced by fibrous tissue
16. The precentral gyrus receives inputs either directly or indirectly from the following areas of the nervous system when voluntary movements are performed, **except** the:
    (a) Superior medullary velum
    (b) Limbic system
    (c) Ascending tracts concerned with pain and touch
    (d) Eyes
    (e) Cerebellum
17. Lesions that are restricted to the corticospinal tracts produce the following clinical signs **except:**
    (a) Absence of superficial abdominal reflexes
    (b) Babinski sign
    (c) Absent cremasteric reflex
    (d) Extensive muscular atrophy
    (e) Loss of fine, skilled voluntary movements
18. Lesions of the descending tracts (other than the corticospinal tracts) produce the following clinical signs **except:**
    (a) Muscle flaccidity
    (b) Paralysis
    (c) Exaggerated knee jerk
    (d) Finger or ankle clonus
    (e) Clasp-knife reaction
19. The knee jerk reflex has the following characteristics **except:**
    (a) It is a muscle stretch reflex
    (b) It is not a response to painful stimulation of the skin
    (c) It involves both afferent fibers and spinal motor neurons
    (d) There are many synapses involved in the reflex arc
    (e) The reflex is very fast
20. The following observations would be consistent with the "gate theory" of pain **except:**
    (a) Vibratory stimulation to the skin could diminish pain sensitivity
    (b) Stimulation of small nonmyelinated nerve fibers could decrease the pain sensitivity
    (c) Stimulation of large myelinated nerve fibers decreases pain sensitivity
    (d) Massage can relieve pain
    (e) Inhibition of pain is thought to take place at the site where the pain fibers enter the central nervous system
21. Corticospinal fibers are found in the following regions of white matter **except:**
    (a) Lateral white column of the spinal cord
    (b) Pyramid of medulla oblongata
    (c) Anterior limb of the internal capsule
    (d) Anterior white column of the spinal cord
    (e) Corona radiata
22. Concerning the reception of pain, the following statements are correct **except:**
    (a) The enkephalins and endorphins may serve to inhibit the release of substance P

(b) Substance P, a peptide, is thought to be the neurotransmitter at the synapses where the first-order neurons terminate on the cells in the posterior gray horn of the spinal cord
(c) Slow conducting C type fibers are responsible for prolonged, burning pain
(d) The lateral spinothalamic tracts conduct the initial, sharp pain
(e) The anterior spinothalamic tracts conduct the deep, blunt pain

23. Following a traumatic hemisection of the spinal cord on the right at the level of C7, the patient presents with the following signs and symptoms **except:**
(a) Right hemiplegia
(b) Right positive Babinski sign
(c) Loss of pain and temperature appreciation on the right below the level of the lesion
(d) Loss of position sense on the right below the level of the lesion
(e) Ipsilateral lower motor neuron paralysis at the level of C7

Directions: Read the case history then answer the question. You will be required to select ONE BEST lettered answer.

A 42-year-old woman was involved in a severe automobile accident resulting in a fracture dislocation of the seventh cervical vertebra. Following the disappearance of the spinal shock, the patient was found to have clinical features indicating the anterior cord syndrome.

24. The following signs and symptoms are consistent with the diagnosis of anterior cord syndrome **except:**
(a) Pressure on the spinal cord from posterior displacement of the seventh cervical vertebral body, as seen on a sagittal MRI.
(b) Bilateral lower motor neuron paralysis at the segment of the cord lesion.
(c) Bilateral spastic paralysis below the level of the cord lesion.
(d) Bilateral loss of pain, temperature, and light touch below the level of the cord lesion.
(e) Bilateral loss of tactile discrimination and vibratory and proprioceptive senses below the level of the cord lesion.

ANSWERS AND EXPLANATIONS

1. B
2. C
3. D
4. B
5. A
6. B
7. A
8. E
9. B
10. C
11. E
12. B
13. C
14. C
15. E. As the muscle fibers atrophy, they are replaced by fibrous tissue.
16. A. There are no known connections between the superior medullary velum and the precentral gyrus, and the function of the velum is not known.
17. D. There is little or no muscular atrophy with lesions of the corticospinal tracts.
18. A. There is spasticity or hypertonicity of the muscles; the lower limb is typically maintained in extension and the upper limb is maintained in flexion.
19. D. It is a monosynaptic reflex arc.
20. B
21. C. The anterior limb of the internal capsule contains frontopontine and thalamocortical fibers.
22. E. The anterior spinothalamic tracts conduct sensations of light touch and pressure.
23. C. The ascending fibers associated with pain and temperature cross over to the opposite side of the spinal cord; thus in this patient there would be loss of pain and temperature on the left side below the level of the lesion.
24. E. In patients with traumatic anterior spinal cord syndrome, tactile discrimination and vibratory and proprioceptive senses are preserved since the posterior white columns on both sides are undamaged.

CHAPTER 8

Brainstem

CHAPTER OUTLINE

SUGGESTED PLAN FOR REVIEW OF CHAPTER 8

1. Learn the general shape and parts of the brainstem so that you can understand the position of the cranial nerve nuclei and how the cranial nerves exit from the brainstem. A three-dimensional picture of the region in your mind will assist you in the visualization of the pathways taken by the various ascending and descending tracts.

SUGGESTED PLAN FOR REVIEW OF CHAPTER 8 (*continued*)

2. Be able to make rough drawings of cross sections of the brainstem at the following levels: the medulla at the levels of the decussation of the pyramids, the decussation of the lemnisci, and the olives; the caudal and cranial parts of the pons; and the midbrain at the levels of the inferior colliculi and the superior colliculi. At each level insert the main structures, including the cranial nerve nuclei and other masses of gray matter, and the main tracts.
3. Understand the Arnold-Chiari phenomenon, the lateral medullary syndrome of Wallenberg, the medial medullary syndrome, Weber's syndrome, and Benedikt's syndrome. Examiners like asking questions on these clinical problems.
4. Learn the significance of blockage of the cerebral aqueduct in the production of hydrocephalus.

INTRODUCTION

The brainstem is made up of the medulla oblongata, the pons, and the midbrain. It is stalklike in shape and connects the narrow spinal cord with the expanded forebrain.

The brainstem participates in three broad functions: (1) It serves as a conduit for the ascending and descending tracts connecting the spinal cord to the different parts of the brain. (2) It contains important reflex centers associated with the control of respiration and the cardiovascular system; it also is associated with the control of consciousness. (3) It contains the important nuclei of cranial nerves III through XII.

The purpose of this chapter is to review the structure of the different parts of the brainstem so that the student can understand the spatial relationships of these parts to one another; the various connections of these parts are dealt with elsewhere as indicated in the text.

MEDULLA OBLONGATA

External Appearance

The medulla oblongata connects the pons superiorly with the spinal cord inferiorly (Fig. 8-1). The junction of the medulla and spinal cord is at the level of the foramen magnum. The medulla oblongata is conical in shape, its broad extremity being directed superiorly. The **central canal** of the spinal cord continues upward into the lower half of the medulla; in the upper half of the medulla it expands as the **cavity of the fourth ventricle** (Fig. 8-1).

On the anterior surface of the medulla is the **anterior median fissure**, which is continuous inferiorly with the **anterior median fissure** of the spinal cord (Fig. 8-1). On each side of the median fissure there is a swelling called the **pyramid**. The pyramids are composed of bundles of corticospinal nerve fibers that originate in large nerve cells in the precentral gyrus of the cerebral cortex. The pyramids taper inferiorly, and it is here that the majority of the descending fibers cross over to the opposite side, forming the **decussation of the pyramids** (Fig. 8-1). Posterolateral to the pyramids are the **olives**, which are oval elevations produced by the underlying **inferior olivary nuclei**. In the groove between the pyramid and the olive emerge the rootlets of the hypoglossal nerve. Posterior to the olives are the **inferior cerebellar peduncles** (Fig. 8-1), which connect the medulla to the cerebellum. In the groove between the olive and the inferior cerebellar peduncle emerge the roots of the glossopharyngeal and vagus nerves and the cranial roots of the accessory nerve (Fig. 8-1).

The posterior surface of the superior half of the medulla oblongata forms the lower part of the **floor of the fourth ventricle** (Fig. 8-1). The posterior surface of the inferior half of the medulla is continuous with the posterior aspect of the spinal cord. On each side of the midline there is an elongated swelling, the **gracile tubercle**, produced by the underlying **gracile nucleus** (Fig. 8-1). Lateral to the gracile tubercle is a similar swelling, the **cuneate tubercle**, produced by the underlying **cuneate nucleus**.

Internal Structure

As in the spinal cord, the medulla oblongata consists of white matter and gray matter, but a study of transverse sections of this region shows that they have been extensively rearranged.

The internal structure of the medulla oblongata will be considered at three levels: (1) level of decussation of pyramids, (2) level of decussation of lemnisci, and (3) level of the olives.

LEVEL OF DECUSSATION OF PYRAMIDS

A transverse section through the inferior half of the medulla oblongata (Fig. 8-2) passes through the **decussation of the pyramids**, the great motor decussation. In the superior part of the medulla the corticospinal fibers occupy and form the pyramid, but inferiorly about three-fourths of the fibers cross the median plane and continue down the spinal cord in the lateral white column as the **lateral corticospinal tract**. As these fibers cross the midline, they sever the continuity between the anterior column of the gray matter of the spinal cord and the gray matter that surrounds the central canal.

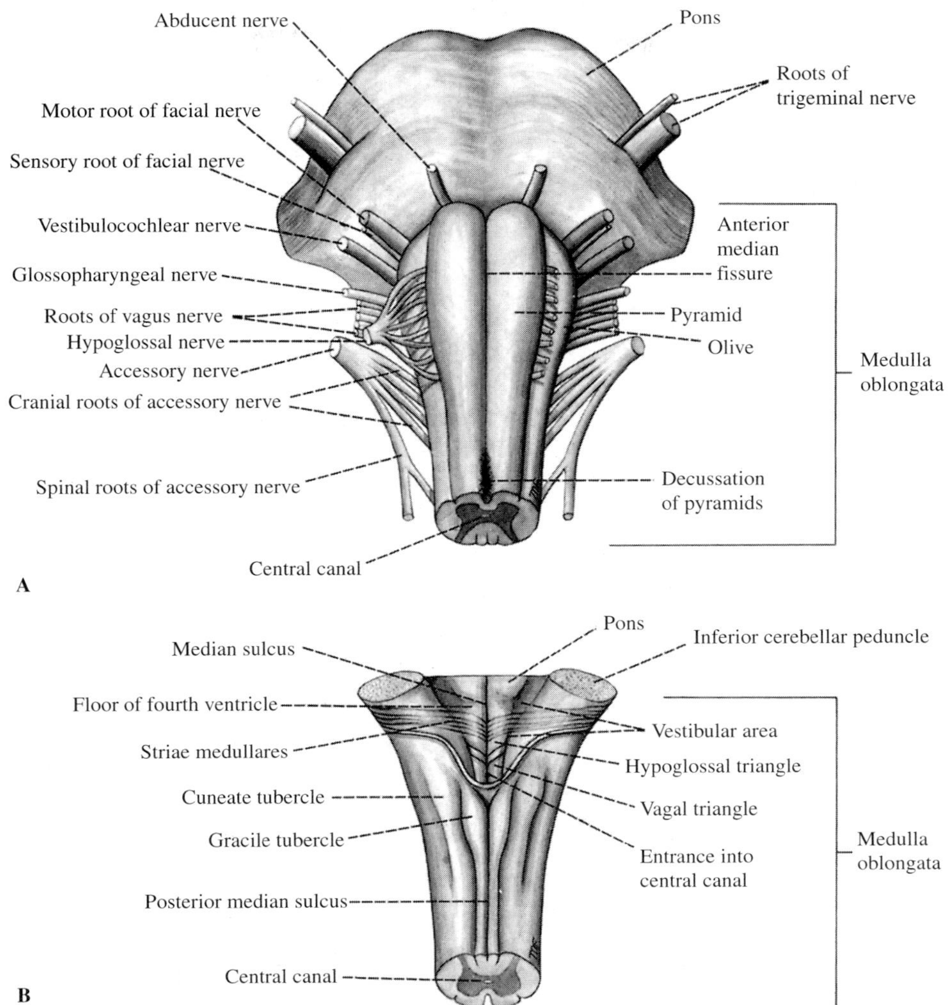

Figure 8–1 Medulla oblongata. **A**. Anterior view. **B**. Posterior view. Note that the roof of the fourth ventricle and the cerebellum have been removed.

The **fasciculus gracilis** and the **fasciculus cuneatus** continue to ascend superiorly posterior to the central gray matter (Fig. 8-2). The **nucleus gracilis** and **the nucleus cuneatus** appear as posterior extensions of the central gray matter.

The **substantia gelatinosa** in the posterior gray column of the spinal cord becomes continuous with the inferior end of the **nucleus of the spinal tract of the trigeminal nerve**. The fibers of the tract of the nucleus are situated between the nucleus and the surface of the medulla oblongata.

The lateral and anterior white columns of the spinal cord are easily identified in these sections and their fiber arrangement is unchanged (Fig. 8-2).

LEVEL OF DECUSSATION OF LEMNISCI

A transverse section through the inferior half of the medulla oblongata, a short distance above the level of the **decussation of the pyramids**, passes through the decussation of lemnisci, the great sensory decussation (Fig. 8-2). The decussation of the lemnisci takes place anterior to the central gray matter and posterior to the pyramids. It should be understood that the lemnisci have been formed from the **internal arcuate fibers**, which have emerged from the anterior aspects of the **nucleus gracilis and nucleus cuneatus**. The internal arcuate fibers travel medially toward the midline, where they decussate with the corresponding fibers of the opposite side (Fig. 8-2).

The **nucleus of the spinal tract of the trigeminal nerve** lies lateral to the internal arcuate fibers. The **spinal tract of the trigeminal nerve** lies lateral to the nucleus (Fig. 8-2).

The **lateral and anterior spinothalamic tracts and the spinotectal tracts** occupy an area lateral to the decussation of the lemnisci and collectively are known as the **spinal lemniscus**. The **spinocerebellar, vestibulospinal,** and the **rubrospinal tracts** are situated in the anterolateral region of the medulla oblongata.

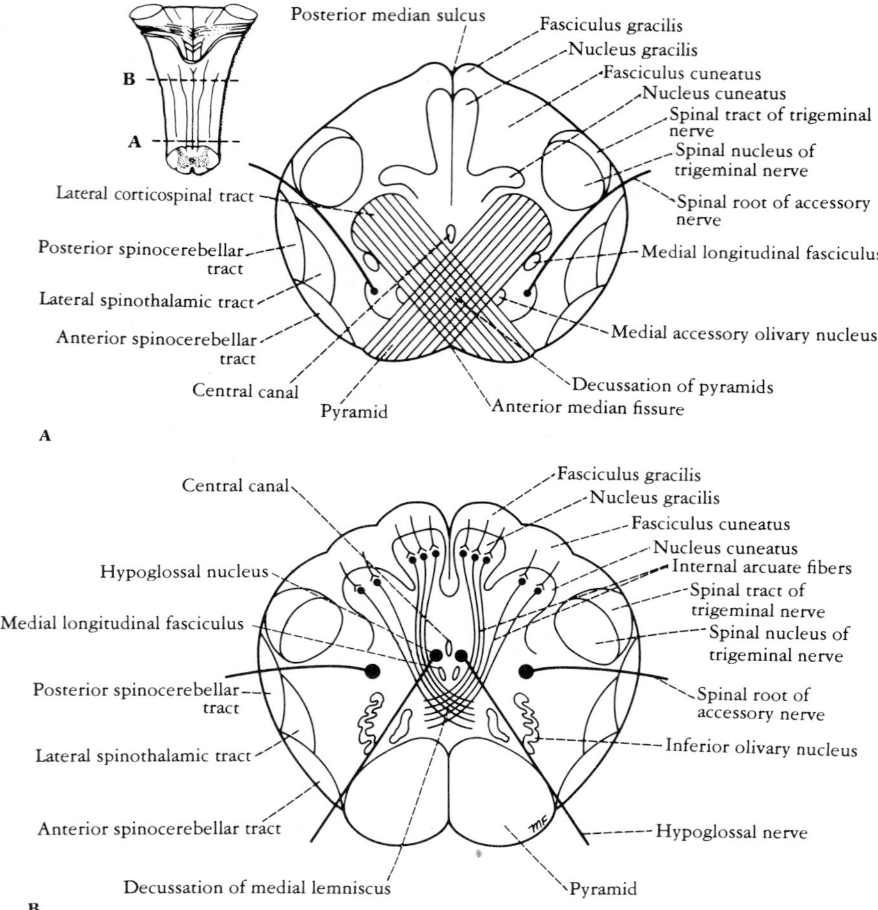

Figure 8–2 Transverse sections of the medulla oblongata. **A**. Level of decussation of the pyramids. **B**. Level of decussation of the medial lemnisci.

LEVEL OF THE OLIVES

A transverse section through the olives passes across the inferior part of the fourth ventricle (Fig. 8-3).

OLIVARY NUCLEAR COMPLEX

This consists of the **inferior olivary nucleus** (Fig. 8-3) and the smaller **dorsal and medial accessory olivary nuclei.** The cells of the inferior olivary nucleus send fibers medially across the midline to enter the cerebellum through the inferior cerebellar peduncle. Afferent fibers reach the inferior olivary nuclei from the spinal cord (the spino-olivary tracts) and from the cerebellum and cerebral cortex. The function of the olivary nuclei is associated with voluntary muscle movement.

VESTIBULOCOCHLEAR NUCLEI

The **vestibular nuclear complex** is made up of the (1) **medial vestibular nucleus**, (2) **inferior vestibular nucleus**, (3) **lateral vestibular nucleus**, and (4) **superior vestibular nucleus**. For connections of these nuclei. The medial and inferior vestibular nuclei can be seen on section at this level (Fig. 8-3).

The **cochlear nuclei** are two in number. The **anterior cochlear nucleus** is situated on the anterolateral aspect of the inferior cerebellar peduncle and the **posterior cochlear nucleus** is situated on the posterior aspect of the peduncle lateral to the floor of the fourth ventricle.

NUCLEUS AMBIGUUS

The nucleus ambiguus consists of large motor neurons and is situated deep within the reticular formation (Fig. 8-3). The emerging nerve fibers join the glossopharyngeal, vagus, and cranial part of the accessory nerve and are distributed to voluntary skeletal muscle.

CENTRAL GRAY MATTER

The central gray matter lies beneath the floor of the fourth ventricle at this level (Fig. 8-3). Passing from medial to lateral, the following important structures may be recognized: (1) the **hypoglossal nucleus**, (2) the **dorsal nucleus of the vagus**, (3) **the nucleus of the tractus solitarius**, and (4) the **medial and inferior vestibular nuclei** (see above). The nucleus ambiguus, referred to earlier, has become deeply placed within the reticular formation (Fig. 8-3).

The **pyramids** containing the corticospinal and some corticonuclear fibers are situated in the anterior part of the medulla (Fig. 8-3); the corticospinal fibers descend to the spinal cord and the corticonuclear fibers are distributed to the motor nuclei of the cranial nerves situated within the medulla.

The **medial lemniscus** forms a flattened tract on each side of the midline posterior to the pyramid (Fig. 8-3). These fibers emerge from the decussation of the lemnisci and convey sensory information to the thalamus.

The **medial longitudinal fasciculus** is situated on each side of the midline posterior to the medial lemniscus and anterior to the hypoglossal nucleus (Fig. 8-3). It consists of ascending and descending fibers.

The **inferior cerebellar peduncle** is situated on the lateral side of the fourth ventricle (Fig. 8-3).

The **spinal tract of the trigeminal nerve and its nucleus** are situated on the anteromedial aspect of the inferior cerebellar peduncle (Fig. 8-3).

The **anterior spinocerebellar tract** is situated near the surface in the interval between the inferior olivary nucleus and the nucleus of the spinal tract of the trigeminal nerve (Fig. 8-3). The **spinal lemniscus**, consisting of the **lateral spinothalamic and spinotectal tracts** and the **rubrospinal tract**, is deeply placed.

The **reticular formation**, consisting of a diffuse mixture of nerve fibers and small groups of nerve cells, is deeply placed posterior to the olivary nucleus (Fig. 8-3). The reticular formation represents, at this level, only a small part of this system, which is also present in the pons and midbrain.

The **glossopharyngeal, vagus**, and **cranial part of the accessory nerves** can be seen running forward and laterally (Fig. 8-3) to emerge between the olives and the inferior cerebellar peduncles. The **hypoglossal nerves** also run anteriorly and laterally to emerge between the pyramids and the olives (Fig. 8-3).

See Table 8-1 for a comparison of the different levels of the medulla oblongata.

Blood Supply of the Medulla Oblongata

The vertebral, anterior and posterior spinal, posterior inferior cerebellar, and basilar arteries all send branches to the medulla oblongata.

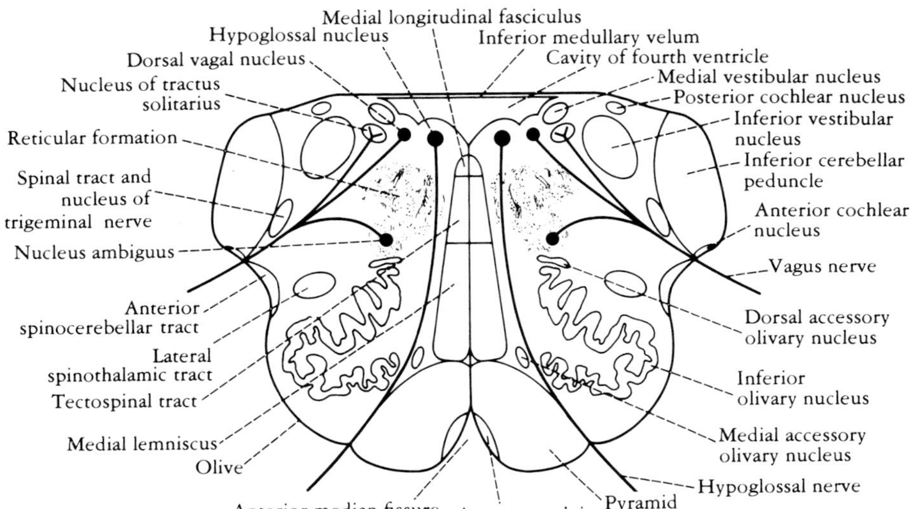

Figure 8–3 Transverse section of the medulla oblongata at the level of the olivary nuclei.

Table 8–1 Comparison of the Different Levels of the Medulla Oblongata Showing the Major Structures at Each Level

Level	Cavity	Nuclei	Motor Tracts	Sensory Tracts
Decussation of pyramids	Central canal	Nucleus gracilis, nucleus cuneatus, spinal nucleus of cranial nerve V, accessory nucleus	Decussation of corticospinal tracts, pyramids	Spinal tract of cranial nerve V, posterior spinocerebellar tract, lateral spinothalamic tract, anterior spinocerebellar tract
Decussation of medial lemnisci	Central canal	Nucleus gracilis, nucleus cuneatus, spinal nucleus of cranial nerve V, accessory nucleus, hypoglossal nucleus	Pyramids	Decussation of medial lemnisci, fasciculus gracilis, fasciculus cuneatus, spinal tract of cranial nerve V, posterior spinocerebellar tract, lateral spinothalamic tract, anterior spinocerebellar tract
Olives, inferior cerebellar peduncle	Fourth ventricle	Inferior olivary nucleus, spinal nucleus of cranial nerve V, vestibular nucleus, glossopharyngeal nucleus, vagal nucleus, hypoglossal nucleus, nucleus ambiguus, nucleus of tractus solitarius	Pyramids	Medial longitudinal fasciculus, tectospinal tract, medial lemniscus, spinal tract of cranial nerve V, lateral spinothalamic tract, anterior spinocerebellar tract

*Note that the reticular formation is present at all levels.

Clinical Notes

Congenital Anomaly

Arnold-Chiari Phenomenon

In this anomaly there is a herniation of the tonsils of the cerebellum and the medulla oblongata through the foramen magnum into the vertebral canal. This results in the blockage of the exits in the roof of the fourth ventricle for cerebrospinal fluid, causing internal hydrocephalus.

Tumors of the Posterior Cranial Fossa

In patients with tumors of the posterior cranial fossa, the intracranial pressure is raised and the cerebellum and the medulla oblongata tend to pushed downward through the foramen magnum. This will produce the symptoms of headache and neck stiffness; paralysis of the glossopharyngeal , vagus, accessory, and hypoglossal nerves may occur due to nerve traction.

Vascular Disorders of the Medulla Oblongata

Lateral Medullary Syndrome of Wallenberg

The lateral part of the medulla oblongata is supplied by the posterior inferior cerebellar artery, which is usually a branch of the vertebral artery. Thrombosis of either of these arteries (Fig. 8-4A) produces the following signs and symptoms: dysphagia and dysarthria due to paralysis of the ipsilateral palatal and laryngeal muscles (innervated by the nucleus ambiguus); analgesia and thermoanesthesia on the ipsilateral side of the face (nucleus and spinal tract of the trigeminal nerve); vertigo, nausea, vomiting, and nystagmus (vestibular nuclei); ipsilateral Horner's syndrome (descending sympathetic fibers); ipsilateral cerebellar signs—gait and limb ataxia (cerebellum or inferior cerebellar peduncle); contralateral loss of sensations of pain and temperature (spinal lemniscus—spinothalamic tract)

Medial Medullary Syndrome

The medial part of the medulla oblongata is supplied by the vertebral artery. Thrombosis of the medullary branch (Fig. 8-4B) produces the following signs and symptoms: contralateral hemiparesis (pyramidal tract); contralateral impaired sensations of position and movement and tactile discrimination (medial lemniscus); ipsilateral paralysis of tongue muscles with deviation of paralyzed side when protruded (hypoglossal nerve)

PONS

External Appearance

The pons is anterior to the cerebellum (Fig. 8-5) and connects the medulla oblongata to the midbrain. It is about 1 inch (2.5 mm) long.

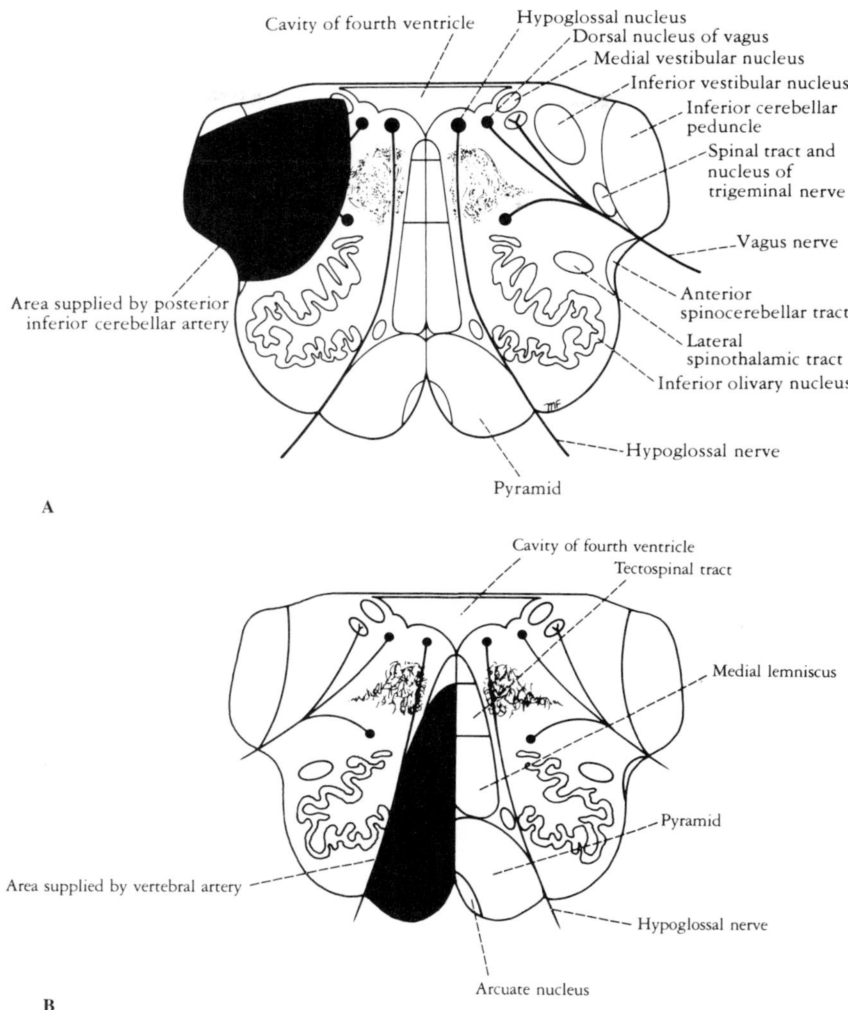

Figure 8–4 Transverse sections of the medulla oblongata. **A.** Shows the lesion that produces the lateral medullary syndrome. **B.** Shows the lesion that produces the medial medullary syndrome.

The anterior surface is convex from side to side and shows many transverse fibers that converge on each side to form the **middle cerebellar peduncle** (Fig. 8-5). The shallow groove in the midline, the **basilar groove**, lodges the basilar artery. On the anterolateral surface of the pons the **trigeminal nerve** emerges on each side. Each nerve consists of a smaller, medial **motor root** and a larger, lateral **sensory root**. In the groove between the pons and the medulla oblongata there emerge, from medial to lateral, the **abducent, facial,** and **vestibulocochlear nerves** (Fig. 8-5).

The posterior surface of the pons is hidden from view by the cerebellum. It forms the upper half of the floor of the fourth ventricle and is triangular (Fig. 8-6). The posterior surface is limited laterally by the **superior cerebellar peduncles** and is divided into symmetrical halves by a **median sulcus**. Lateral to this sulcus is an elongated elevation, the **medial eminence**, which is bounded laterally by a sulcus, the **sulcus limitans** (Fig. 8-6). The inferior end of the medial eminence is slightly expanded to form the **facial colliculus**, which is produced by the root of the facial nerve winding around the nucleus of the abducent nerve (Fig. 8-7). The floor of the superior part of the **sulcus limitans** is bluish-gray and is called the **substantia ferruginea**; it owes its color to a group of deeply pigmented nerve cells. Lateral to the sulcus limitans is the **area vestibuli** produced by the underlying vestibular nuclei (Fig. 8-6).

Internal Structure

The pons is divided into a posterior part, the **tegmentum**, and an anterior **basal part** by the transversely running fibers of the **trapezoid body** (Fig. 8-7).

The structure of the pons can be studied at two levels: (1) transverse section through the caudal part, passing through the facial colliculus, and (2) transverse section through the cranial part, passing through the trigeminal nuclei.

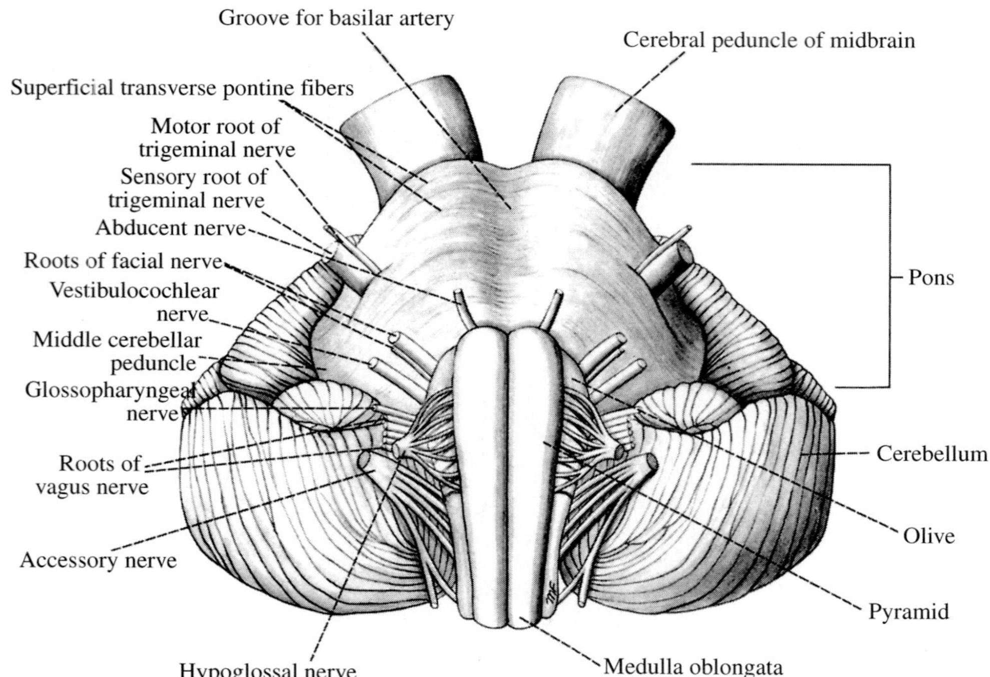

Figure 8–5 Anterior surface of the brainstem showing the pons.

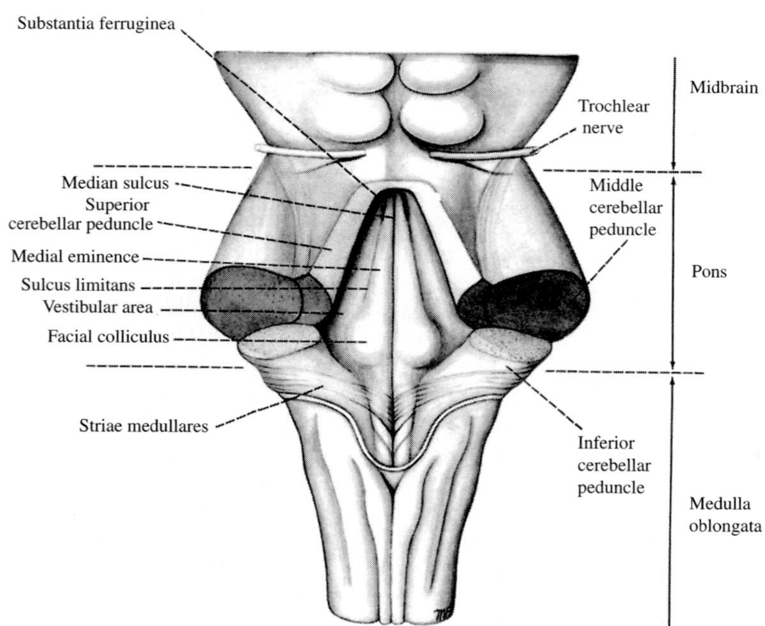

Figure 8–6 Posterior surface of the brainstem showing the pons. The cerebellum has been removed.

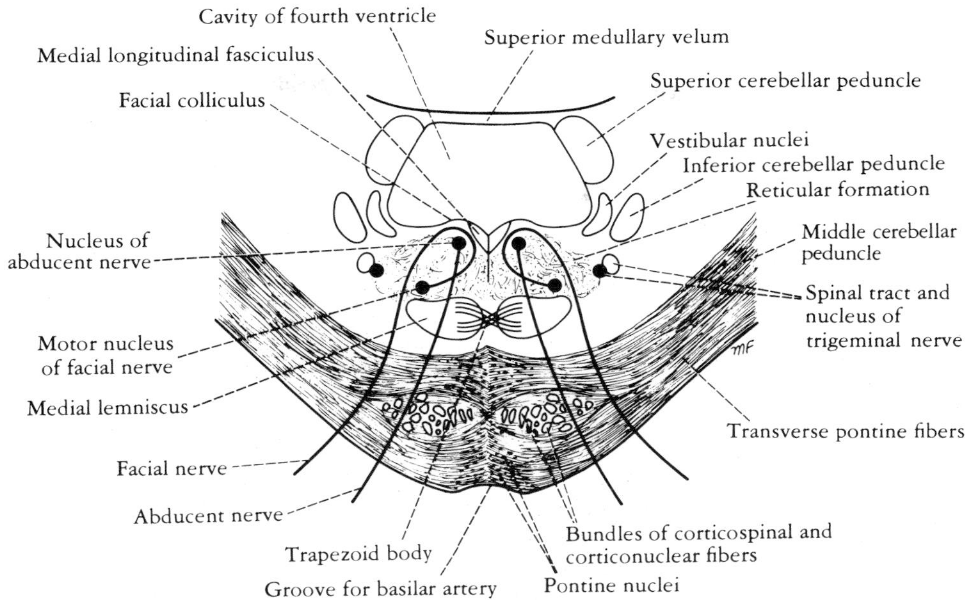

Figure 8–7 Transverse section of the caudal part of the pons at the level of the facial colliculus.

TRANSVERSE SECTION THROUGH THE CAUDAL PART OF THE PONS

The **medial lemniscus** rotates as it passes from the medulla into the pons. It is situated in the most anterior part of the tegmentum with its long axis running transversely (Fig. 8-7).

The **facial nucleus** lies posterior to the lateral part of the medial lemniscus. The fibers of the facial nerve wind around the **nucleus of the abducent nerve**, producing the **facial colliculus** (Fig. 8-7).

The medial longitudinal fasciculus is situated beneath the floor of the fourth ventricle on either side of the midline (Fig. 8-7). The medial longitudinal fasciculus is the main pathway that connects the vestibular and cochlear nuclei with the nuclei controlling the extraocular muscles (oculomotor, trochlear, and abducent nuclei).

The **medial vestibular nucleus** is situated lateral to the abducent nucleus (Fig. 8-7). The **superior vestibular nucleus** and the **posterior and anterior cochlear nuclei** are also found at this level.

The **spinal nucleus of the trigeminal nerve** and its tract lie on the anteromedial aspect of the inferior cerebellar peduncle (Fig. 8-7).

The **trapezoid body** is made up of fibers derived from the cochlear nuclei and the nuclei of the trapezoid body. They run transversely (Fig. 8-7) in the anterior part of the tegmentum (see p. 262).

The basilar part of the pons, at this level, contains small masses of nerve cells called **pontine nuclei** (Fig. 8-7). The **corticopontine fibers** of the crus cerebri of the midbrain terminate in the pontine nuclei. The axons of these cells give origin to the **transverse fibers** of the pons, which cross the midline and intersect the corticospinal and corticonuclear tracts, breaking them up into small bundles. The transverse fibers of the pons enter the middle cerebellar peduncle and are distributed to the cerebellar hemisphere. This connection forms the main pathway linking the cerebral cortex to the cerebellum.

TRANSVERSE SECTION THROUGH THE CRANIAL PART OF THE PONS

The internal structure of the pons is similar to that seen at the caudal level (Fig. 8-8), but it now contains the motor and principal sensory nuclei of the trigeminal nerve.

The **motor nucleus of the trigeminal nerve** is situated beneath the lateral part of the fourth ventricle (Fig. 8-8). The emerging motor fibers travel anteriorly and exit on the anterior surface.

The **principal sensory nucleus of the trigeminal nerve** is situated on the lateral side of the motor nucleus (Fig. 8-8); it is continuous inferiorly with the nucleus of the spinal tract. The entering sensory fibers lie lateral to the motor fibers (Fig. 8-8).

The **superior cerebellar peduncle** is situated posterolateral to the motor nucleus of the trigeminal nerve (Fig. 8-8). It is joined by the **anterior spinocerebellar tract**.

The **trapezoid body** and the **medial lemniscus** are situated in the same position as they were in the previous section (Fig. 8-8). The **spinal and lateral lemnisci** lie at the lateral extremity of the medial lemniscus (Fig. 8-8).

See Table 8-2 for a comparison of the two levels of the pons.

BLOOD SUPPLY OF THE PONS

The pons is supplied by the basilar artery and the anterior, inferior, and superior cerebellar arteries.

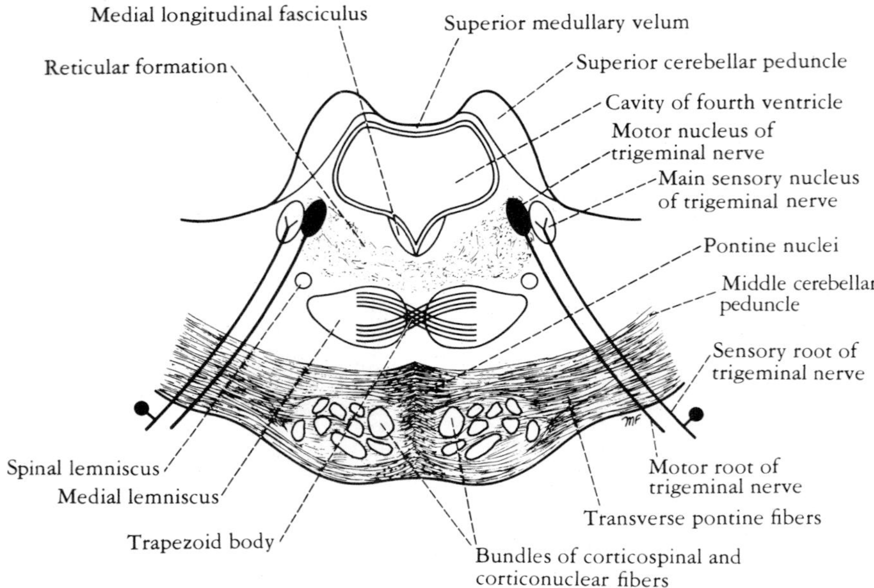

Figure 8–8 Transverse section of the pons at the level of the trigeminal nuclei.

Table 8–2 Comparison of Different Levels of the Pons Showing the Major Structures at Each Level*

Level	Cavity	Nuclei	Motor Tracts	Sensory Tracts
Facial colliculus	Fourth ventricle	Facial nucleus, abducent nucleus, medial vestibular nucleus, spinal nucleus of cranial nerve V, pontine nuclei, trapezoid nuclei	Corticospinal and corticonuclear tracts, transverse pontine fibers, medial longitudinal fasciculus	Spinal tract of cranial nerve V, lateral, spinal, and medial lemnisci
Trigeminal nuclei	Fourth ventricle	Main sensory and motor nuclei of cranial nerve V, pontine nuclei, trapezoid nuclei	Corticospinal and corticonuclear tracts, transverse pontine fibers, medial longitudinal fasciculus	Lateral, spinal, and medial lemnisci

*Note that the reticular formation is present at all levels.

Clinical Notes

Tumors of the Pons

The symptoms and signs are those of ipsilateral cranial nerve paralysis and contralateral hemiparesis: weakness of the facial muscles on the same side (facial nerve nucleus), weakness of the lateral rectus muscle on one or both sides (abducent nerve nucleus), nystagmus (vestibular nucleus), weakness of the jaw muscles (trigeminal nerve nucleus), impairment of hearing (cochlear nuclei), contralateral hemiparesis, quadriparesis (corticospinal fibers), anesthesia to light touch with the preservation of appreciation of pain over the skin of the face (principal sensory nucleus of trigeminal nerve involved, with sparing of the spinal nucleus and tract of the trigeminal nerve), and contralateral sensory defects of the trunk and limbs (medial and spinal lemnisci). Involvement of the corticopontocerebellar tracts may cause ipsilateral cerebellar signs and symptoms. There may be impairment of conjugate deviation of the eyeballs due to involvement of the medial longitudinal fasciculus, which connects the oculomotor, trochlear, and abducent nerve nuclei.

Pontine Hemorrhage

Unilateral hemorrhage may result in the following signs and symptoms: facial paralysis on the same side of the lesion (facial nerve nucleus), paralysis of the limbs of the opposite side (corticospinal fibers), and paralysis of conjugate ocular deviation (abducent nerve nucleus and medial longitudinal fasciculus).

MIDBRAIN

External Appearance

The midbrain measures about 0.8 inch (2 cm) in length and connects the pons and cerebellum with the forebrain. The midbrain is traversed by a narrow channel, the **cerebral aqueduct**, which is filled with cerebrospinal fluid (Fig. 8-9).

On the posterior surface are four **colliculi** (corpora quadrigemina). These are rounded eminences that are divided into superior and inferior pairs by a vertical and a transverse groove. The superior colliculi are centers for visual reflexes, and the inferior are lower auditory centers. In the midline below the inferior colliculi, the **trochlear nerves** emerge (Fig. 8-9). These are delicate nerves that wind around the lateral aspect of the midbrain to enter the lateral wall of the cavernous sinus.

On the lateral aspect of the midbrain, the superior and inferior brachia ascend in an anterolateral direction. The **superior brachium** passes from the superior colliculus to the lateral geniculate body and the optic tract. The **inferior brachium** connects the inferior colliculus to the **medial geniculate body**.

On the anterior aspect of the midbrain (Fig. 8-9) there is a deep depression in the midline, the **interpeduncular fossa**, which is bounded on either side by the **crus cerebri**. The **oculomotor nerve** emerges from the medial side of the crus cerebri and passes forward in the lateral wall of the cavernous sinus (Fig. 8-9).

Internal Structure

The midbrain is comprised of two lateral halves, called the **cerebral peduncles**; each of these is divided into an anterior part, the **crus cerebri**, and a posterior part, the **tegmentum**, by a pigmented band of gray matter, the **substantia nigra** (Fig. 8-9). The narrow cavity of the midbrain

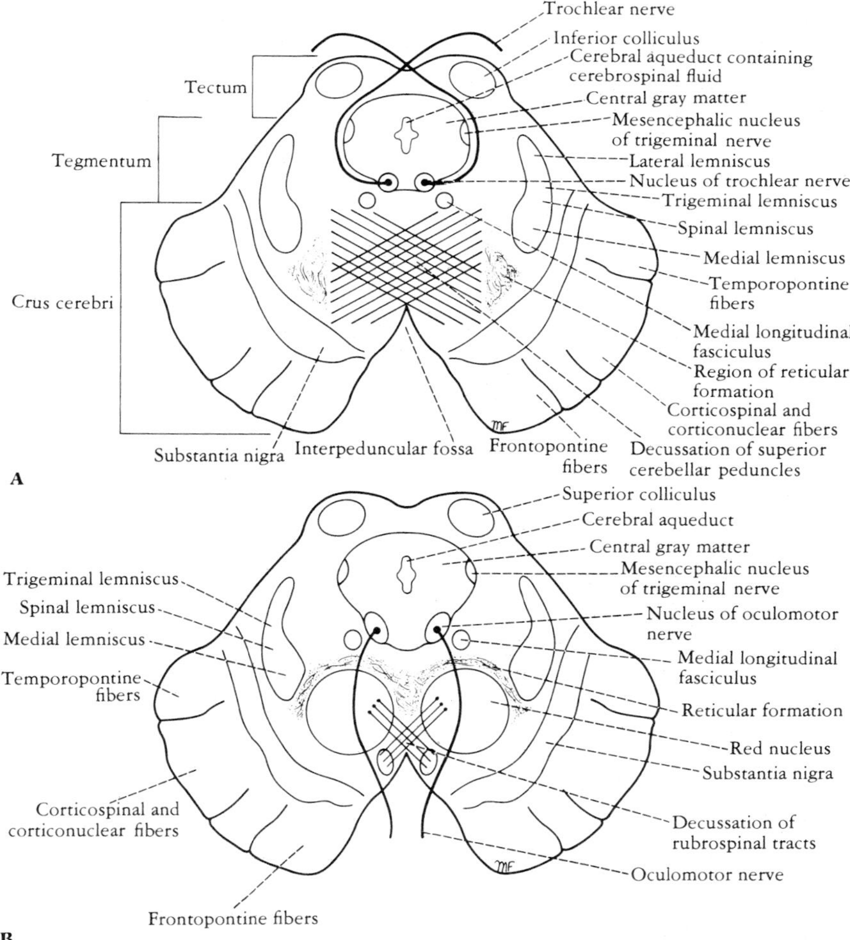

Figure 8–9 Transverse sections of the midbrain. **A.** At the level of the inferior colliculus. **B.** At the level of the superior colliculus.

is the **cerebral aqueduct**, which connects the third and fourth ventricles. The **tectum** is the part of the midbrain posterior to the cerebral aqueduct; it has four small surface swellings referred to previously: the **two superior** and **two inferior colliculi** (Fig. 8-9). The cerebral aqueduct is lined by ependyma and is surrounded by the **central gray matter**.

TRANSVERSE SECTION OF THE MIDBRAIN AT THE LEVEL OF THE INFERIOR COLLICULI

The **inferior colliculus**, consisting of a large nucleus of gray matter, lies beneath the corresponding surface elevation and forms part of the auditory pathway (Fig. 8-9). It receives many of the terminal fibers of the lateral lemniscus. The pathway then continues through the inferior brachium to the medial geniculate body.

The **trochlear nucleus** is situated in the central gray matter close to the median plane just posterior to the **medial longitudinal fasciculus**. The emerging fibers of the trochlear nucleus pass laterally and posteriorly around the central gray matter and leave the midbrain just below the inferior colliculi. The fibers of the trochlear nerve now **decussate completely** in the **superior medullary velum.** The **mesencephalic nuclei of the trigeminal nerve** are lateral to the cerebral aqueduct (Fig. 8-9). The **decussation of the superior cerebellar peduncles** occupies the central part of the tegmentum anterior to the cerebral aqueduct. The **reticular formation** is smaller than that of the pons and is situated lateral to the decussation.

The **medial lemniscus** ascends posterior to the substantia nigra; the **spinal** and **trigeminal lemnisci** are situated lateral to the medial lemniscus (Fig. 8-9). The **lateral lemniscus** is located posterior to the trigeminal lemniscus.

The **substantia nigra** (Fig. 8-9) is a large motor nucleus situated between the tegmentum and the crus cerebri and is found throughout the midbrain. The nucleus is composed of medium-sized multipolar neurons that possess inclusion granules of melanin pigment within their cytoplasm. The substantia nigra is concerned with muscle tone and is connected to the cerebral cortex, spinal cord, hypothalamus, and basal nuclei.

The **crus cerebri** contains important descending tracts and is separated from the tegmentum by the substantia nigra (Fig. 8-9). The corticospinal and corticonuclear fibers occupy the middle two-thirds of the crus. The frontopontine fibers occupy the medial part of the crus and the temporopontine fibers occupy the lateral part of the crus (Fig. 8-9). These descending tracts connect the cerebral cortex to the anterior gray column cells of the spinal cord, the cranial nerve nuclei, the pons, and the cerebellum.

TRANSVERSE SECTION OF THE MIDBRAIN AT THE LEVEL OF THE SUPERIOR COLLICULI

The **superior colliculus** (Fig. 8-9), a large nucleus of gray matter that lies beneath the corresponding surface elevation, forms part of the visual reflexes. It is connected to the lateral geniculate body by the superior brachium. It receives afferent fibers from the optic nerve, the visual cortex, and the spinotectal tract. The efferent fibers form the tectospinal and tectobulbar tracts, which are probably responsible for the reflex movements of the eyes, head, and neck in response to visual stimuli. The afferent pathway for the **light reflex** ends in the **pretectal nucleus**. This small group of neurons is situated close to the lateral part of the superior colliculus. After relaying in the pretectal nucleus, the fibers pass to the parasympathetic nucleus of the oculomotor nerve (Edinger-Westphal nucleus). The emerging fibers then pass to the oculomotor nerve. The **oculomotor nucleus** is situated in the central gray matter close to the median plane, just posterior to the **medial longitudinal fasciculus** (Fig. 8-9). The fibers of the oculomotor nucleus pass anteriorly through the red nucleus to emerge on the medial side of the crus cerebri in the interpeduncular fossa.

The **medial, spinal, and trigeminal lemnisci** form a curved band posterior to the substantia nigra but the **lateral lemniscus** does not extend superiorly to this level (Fig. 8-9).

Table 8–3 Comparison of Two Levels of the Midbrain Showing the Major Structures at Each Level*

Level	Cavity	Nuclei	Motor Tracts	Sensory Tracts
Inferior colliculi	Cerebral aqueduct	Inferior colliculus, substantia nigra, trochlear nucleus, mesencephalic nuclei of cranial nerve V	Corticospinal and corticonuclear tracts, temporopontine fibers, frontopontine fibers, medial longitudinal fasciculus	Lateral, trigeminal, spinal, and medial lemnisci, decussation of superior cerebellar peduncles
Superior colliculi	Cerebral aqueduct	Superior colliculus, substantia nigra, oculomotor nucleus, Edinger-Westphal nucleus, red nucleus, mesencephalic nucleus of cranial nerve V	Corticospinal and corticonuclear tracts, temporopontine fibers, frontopontine fibers, medial longitudinal fasciculus, decussation of rubrospinal tract	Trigeminal, spinal, and medial lemnisci

*Note that the reticular formation is present at all levels.

The **red nucleus** (Fig. 8-9) is a rounded mass of gray matter situated between the cerebral aqueduct and the substantia nigra. Afferent fibers reach the red nucleus from (1) the cerebral cortex through the corticospinal fibers, (2) the cerebellum through the superior cerebellar peduncle, and (3) the lentiform nucleus, subthalamic and hypothalamic nuclei, substantia nigra, and spinal cord. Efferent fibers leave the red nucleus and pass to (1) the spinal cord through the rubrospinal tract (as this tract descends, it decussates), (2) the reticular formation through the rubroreticular tract, (3) the thalamus, and (4) the substantia nigra.

The **reticular formation** is situated in the tegmentum lateral and posterior to the red nucleus (Fig. 8-9).

The **crus cerebri** contains the identical important descending tracts, the **corticospinal, corticonuclear,** and **corticopontine fibers**, that are present at the level of the inferior colliculus.

See Table 8-3 for a comparison of the two levels of the midbrain.

The continuity of the various cranial nerve nuclei through the different regions of the brainstem is shown in Figure 8-10.

BLOOD SUPPLY OF THE MIDBRAIN

The midbrain is supplied by the posterior cerebral, the superior cerebellar, and the basilar arteries.

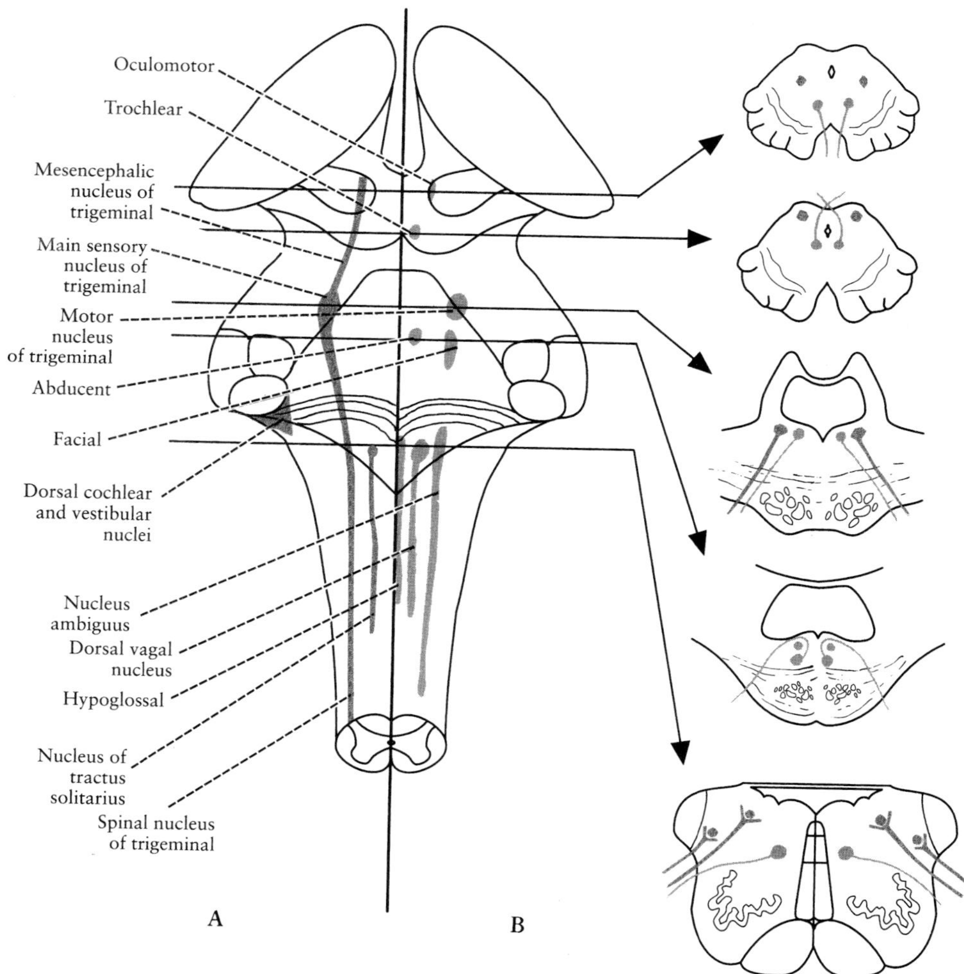

Figure 8–10 Diagram showing the continuity of the various cranial nerve nuclei through the different regions of the brainstem. Side **A** shows the sensory nuclei and side **B** shows the motor nuclei. Cross sections at the level of the nuclei are also shown.

Clinical Notes

Trauma to the Midbrain

As the result of the sudden movement of the head, the cerebral peduncles may impinge against the sharp edge of the tentorium cerebelli. This may result in injury to the oculomotor and or the trochlear nuclei.

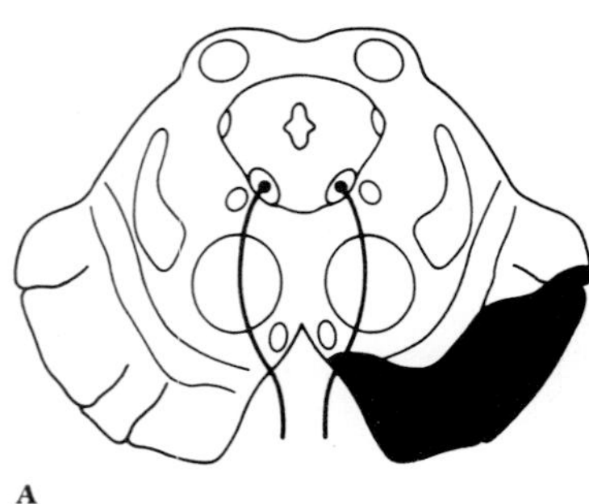

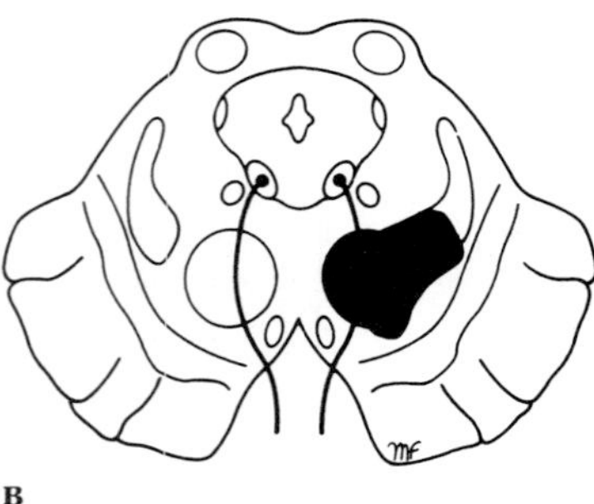

Figure 8–11 Vascular disorders of the midbrain. **A.** Weber's syndrome, involving the oculomotor nerve and the crus cerebri. **B.** Benedikt's syndrome, involving the red nucleus and the medial lemniscus.

Blockage of the Cerebral Aqueduct

The cerebral aqueduct is one of the narrower parts of the ventricular system. Normally, cerebrospinal fluid that has been produced in the lateral and third ventricles passes through this channel to enter the fourth ventricle and so escapes through the foramina in its roof to enter the subarachnoid space. In congenital hydrocephalus, the cerebral aqueduct may be blocked. A tumor of the midbrain or pressure on the midbrain from a tumor arising outside the midbrain may compress the aqueduct and produce hydrocephalus.

Vascular Disorders of the Midbrain

Weber's Syndrome

Weber's syndrome (Fig. 8-11A) is commonly produced by occlusion of a branch of the posterior cerebral artery that supplies the midbrain, and results in the necrosis of brain tissue involving the oculomotor nerve and the crus cerebri. There is ipsilateral ophthalmoplegia and contralateral paralysis of the lower part of the face, the tongue, and the arm and leg. The eyeball is deviated laterally because of the paralysis of the medial rectus muscle; there is drooping (ptosis) of the upper lid, and the pupil is dilated and fixed to light and accommodation.

Benedikt's Syndrome

Benedikt's syndrome (Fig. 8-11B) is similar to Weber's syndrome, but the necrosis involves the medial lemniscus and red nucleus, producing contralateral hemianesthesia and involuntary movements of the limbs of the opposite side.

REVIEW QUESTIONS

Directions: Each of the incomplete statements in this section is followed by completions of the statement. Select the ONE lettered completion that is BEST in each case.

1. On the anterior surface of the medulla oblongata are:
   (a) three swellings called the pyramids
   (b) the hypoglossal nerves emerging between the olives and the inferior cerebellar peduncle
   (c) glossopharyngeal nerves emerging between the olives and the inferior cerebellar peduncles
   (d) two small swellings produced by the underlying cuneate and gracile nuclei
   (e) cranial part of the accessory nerves emerging between the pyramids and the olives
2. The pons has on its anterior surface the:
   (a) superior medullary velum
   (b) emerging trigeminal nerve
   (c) grooves for the two posterior cerebral arteries
   (d) colliculus facialis
   (e) medial eminence
3. The posterior surface of the midbrain shows:
   (a) five swellings called colliculi
   (b) the emerging oculomotor nerve
   (c) the emerging trochlear nerve
   (d) the interpeduncular fossa
   (e) the decussation of the pyramids

For questions 4-8 study, Figure 8-12, showing a transverse section of the medulla oblongata.

4. Structure number 1 is the:
   (a) inferior cerebellar peduncle
   (b) inferior olivary nucleus
   (c) pyramid
   (d) medial vestibular nucleus
   (e) nucleus ambiguus
5. Structure number 2 is the:
   (a) reticular formation
   (b) pyramid
   (c) medial longitudinal bundle
   (d) inferior olivary nucleus
   (e) sensory nucleus of trigeminal nerve
6. Structure number 3 is the:
   (a) medial lemniscus
   (b) tectospinal tract
   (c) pyramid
   (d) arcuate nucleus
   (e) spinal tract of the trigeminal nerve
7. Structure number 4 is the:
   (a) medial longitudinal bundle
   (b) tectospinal tract
   (c) lateral spinal thalamic tract
   (d) medial lemniscus
   (e) lateral spinothalamic tract
8. Structure number 5 is the:
   (a) tectospinal tract
   (b) pyramid
   (c) medial longitudinal bundle
   (d) reticular formation
   (e) posterior spinocerebellar tract

For questions 9-13, study Figure 8-13, showing a transverse section of the pons.

9. Structure number 1 is the:
   (a) inferior cerebellar peduncle
   (b) superior medullary velum
   (c) main sensory nucleus of the trigeminal nerve
   (d) medial longitudinal fasciculus
   (e) superior cerebellar peduncle
10. Structure number 2 is the:
   (a) middle cerebellar peduncle
   (b) medial lemniscus
   (c) transverse pontine fibers
   (d) spinal lemniscus
   (e) reticular formation
11. Structure number 3 is the:
   (a) pyramids
   (b) trapezoid body
   (c) medial longitudinal fasciculus
   (d) transverse pontine fibers
   (e) decussation of the superior cerebellar peduncles
12. Structure number 4 is the:
   (a) bundles of corticospinal fibers
   (b) reticular formation
   (c) medial lemniscus
   (d) medial longitudinal fasciculus
   (e) spinal lemniscus
13. Structure number 5 is the:
   (a) sensory nucleus of the trigeminal nerve
   (b) nucleus ambiguus
   (c) motor nucleus of the trigeminal nerve
   (d) nucleus of the abducent nerve
   (e) motor nucleus of the facial nerve

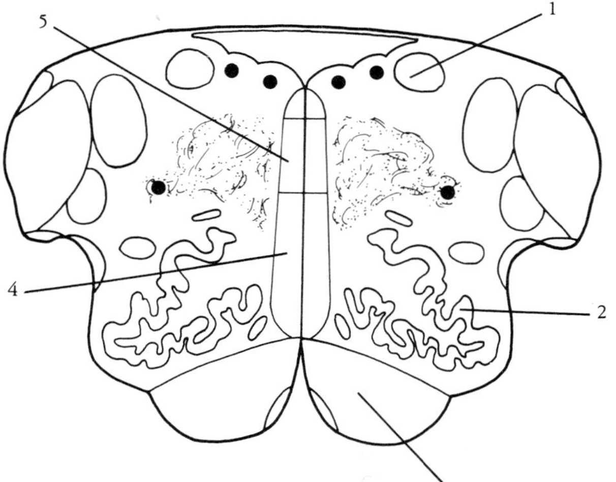

Figure 8–12 Transverse section of the medulla oblongata.

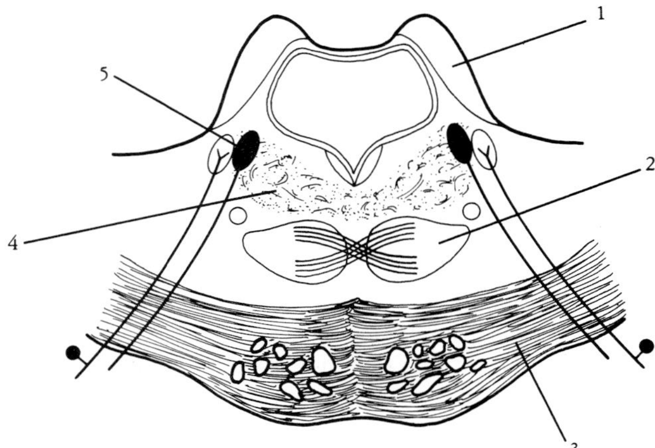

Figure 8–13 Transverse section of the pons.

For questions 14-18, study Figure 8-14, showing a transverse section of the midbrain.

14. Structure number 1 is the:
    (a) oculomotor nerve nucleus
    (b) trochlear nerve nucleus
    (c) mesencephalic nucleus
    (d) superior colliculus
    (e) red nucleus
15. Structure number 2 is the:
    (a) spinal lemniscus
    (b) decussation of the rubrospinal tract
    (c) substantia nigra
    (d) oculomotor nucleus
    (e) red nucleus
16. Structure number 3 is the:
    (a) decussation of the rubrospinal tract
    (b) decussation of the trochlear nerve
    (c) reticular formation
    (d) decussation of the superior cerebellar peduncle
    (e) medial longitudinal fasciculus
17. Structure number 4 is the:
    (a) frontopontine fibers
    (b) temporopontine fibers
    (c) corticonuclear fibers
    (d) medial lemniscus
    (e) substantia nigra
18. Structure number 5 is the:
    (a) mesencephalic nucleus
    (b) superior colliculus
    (c) inferior colliculus
    (d) superior cerebellar peduncle
    (e) red nucleus

For questions 19-23, study Figure 8-15, showing a coronal MRI of the head.

19. Structure number 1 is the:
    (a) fourth ventricle
    (b) cerebral aqueduct
    (c) lateral ventricle
    (d) third ventricle
    (e) middle cerebral artery
20. Structure number 2 is the:
    (a) superior cerebellar peduncle
    (b) cerebral peduncle
    (c) midbrain
    (d) middle cerebellar peduncle
    (e) inferior cerebellar peduncle
21. Structure number 3 is the:
    (a) falx cerebri
    (b) basilar artery
    (c) cerebral aqueduct
    (d) straight sinus
    (e) central canal
22. Structure number 4 is the:
    (a) fourth ventricle
    (b) foramen of Magendie
    (c) foramen magnum
    (d) lateral ventricle
    (e) cerebral aqueduct
23. Structure number 5 is the:
    (a) occipital lobe of the cerebral hemisphere
    (b) temporal lobe of the cerebral hemisphere
    (c) petrous part of the temporal bone
    (d) cerebellar hemisphere
    (e) vermis of the cerebellum

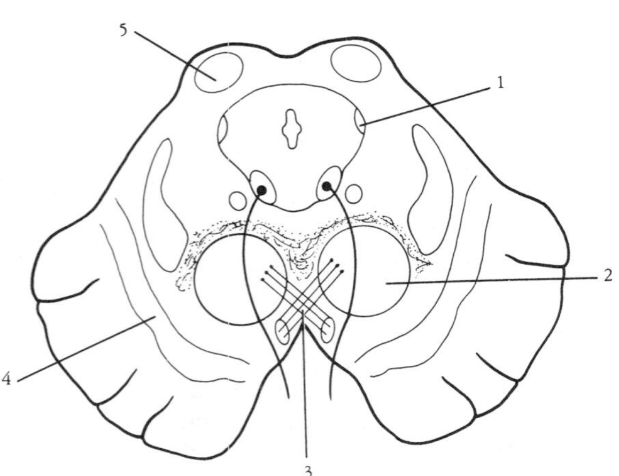

Figure 8–14 Transverse section of the midbrain.

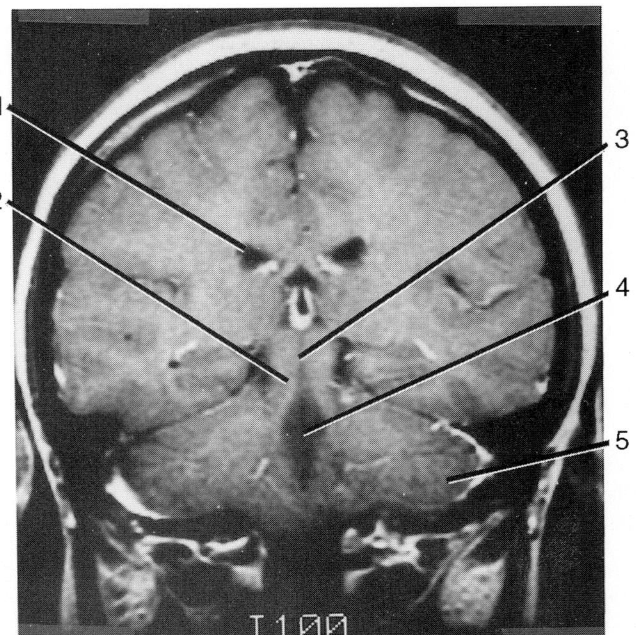

Figure 8–15 Coronal MRI of the head.

Directions: Each of the numbered items in this section is followed by answers that are positively phrased.. Select the ONE lettered answer that is an EXCEPTION.

24. The following statements concerning the interior of the lower part of the medulla are correct **except:**
    (a) It contains the central canal.
    (b) About three-fourths of the corticospinal fibers cross the median plane.
    (c) The substantia gelatinosa of the spinal cord becomes continuous with the nucleus of the spinal tract of the trigeminal nerve.
    (d) The medial lemniscus is formed by nerve fibers entering the hypoglossal nucleus.
    (e) The nucleus gracilis lies lateral to the posterior median sulcus.
25. The following statements concerning the interior of the upper part of the medulla are correct **except:**
    (a) The medial longitudinal fasciculus lies on either side of the midline.
    (b) The dorsal nucleus of the vague nerve lies between the pyramid and the olive.
    (c) The hypoglossal nucleus lies just beneath the floor of the fourth ventricle.
    (d) The nucleus ambiguus is situated within the reticular formation.
    (e) The inferior cerebellar peduncle is located along the lateral border of this part of the medulla.
26. The following statements concerning a transverse section through the caudal part of the pons are correct **except:**
    (a) All the transverse pontine fibers cross the pons posterior to the corticospinal fibers.
    (b) The motor nucleus of the facial nerve lies posterior to the medial lemniscus.
    (c) The trapezoid body is present.
    (d) The cavity of the fourth ventricle is roofed over by the superior medullary velum.
    (e) The spinal tract and nucleus of the trigeminal nerve are present.
27. The following statements concerning a transverse section through the midbrain at the level of the superior colliculus are correct **except:**
    (a) The nucleus of the oculomotor nerve is present in the central gray matter.
    (b) The red nucleus is traversed by the emerging fibers of the third cranial nerve.
    (c) The medial lemniscus lies anterior to the substantia nigra.
    (d) The spinal lemniscus lies a short distance lateral to the medial longitudinal bundle.
    (e) The rubrospinal tracts decussate at this level of the brainstem.
28. The following statements concerning a transverse section of the midbrain at the level of the inferior colliculus are correct **except:**
    (a) The frontopontine fibers are situated lateral to the temporopontine fibers.
    (b) The superior cerebellar peduncles decussate at this level.
    (c) The nucleus of the trochlear nerve lies in the central gray matter.
    (d) The reticular formation lies posterior to the substantia nigra.
    (e) The tectum lies posterior to the cerebral aqueduct.
29. The following statements concerning the medulla oblongata are correct **except:**
    (a) The central canal is continuous below with the central canal of the spinal cord.
    (b) The inferior medullary velum stretches between the inferior cerebellar peduncles.
    (c) The floor of the fourth ventricle is lined with ependyma.
    (d) The blood supply is derived from the vertebral, anterior and posterior spinal, posterior inferior cerebellar, and basilar arteries.
    (e) The posterior median fissure lies between the pyramids.
30. The following statements concerning the pons are correct **except:**
    (a) The pontine nuclei have no relationship to the transverse pontine fibers.
    (b) The pons lies anterior to the cerebellum.
    (c) The basilar artery lies on the anterior surface, producing a groove.
    (d) The posterior surface of the pons forms part of the floor of the fourth ventricle.
    (e) The posterior part of the pons is often referred to as the tegmentum.
31. The following statements concerning the midbrain are correct **except:**
    (a) It is surrounded by cerebrospinal fluid.
    (b) The crus cerebri forms the posterior part of the cerebral peduncles.
    (c) The inferior colliculi are concerned with auditory reflexes.
    (d) The inferior brachium connects the inferior colliculus with the medial geniculate body.
    (e) The midbrain is covered with pia mater.
32. The following statements concerning the lateral medullary syndrome of Wallenberg are correct **except:**
    (a) The syndrome can be caused by thrombosis of the posterior inferior cerebellar artery.
    (b) The patient experiences analgesia and thermoanesthesia on the ipsilateral side of the face.
    (c) There is ipsilateral Horner's syndrome.
    (d) Paralysis of the contralateral palatal and laryngeal muscles occurs.
    (e) There is contralateral loss of pain and temperature sensations.
33. The following signs and symptoms concerning the medial medullary syndrome are correct **except:**
    (a) There are contralateral impaired sensations of position and movement.
    (b) Contralateral hemiparesis occurs.
    (c) There is ipsilateral loss of tactile discrimination.
    (d) There is ipsilateral paralysis of the tongue.
    (e) The syndrome can be caused by a thrombosis of the medullary branch of the vertebral artery.

34. The following facts concerning the Arnold-Chiari phenomenon are correct **except:**
    (a) It is a congenital anomaly.
    (b) There is herniation of part of the cerebellum through the foramen magnum.
    (c) The apertures in the roof of the fourth ventricle become blocked.
    (d) Internal hydrocephalus occurs.
    (e) The medulla oblongata is unaffected.
35. The following statements concerning the cerebral aqueduct are correct **except:**
    (a) It is lined by ependyma.
    (b) It is continuous above with the third ventricle.
    (c) It drains into the fourth ventricle.
    (d) It is one of the narrowest parts of the ventricular system of the brain.
    (e) It is not surrounded by gray matter.
36. The following statements concerning Weber's syndrome are correct **except:**
    (a) There is ptosis of the contralateral upper eyelid.
    (b) It results in necrosis of the brain tissue involving the oculomotor nerve.
    (c) There is ipsilateral ophthalmoplegia.
    (d) There is contralateral paralysis of the upper and lower limbs.
    (e) There is contralateral paralysis of the lower part of the face.

Directions: Read the case history then answer the question. You will be required to select ONE BEST lettered answer.

An 8-year-old boy was seen by a neurologist because of right-sided facial weakness and medial strabismus of the right eye. Examination also revealed slight weakness of the muscles of the left upper and lower limbs. An MRI revealed a tumor of the pons.

37. The following facts concerning this patient are correct **except:**
    (a) The right unilateral weakness of the face is due to destruction of the right facial nucleus by the tumor.
    (b) The medial strabismus of the right eye is due to paralysis of the right lateral rectus muscle.
    (c) The right lateral rectus muscle is innervated by the right abducent nerve, and the expanding tumor is pressing on the abducent nerve nucleus on that side.
    (d) The weakness of the muscles of the upper and lower limbs is due to the involvement of the corticospinal fibers as they pass down through the pons.
    (e) The majority of the corticospinal fibers cross the midline at the decussation of the pyramids in the medulla, so that the left corticospinal fibers are involved in the pons in this patient.

ANSWERS AND EXPLANATIONS

1. C
2. B
3. C
4. D
5. D
6. C
7. D
8. A
9. E
10. B
11. D
12. B
13. C
14. C
15. E
16. A
17. E
18. B
19. C
20. C
21. C
22. A
23. D
24. D. The medial lemniscus is formed from the internal arcuate fibers that have emerged from the nucleus gracilis and nucleus cuneatus.
25. B. The dorsal nucleus of the vagus nerve lies beneath the floor of the fourth ventricle just lateral to the hypoglossal nucleus.
26. A. The corticospinal and corticonuclear fibers lie among the transverse pontine fibers.
27. C. The medial lemniscus lies posterior to the substantia nigra.
28. A. The frontopontine fibers lie medial to the temporopontine fibers.
29. E. The anterior median fissure lies between the pyramids.
30. A. The pontine nuclei give rise to the transverse pontine fibers.
31. B. The crus cerebri forms the anterior part of the cerebral peduncle.
32. D. There is paralysis of the ipsilateral palatal and laryngeal muscles. The lateral medullary syndrome of Wallenberg is described on page 96.
33. C. There is contralateral loss of tactile discrimination. The medial medullary syndrome is described on page 96.
34. E. The medulla oblongata becomes elongated and is herniated through the foramen magnum.
35. E. The cerebral aqueduct is surrounded by gray matter in which are located the nuclei of the third and fourth cranial nerves.
36. A. Ptosis occurs on the same side as the lesion and is caused by paralysis of the levator palpebrae superioris due to involvement of the oculomotor nerve.
37. E. The weakness of the muscles of the left upper and lower limbs is due to destruction of the right corticospinal fibers as they descend through the pons; these fibers cross the midline at the decussation of the pyramids at the lower end of the medulla oblongata.

CHAPTER 9

Cerebellum

CHAPTER OUTLINE

SUGGESTED PLAN FOR REVIEW OF CHAPTER 9

1. Learn the structure of the gray matter of the cerebellar cortex and the arrangement of the intracerebellar nuclei. Memorize the connections of the cells of the cerebellar cortex. Examiners are fond of asking questions about the Purkinje cells.
2. Understand the difference between the climbing and the mossy fibers. Where do these fibers terminate in the cerebellar cortex?
3. Learn the main connections between the cerebellum and the remainder of the nervous system. Do not just commit connections to memory but understand the functions of the various connections. You will find that this approach helps you to retain the material.

SUGGESTED PLAN FOR REVIEW OF CHAPTER 9 (continued)

4. Know the functions of the cerebellum and understand what happens when the cerebellum fails to function because of disease. Remember that each cerebellar hemisphere controls muscular movement on the same side of the body. Also note that the cerebellum has no direct pathway to the lower motor neurons but exerts its control via the cerebral cortex and the brainstem.

INTRODUCTION

The cerebellum lies in the posterior cranial fossa of the skull and forms the roof of the fourth ventricle. It is joined to the brainstem by three pairs of peduncles: the superior, middle, and inferior peduncles.

The essential function of the cerebellum is to coordinate, by synergistic action, all reflex and voluntary muscular activity. It thus graduates and harmonizes muscle tone and maintains normal body posture. It permits voluntary movements to take place with precision and economy of effort.

EXTERNAL APPEARANCES

The cerebellum is somewhat ovoid in shape and constricted in its median part. It consists of two **cerebellar hemispheres** joined by a narrow median vermis (Figs. 9-1 and 9-2).

The cerebellum is divided into three main lobes: the **anterior lobe**, the **middle lobe**, and the **flocculonodular lobe**. The **anterior lobe** may be seen on the superior surface of the cerebellum and is separated from the middle lobe by a wide V-shaped fissure called the **primary fissure** (Fig. 9-2). The **middle lobe** (sometimes called the posterior lobe), which is the largest part of the cerebellum, is situated between the primary and **uvulonodular fissures**. The **flocculonodular lobe** is situated posterior to the uvulonodular fissure. A deep **horizontal fissure** that is found along the margin of the cerebellum separates the superior from the inferior surfaces; it is of no morphological or functional significance (Fig. 9-2).

INTERNAL STRUCTURE

The cerebellum is composed of an outer covering of gray matter called the **cortex** and inner white matter. Embedded

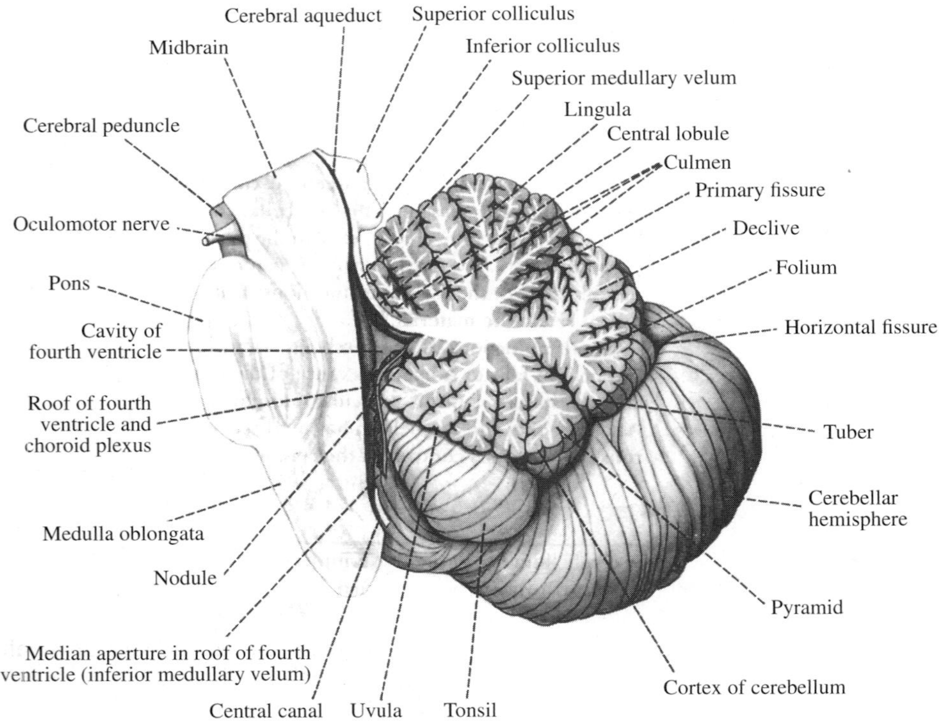

Figure 9–1 Sagittal section through the brainstem and the cerebellum.

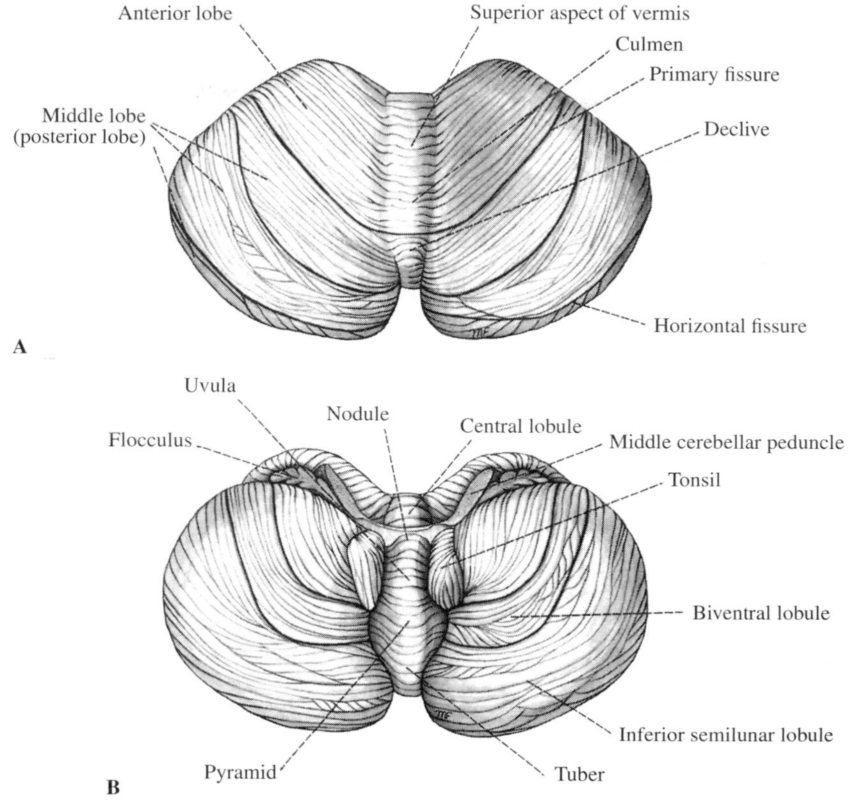

Figure 9–2 Cerebellum. **A**. Superior view. **B**. Inferior view.

in the white matter of each hemisphere are three masses of gray matter forming the **intracerebellar nuclei.**

Gray Matter of the Cerebellum

CEREBELLAR CORTEX

The cortex of the cerebellum is folded into the **cerebellar folia** (Fig. 9-1). Each folium contains a core of white matter covered superficially by gray matter. A section made through the cerebellum parallel with the median plane divides the folia at right angles, and the cut surface has a branched appearance, called the **arbor vitae** (Fig. 9-1).

The cerebellar cortex throughout its extent has a uniform structure and can be divided into three layers: (1) an external layer, the **molecular layer**; (2) a middle layer, the **Purkinje cell layer**; and (3) an internal layer, the **granular layer** (Fig. 9-3).

Molecular Layer

The molecular layer contains two types of neurons: the outer **stellate cell** and the inner **basket cell** (Fig. 9-3). These neurons are scattered among the dendrites and axons that run parallel to the long axis of the folia.

Purkinje Cell Layer

The Purkinje cells are larger Golgi type I neurons. They are flask-shaped and are arranged in a single layer (Fig. 9-3). In a plane transverse to the folium, the dendrites of these cells pass into the molecular layer, where they undergo profuse branching. The distal branches are covered by short, thick **dendritic spines** that form synaptic contacts with the parallel fibers derived from the granule cell axons.

The axon of the Purkinje cell passes through the granular layer to enter the white matter where it acquires a myelin sheath and terminates by synapsing with cells of one of the intercerebellar nuclei. Collateral branches of the Purkinje axon make synaptic contacts with the dendrites of basket and stellate cells of the granular layer. A few of the Purkinje cell axons pass directly to end in the vestibular nuclei of the brainstem.

Granular Layer

The granular layer is packed with small cells with densely staining nuclei and scanty cytoplasm (Fig. 9-3). Each cell gives rise to four or five dendrites, which have synaptic contact with mossy fiber input. The axon of each granule cell passes into the molecular layer, where it bifurcates at a T junction, the branches running parallel to the long axis of

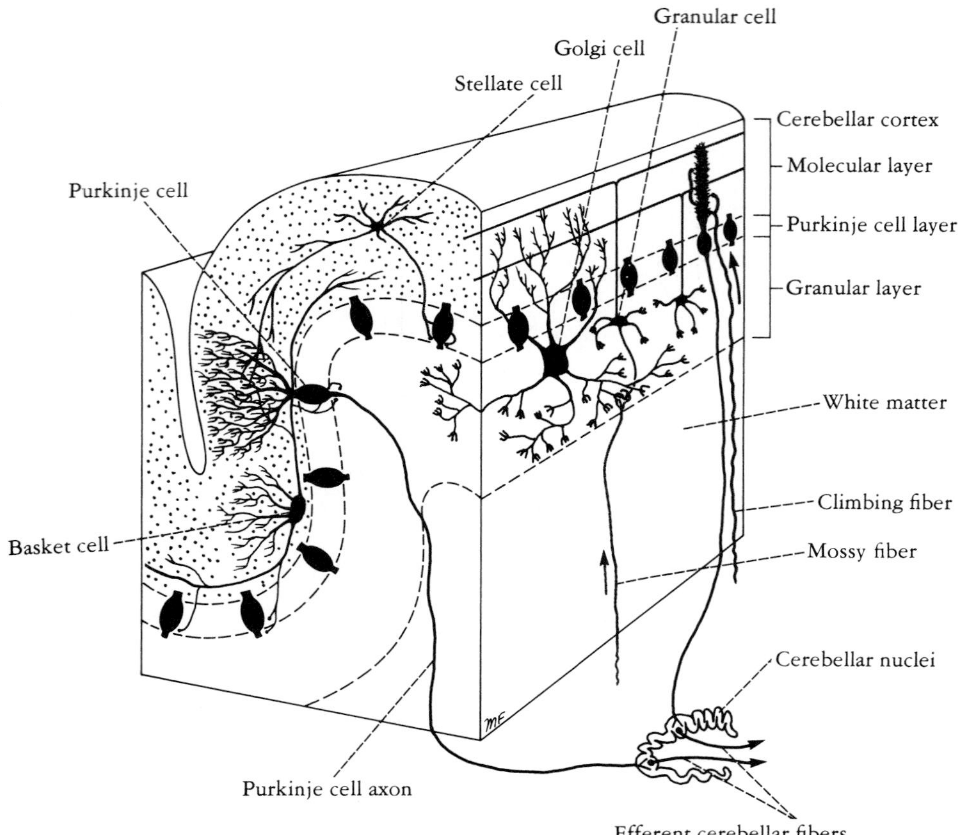

Figure 9–3 Cellular organization of the cerebellar cortex with the afferent and efferent fibers.

the cerebellar folium. The majority of the parallel fibers make synaptic contacts with the dendrites of the Purkinje cells. Scattered throughout the granular layer are Golgi cells (Fig. 9-3). Their dendrites ramify in the molecular layer and their axons synapse with the dendrites of the granular cells.

INTRACELLULAR NUCLEI

Four masses of gray matter are embedded in the white matter of the cerebellum on each side of the midline. From lateral to medial these nuclei are the **dentate**, the **emboliform**, the **globose**, and the **fastigial**.

The **dentate nucleus**, the largest of the cerebellar nuclei, has the shape of a crumpled bag with the opening facing medially (Fig. 9-4). The interior of the bag is filled with white matter made up of efferent fibers that leave the nucleus to form a large part of the superior cerebellar peduncle.

The **emboliform nucleus** is oval and situated medial to the dentate nucleus (Fig. 9-4).

The **globose nucleus** lies medial to the emboliform nucleus (Fig. 9-4).

The **fastigial nucleus** lies near the midline in the vermis and close to the roof of the fourth ventricle (Fig. 9-4).

The intracerebellar nuclei are composed of large, multipolar neurons whose axons form the cerebellar outflow in the superior and inferior cerebellar peduncles.

White Matter of the Cerebellum

The white matter is made up of three groups of fibers: (1) intrinsic, (2) afferent, and (3) efferent.

The **intrinsic fibers** do not leave the cerebellum but connect different folia of the cerebellar cortex and vermis on the same side, while others connect the two cerebellar hemispheres together.

The **afferent fibers** form the greater part of the white matter and proceed to the cerebellar cortex. Here, they lose their myelin sheath and end as either **climbing** or **mossy fibers** (Fig. 9-3). The afferent fibers enter the cerebellum mainly through the inferior and middle cerebellar peduncles.

The **efferent fibers** constitute the output of the cerebellum and commence as the axons of the Purkinje cells of the cerebellar cortex. The great majority of the Purkinje cell axons pass to and synapse with the neurons of the cerebellar nuclei (fastigial, globose, emboliform, and dentate). The axons of the neurons then leave the cerebellum. A few

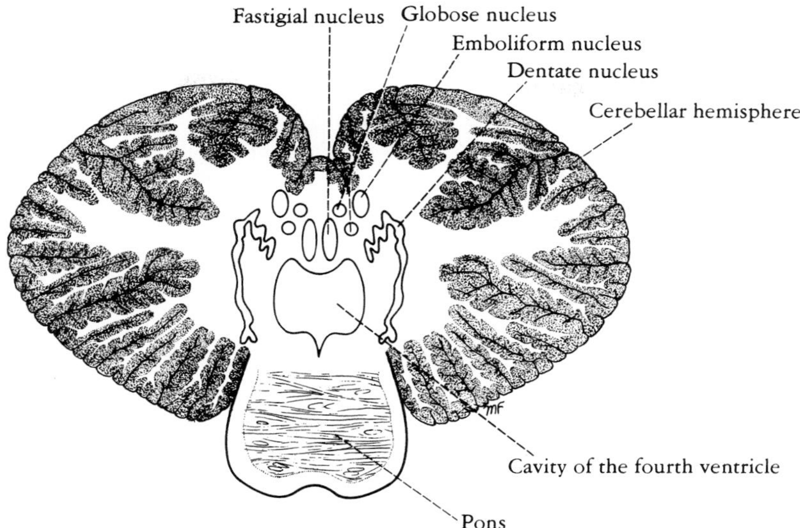

Figure 9–4 Coronal section through the cerebellum and pons showing the intracerebellar nuclei.

Purkinje cell axons in the flocculonodular lobe and in parts of the vermis bypass the cerebellar nuclei and leave the cerebellum without synapsing.

Fibers from the dentate, emboliform, and globose nuclei leave the cerebellum through the superior cerebellar peduncle. Fibers from the fastigial nucleus leave through the inferior cerebellar peduncle.

CEREBELLAR PEDUNCLES

The efferent and afferent fibers of the cerebellum are grouped together on each side into three large bundles, or peduncles.

The **inferior cerebellar peduncle** arises from the superior half of the medulla oblongata. The two peduncles diverge as they ascend and pass into their respective cerebellar hemispheres.

The **middle cerebellar peduncle** is the largest of the three peduncles. It arises from the pons and enters the cerebellar hemisphere on each side.

The **superior cerebellar peduncle** runs superiorly, lateral to the upper half of the fourth ventricle, to enter the lower part of the midbrain on each side.

INTERCONNECTIONS OF THE NEURONS OF THE CEREBELLAR CORTEX

Two types of afferent fibers enter the cerebellar cortex, the **climbing fibers** and the **mossy fibers**. The climbing fibers are the terminal fibers of the olivocerebellar tracts (Fig. 9-3). They enter the molecular layer of the cortex, where they branch and make multiple synaptic contacts with one Purkinje cell. A few side branches leave each climbing fiber and synapse with adjacent stellate and basket cells.

The mossy fibers are the terminal fibers of all other cerebellar afferent tracts. They have multiple branches, so a single mossy fiber may stimulate thousands of Purkinje cells through the granule cells (Fig. 9-3).

CEREBELLAR AFFERENT FIBERS FROM THE CEREBRAL CORTEX

The cerebral cortex sends information to the cerebellum by three pathways: (1) the corticopontocerebellar pathway, (2) the cerebro-olivocerebellar pathway, and (3) the cerebroreticulocerebellar pathway.

Corticopontocerebellar Pathway

The corticopontine fibers arise from nerve cells in the frontal, parietal, temporal, and occipital lobes of the cerebral cortex and descend through the corona radiata and internal capsule and terminate on the pontine nuclei (Fig. 9-5). The pontine nuclei give rise to the **transverse fibers of the pons,** which cross the midline and enter the opposite cerebellar hemisphere as the middle cerebellar peduncle.

Cerebro-olivocerebellar Pathway

The cortico-olivary fibers arise from nerve cells in the frontal, parietal, temporal, and occipital lobes of the cerebral cortex and descend through the corona radiata and internal capsule to terminate bilaterally on the inferior olivary nuclei (Fig. 9-5). The inferior olivary nuclei give rise to fibers that cross the midline and enter the opposite cerebellar hemisphere through the inferior cerebellar

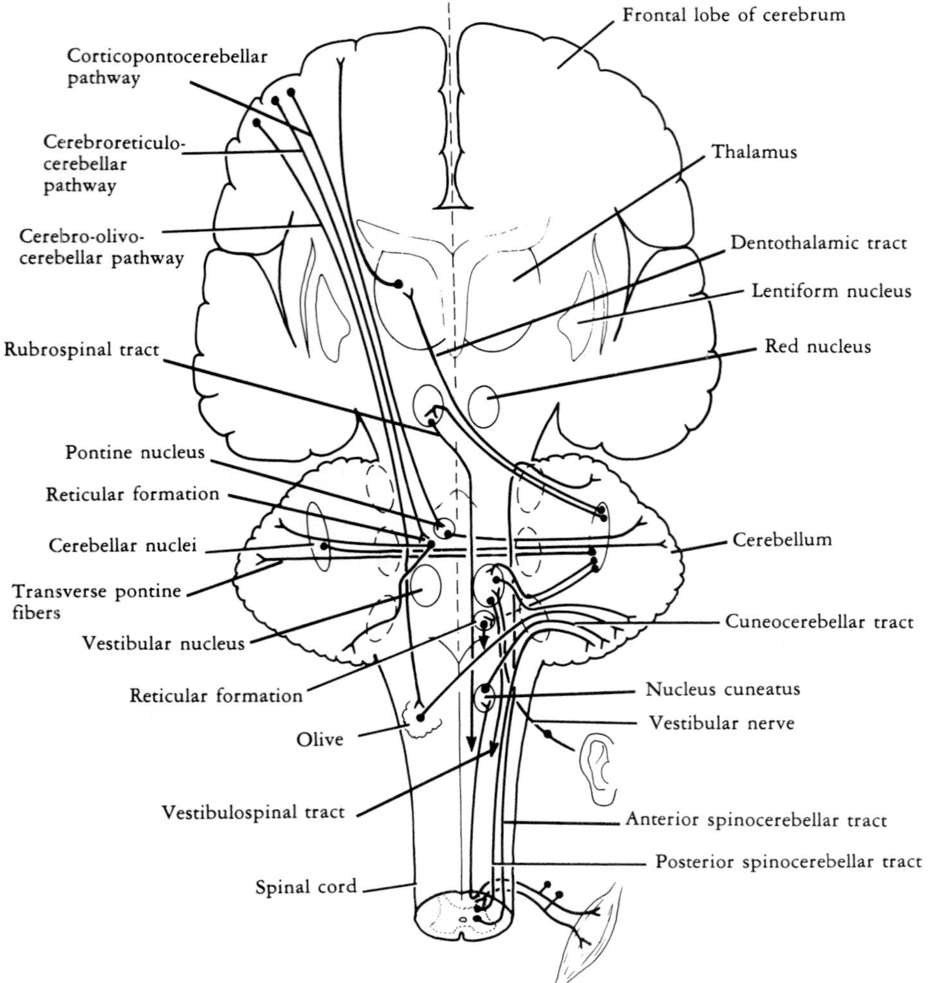

Figure 9–5 Main connections of the cerebellum; the cerebellar peduncles are shown as ovoid dashes.

peduncle. These fibers terminate as the climbing fibers in the cerebellar cortex.

Cerebroreticulocerebellar Pathway

The corticoreticular fibers arise from nerve cells from many areas of the cerebral cortex, particularly the sensorimotor areas. They descend to terminate in the reticular formation on the same side and on the opposite side in the pons and medulla (Fig. 9-5). The cells in the reticular formation give rise to the reticulocerebellar fibers that enter the cerebellar hemisphere on the same side through the inferior and middle cerebellar peduncles.

This connection between the cerebrum and the cerebellum is important in the control of voluntary movement. Information regarding the initiation of movement in the cerebral cortex is probably transmitted to the cerebellum so that the movement can be monitored and appropriate adjustments in the muscle activity can be made.

CEREBELLAR AFFERENT FIBERS FROM THE SPINAL CORD

The spinal cord sends information to the cerebellum by three pathways: (1) the anterior spinocerebellar tract, (2) the posterior spinocerebellar tract, and (3) the cuneocerebellar tract.

Anterior Spinocerebellar Tract

The axons entering the spinal cord from the posterior root ganglion terminate by synapsing with the neurons in the **nucleus dorsalis** (Clark's column) at the base of the posterior gray column. The majority of the axons of these neurons cross to the opposite side and ascend as the **anterior spinocerebellar tract** in the contralateral white column; the minority of the axons ascend as the anterior spinocerebellar tract in the lateral white column of the same side (Fig. 9-5). The fibers enter the cerebellum through the superior cerebellar peduncle and terminate as mossy fibers in the cerebellar cortex. Collateral branches that end in the deep cerebellar nuclei are also given off. It is believed that those fibers that crossed over to the opposite side in the spinal cord cross back within the cerebellum.

The anterior spinocerebellar tract is found at all segments of the spinal cord and its fibers convey muscle joint information from the muscle spindles, tendon organs, and joint receptors of the upper and lower limbs. It is also believed that the cerebellum receives information from the skin and superficial fascia by this tract.

Posterior Spinocerebellar Tract

The axons entering the spinal cord from the posterior root ganglion enter the posterior gray column and terminate by synapsing on the neurons at the base of the posterior gray column. These neurons are known collectively as the nucleus dorsalis (Clark's column). The axons of these neurons enter the posterolateral part of the lateral white column on the same side and ascend as the **posterior spinocerebellar tract** to the medulla oblongata (Fig. 9-5). Here the tract enters the cerebellum through the inferior cerebellar peduncle and terminates as mossy fibers in the cerebellar cortex. Collateral branches that end in the deep cerebellar nuclei are also given off. The posterior spinocerebellar tract receives muscle joint information from the muscle spindles, tendon organs, and joint receptors of the trunk and lower limbs.

Cuneocerebellar Tract

These fibers originate in the nucleus cuneatus of the medulla oblongata and enter the cerebellar hemisphere on the same side through the inferior cerebellar peduncle (Fig. 9-5). The fibers terminate as mossy fibers in the cerebellar cortex. Collateral branches that end in the deep cerebellar nuclei are also given off. The cuneocerebellar tract receives muscle joint information from the muscle spindles, tendon organs, and joint receptors of the upper limb and upper part of the thorax.

CEREBELLAR AFFERENT FIBERS FROM THE VESTIBULAR NERVE

The vestibular nerve sends many afferent fibers directly to the cerebellum through the inferior cerebellar peduncle on the same side. Other vestibular afferent fibers pass first to the vestibular nuclei in the brainstem, where they synapse and are relayed to the cerebellum (Fig. 9-5). They enter the cerebellum through the inferior cerebellar peduncle on the same side. All the afferent fibers from the inner ear terminate as mossy fibers in the flocculonodular lobe of the cerebellum.

OTHER AFFERENT FIBERS

In addition, the cerebellum receives small bundles of afferent fibers from the red nucleus and the tectum.

The afferent cerebellar pathways are summarized in Table 9-1.

CEREBELLAR EFFERENT FIBERS

The entire output of the cerebellar cortex is through the axons of the Purkinje cells. The majority of the axons of the Purkinje cells end by synapsing on the neurons of the deep cerebellar nuclei (Fig. 9-3). The axons of the neurons that form the cerebellar nuclei constitute the efferent outflow from the cerebellum. A few Purkinje cell axons pass directly out of the cerebellum to the lateral vestibular nucleus. The efferent fibers from the cerebellum connect with the red nucleus, thalamus, vestibular complex, and reticular formation.

Globose-Emboliform-Rubral Pathway

Axons of neurons in the globose and emboliform nuclei travel through the superior cerebellar peduncle and cross the midline to the opposite side in the **decussation of the superior cerebellar peduncles** (Fig. 9-5). The fibers end by synapsing with cells of the contralateral red nucleus, which give rise to axons of the **rubrospinal tract** (Fig. 9-5). Thus it is seen that this pathway crosses twice, once in the decussation of the superior cerebellar peduncle, and again in the rubrospinal tract close to its origin. By this means, the globose and emboliform nuclei influence motor activity on the same side of the body.

Dentothalamic Pathway

Axons of neurons in the dentate nucleus travel through the superior cerebellar peduncle and cross the midline to the opposite side in the **decussation of the superior cerebellar peduncle** (Fig. 9-5). The fibers end by synapsing with cells in the contralateral **ventrolateral nucleus of the thalamus**. The axons of the thalamic neurons ascend through the internal capsule and corona radiata and terminate in the primary motor area of the cerebral cortex. By this pathway, the dentate nucleus can influence motor activity by acting on the motor neurons of the opposite cerebral cortex; impulses from the motor cortex are transmitted to spinal segmental levels through the corticospinal tract. The majority of the fibers of the corticospinal tract cross to the opposite side in the decussation of the pyramids or later at the spinal segmental levels. The dentate nucleus thus is able to coordinate muscle activity on the same side of the body.

Fastigial Vestibular Pathway

The axons of neurons in the fastigial nucleus travel through the inferior cerebellar peduncle and end by projecting on the neurons of the **lateral vestibular nucleus** on both sides (Fig. 9-5). It will be remembered that some Purkinje cell axons project directly to the lateral vestibular nucleus. The neurons of the lateral vestibular nucleus form the **vestibulospinal tract**. The fastigial nucleus exerts a facilitatory influence mainly on the ipsilateral extensor muscle tone.

Fastigial Reticular Pathway

The axons of neurons in the fastigial nucleus travel through the inferior cerebellar peduncle and end by synapsing with neurons of the reticular formation (Fig. 9-5). Axons of these

Table 9–1 Summary of the Afferent Cerebellar Pathways

Pathway	Function	Origin	Destination
Corticopontocerebellar	Control from cerebral cortex	Frontal, parietal, temporal, and occipital lobes	Via pontine nuclei and mossy fibers to cerebellar cortex
Cerebro-olivocerebellar	Control from cerebral cortex	Frontal, parietal, temporal, and occipital lobes	Via inferior olivary nuclei and climbing fibers to cerebellar cortex
Cerebroreticulocerebellar	Control from cerebral cortex	Sensorimotor areas	Via reticular formation
Anterior spinocerebellar	Conveys information from muscles and joints	Muscle spindles, tendon organs, joint receptors	Via mossy fibers to cerebellar cortex
Posterior spinocerebellar	Conveys information from muscles and joints	Muscle spindles, tendon organs, joint receptors	Via mossy fibers to cerebellar cortex
Cuneocerebellar	Conveys information from muscles and joints of upper limb	Muscle spindles, tendon organs, joint receptors	Via mossy fibers to cerebellar cortex
Vestibular nerve	Conveys information of head position and movement	Utricle, saccule, semicircular canals	Via mossy fibers to cortex of flocculonodular lobe
Other afferents	Conveys information from midbrain	Red nucleus, tectum	Cerebellar cortex

neurons influence spinal segmental motor activity through the reticulospinal tract.

The efferent cerebellar pathways are summarized in Table 9-2.

CEREBELLAR CORTICAL MECHANISMS

Certain basic mechanisms have been attributed to the cerebellar cortex. The climbing and the mossy fibers constitute the two main lines of input to the cortex and are excitatory to the Purkinje cells. The climbing fibers pass through the granular layer of the cortex and terminate by dividing repeatedly. Each climbing fiber makes a large number of synaptic contacts with the dendrites of a single Purkinje cell. A few side branches leave each climbing fiber and synapse with the stellate cells and basket cells. The mossy fibers, on the other hand, exert a much more diffuse excitatory effect, so that a single mossy fiber may stimulate thousands of Purkinje cells through the granule cells. The Purkinje cells, by means of their axons, exert an inhibitory effect on the intracerebellar and vestibular nuclei. The remaining cells of the cerebellar cortex, namely, the stellate, basket, and Golgi cells, serve as inhibitory interneurons. It is believed that they not only limit the area of cortex excited but also influence the degree of Purkinje cell excitation produced by the climbing and mossy fiber input. By this means, fluctuating inhibitory impulses are transmitted by the Purkinje cells to the intracerebellar nuclei, which in turn modify muscular activity through the motor control areas of the brainstem and cerebral cortex.

FUNCTIONS OF THE CEREBELLUM

The cerebellum receives afferent information concerning voluntary movement from the cerebral cortex and from the muscles, tendons, and joints. It also receives information concerning balance from the vestibular nerve and possibly concerning sight through the tectocerebellar tract. All this information is fed into the cerebellar cortical circuitry by the mossy fibers and the climbing fibers (Fig. 9-3). After several synaptic relays in the cerebellar cortex, the afferent impulses converge on the Purkinje cells. The axons of the Purkinje cells project with few exceptions on the deep cerebellar nuclei. The output of the lateral cerebellar hemisphere projects to the dentate nucleus, the vermis projects to the fastigial nucleus, and the intermediate regions of the cortex project to the globose and emboliform nuclei. A few Purkinje cell axons pass directly out of the cerebellum and end on the lateral vestibular nucleus in the brainstem. Now it is generally believed that the Purkinje axons exert an inhibitory influence on the neurons of the cerebellar nuclei and the lateral vestibular nuclei.

The cerebellar output is conducted to the sites of origin of the descending pathways that influence motor activity at the segmental spinal level. In this respect, it is interesting to note that **the cerebellum has no direct neuronal connections with the lower motor neurons but exerts its influence indirectly through the cerebral cortex and brainstem**.

The cerebellum functions unconsciously as a coordinator of precise movements by continually comparing the output of the motor area of the cerebral cortex with the proprioceptive information received from the site of muscle action; it is then able to bring about the necessary adjustments by influencing the activity of the lower motor neurons. This is accomplished by controlling the sequence of firing of the alpha and gamma motor neurons. It is also believed that the cerebellum can send back information to the motor cerebral cortex, to inhibit the agonist muscles and stimulate the antagonist muscles, thus limiting the extent of voluntary movement.

Table 9–2 Summary of the Efferent Cerebellar Pathways

Pathway	Function	Origin	Destination
Globose-emboliform-rubral	Influences ipsilateral motor activity	Globose and emboliform nuclei	To contralateral red nucleus, then via crossed rubrospinal tract to ipsilateral motor neurons in spinal cord
Dentothalamic	Influences ipsilateral motor activity	Dentate nucleus	To contralateral ventrolateral nucleus of thalamus, then to contralateral motor cerebral cortex; corticospinal tract crosses midline and controls ipsilateral motor neurons in spinal cord
Fastigial vestibular	Influences ipsilateral extensor muscle tone	Fastigial nucleus	Mainly to ipsilateral and to contralateral lateral vestibular nuclei; vestibulospinal tract to ipsilateral motor neurons in spinal cord
Fastigial reticular	Influences ipsilateral muscle tone	Fastigial nucleus	To neurons of reticular formation; reticulospinal tract to ipsilateral motor neurons to spinal cord

Note that each cerebellar hemisphere influences the voluntary muscle tone on the same side of the body.

CLINICAL NOTES

CEREBELLAR DYSFUNCTION

There are two neuroanatomical features concerning the cerebellum that are of great clinical significance. First, the cortex of the cerebellum, unlike that of the cerebrum, has a uniform microscopic structure. Second, each cerebellar hemisphere is connected by nervous pathways principally with the same side of the body, so that a lesion in one cerebellar hemisphere gives rise to signs and symptoms that are limited to the same side of the body.

The classic signs and symptoms of cerebellar disease include **hypotonia, alteration of gait** with a tendency to stagger toward the affected side, **intention tremor, decomposition of movement, pendular knee jerk, nystagmus,** and **dysarthria**.

COMMON DISEASES INVOLVING THE CEREBELLUM

The following conditions frequently involve the cerebellum: congenital agenesis or hypoplasia, trauma, infections, tumors, multiple sclerosis, alcoholism, vascular disorders such as thrombosis of the cerebellar arteries, and poisoning with heavy metals.

REVIEW QUESTIONS

Directions: Each of the incomplete statements in this section is followed by completions of the statement. Select the ONE lettered completion that is BEST in each case.

1. The cerebellum has a:
   (a) location in the posterior cranial fossa above the tentorium cerebelli
   (b) position anterior to the fourth ventricle
   (c) horizontal fissure that separates the anterior lobe from the middle lobe
   (d) anterior lobe, a middle lobe, and a flocculonodular lobe
   (e) vermis that lies on either side in the cerebellar hemisphere
2. The cerebellum has a:
   (a) cortex that differs in structure from one lobe to another
   (b) cuneocerebellar tract that is located in the middle cerebellar peduncle
   (c) posterior spinocerebellar tract that is located in the superior cerebellar peduncle
   (d) anterior spinocerebellar tract that is located in the inferior cerebellar peduncle
   (e) cortico pontocerebellar tract that is located in the middle cerebellar peduncle
3. The cerebellar nuclei receive direct input from the:
   (a) granule cells
   (b) Golgi cells
   (c) Purkinje cells
   (d) vestibular nuclei
   (e) red nucleus
4. The cerebellum is inhibited by:
   (a) Purkinje cell axons
   (b) climbing fibers
   (c) mossy fibers
   (d) granule cell efferent fibers
   (e) neuroglial cells

5. The pontocerebellar tract enters the cerebellum via the:
   (a) superior cerebellar peduncle
   (b) superior medullary velum
   (c) middle cerebellar peduncle
   (d) inferior medullary velum
   (e) inferior cerebellar peduncle
6. The dentorubral tract leaves the cerebellum via the:
   (a) inferior cerebellar peduncle
   (b) middle cerebellar peduncle
   (c) superior cerebellar peduncle
   (d) cerebral peduncle
   (e) reticular formation
7. The dentothalamic tract leaves the cerebellum via the:
   (a) medial lemniscus
   (b) middle cerebellar peduncle
   (c) inferior cerebellar peduncle
   (d) superior cerebellar peduncle
   (e) vermis
8. The vestibulocerebellar tract enters the cerebellum via the:
   (a) inferior cerebellar peduncle
   (b) superior cerebellar peduncle
   (c) Middle cerebellar peduncle
   (d) internal arcuate fibers
   (e) tectum

Directions: Each of the numbered items in this section is followed by answers that are positively phrased. Select the ONE lettered answer that is an EXCEPTION.

9. The following statements concerning the cerebellum are correct **except:**
   (a) Each cerebellar hemisphere principally influences movement on the same side of the body.
   (b) The middle cerebellar peduncle contains axons that arise from the pontine nuclei.
   (c) The Purkinje cells are found in the most superficial layer of the cortex.
   (d) The inferior cerebellar peduncles join the cerebellum to the medulla oblongata.
   (e) The Golgi cells are found in the deepest layer of the cerebellar cortex.
10. The following statements concerning the intracerebellar nuclei are correct **except:**
   (a) The nuclei are named from lateral to medial, fastigial, globose, emboliform, and dentate.
   (b) Their axons form the main efferent outflow of the cerebellum.
   (c) They are embedded in the white matter.
   (d) They are located above the cavity of the fourth ventricle.
   (e) The nuclei are made up of nerve cells supported by neuroglia.
11. The following statements concerning the functions of the cerebellum are correct **except:**
   (a) It does not influence the tone of smooth muscle.
   (b) It influences the tone of skeletal muscle.
   (c) It does not influence the tone of cardiac muscle.
   (d) It coordinates the force and extent of contraction of voluntary movements.
   (e) The cerebellum functions consciously as a coordinator of precise movements.
12. The following signs and symptoms are indicative of a cerebellar lesion **except:**
   (a) Resting tremor
   (b) Intention tremor
   (c) Ataxia
   (d) Dysdiadochokinesis
   (e) The shoulder on the side of the lesion may be lower than the shoulder on the normal side
13. Efferent fibers leaving the deep cerebellar nuclei may synapse with the following **except:**
   (a) Cells of the red nucleus
   (b) Anterior gray horn cells in the spinal cord
   (c) Cells in the ventral lateral nucleus of the thalamus
   (d) Vestibular nucleus
   (e) Cells in the reticular formation
14. The following statements concerning the superior cerebellar peduncle are correct **except:**
   (a) It contains fibers that synapse in the ventral lateral nucleus of the thalamus.
   (b) It contains fibers that originate in the dentate nucleus.
   (c) It conveys nervous impulses regulating skilled motor movements.
   (d) It contributes fibers to the medial longitudinal fasciculus.
   (e) It forms the lateral boundary to the upper part of the fourth ventricle.
15. The following statements concerning the structure and function of the cerebellum are correct **except:**
   (a) The mossy fibers end by synapsing with the granular cells in the granular layer of the cortex.
   (b) The structure of the cerebellar cortex differs completely from that of the cerebral cortex.
   (c) A tumor of the right cerebellar hemisphere causes the patient to lurch to the right while walking.
   (d) Stimulation of the cerebellar cortex produces a sensory response.
   (e) The cerebellum plays no part in modulating the sensation of pain.
16. The following statements concerning the structure and function of the cerebellum are correct **except:**
   (a) The axons of the granular cells bifurcate in the molecular layer of the cortex and run parallel to the long axis of the cerebellar folium.
   (b) A lesion of the cerebellum does not cause muscular paralysis.
   (c) Afferent fibers from muscles originate in the muscle spindles.
   (d) The tendon spindles provide the cerebellum with information.
   (e) No afferent fibers from the joints influence the activity of the cerebellum.

Directions: Read the case history then answer the question. You will be required to select the ONE BEST lettered answer.

A 26-year-old woman noticed that she had clumsiness of her right arm. She also noticed that her right hand had a tremor when she attempted to insert the key into her car door. Her friend noticed that when walking on the sidewalk, she tended to reel to the right and repeatedly bumped into her. On physical examination, the physician noted that her right shoulder was held lower than her left. There was evidence of hypotonia and looseness on the right side when her arms and legs were passively moved. When she was asked to touch her nose with her right index finger, the right hand displayed tremor and the finger overshot the target.

17. The clumsiness, tremor, muscle incoordination, and hypotonia involving the muscles on the right side can be explained by the following facts **except:**
    (a) The right cerebellar hemisphere is involved by disease.
    (b) The voluntary muscles on the right side of the body are not receiving the correct nervous control.
    (c) The sequence of firing of the alpha and gamma motor neurons controlling the muscles on the right side is not normal.
    (d) The efferent axons, which pass directly from the cerebellum to the lower motor neurons, are not functioning.
    (e) The cerebellum is not sending information to the motor cerebral cortex to inhibit the agonist muscles and stimulate the antagonist muscles.

ANSWERS AND EXPLANATIONS

1. D
2. E
3. C
4. A
5. C
6. C
7. D
8. A
9. C. The Purkinje cells lie in the middle layer of the cerebellar cortex.
10. A. The intracerebellar nuclei are named from medial to lateral, fastigial, globose, emboliform, and dentate.
11. E. The activities of the cerebellum do not reach consciousness.
12. A. Resting tremor does not occur with cerebellar disease; it is characteristic of Parkinson's disease.
13. B. The cerebellum, unlike the cerebrum, has no direct pathway to the lower motor neurons in the spinal cord.
14. D
15. D. The function of the cerebellum is to control or influence motor, not sensory activities.
16. E. Stretch receptors in the joint capsule and ligaments provide the cerebellum with afferent information concerning movements.
17. D. The cerebellum has no direct neuronal connections with the lower motor neurons, but exerts its influence indirectly through the cerebral cortex and brainstem.

CHAPTER 10

Reticular Formation

CHAPTER OUTLINE

SUGGESTED PLAN FOR REVIEW OF CHAPTER 10

1. Understand that the reticular formation consists of a network of nerve cells and fibers that extends from the spinal cord up through the brain to the cerebrum.
2. Appreciate that throughout its length the reticular formation has connections to all parts of the central nervous system including the cerebral cortex and the cerebellum.
3. Learn the main afferent and efferent connections.
4. Learn the six main functions of the reticular formation outlined in this chapter.

INTRODUCTION

The reticular formation, as its name would suggest, resembles a net (reticular) that is made up of nerve cells and nerve fibers. The net extends up through the axis of the central nervous system from the spinal cord to the cerebrum. It receives input from most of the sensory systems and has efferent fibers that descend and influence nerve cells at all levels of the central nervous system. The exceptionally long dendrites of the neurons of the reticular formation permit input from widely placed ascending and descending pathways. Through its many connections it can influence skeletal muscle activity, somatic and visceral sensations, the autonomic and endocrine systems, and even the level of consciousness. The purpose of this chapter is to provide a brief overview of the structure and functions of the reticular formation.

GENERAL ARRANGEMENT

The reticular formation consists of a deeply placed continuous network of nerve cells and fibers that extends from the spinal cord, through the medulla, the pons, the midbrain, the subthalamus, the hypothalamus, and the thalamus. The diffuse network can be divided into three longitudinal columns: the first occupying the **median plane**, called the **median column**; the second called the medial column; and the third or **lateral column** (Fig. 10-1).

The groups of neurons are poorly defined and it is difficult to trace an anatomical pathway through the network. However, with the new techniques of neurochemistry and cytochemical localization, the reticular formation is shown to contain highly organized groups of transmitter-specific cells that can influence functions in specific areas of the central nervous system. The monoaminergic groups of cells, for example, are located in well-defined areas throughout the reticular formation. Polysynaptic pathways exist and both crossed and uncrossed ascending and descending pathways are present, involving many neurons that serve both somatic and visceral functions.

Inferiorly, the reticular formation is continuous with the interneurons of the gray matter of the spinal cord, while superiorly impulses are relayed to the whole cerebral cortex; a substantial projection of fibers also leaves the reticular formation to enter the cerebellum.

AFFERENT PROJECTIONS

Many different afferent pathways project onto the reticular formation from most parts of the central nervous system. From the spinal cord there are the spinoreticular tracts, the spinothalamic tracts, and the medial lemniscus. From the cranial nerve nuclei there are ascending afferent tracts that include the vestibular, acoustic, and visual pathways. From the cerebellum, there is the cerebelloreticular pathway. From the subthalamic, hypothalamic, and thalamic nuclei, and from the corpus striatum and the limbic system, there are further afferent tracts. Other important afferent fibers arise in the primary motor cortex of the frontal lobe and from the somesthetic cortex of the parietal lobe.

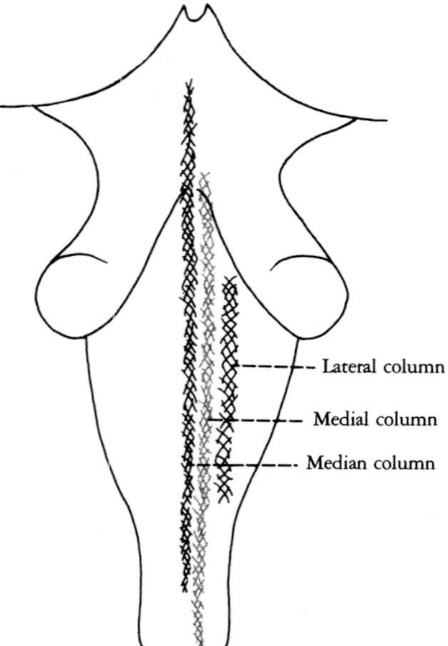

Figure 10–1 Diagram showing the approximate positions of the median, medial, and lateral columns of the reticular formation in the brainstem.

EFFERENT PROJECTIONS

Multiple efferent pathways extend down to the brainstem and spinal cord through the reticulobulbar and reticulospinal tracts to neurons in the motor nuclei of the cranial nerves and the anterior horn cells of the spinal cord. Other descending pathways extend to the sympathetic outflow and the craniosacral parasympathetic outflow of the autonomic nervous system. Additional pathways extend to the corpus striatum, the cerebellum, the red nucleus, the substantia nigra, the tectum, and the nuclei of the thalamus, subthalamus, and hypothalamus. Most regions of the cerebral cortex also receive efferent fibers.

FUNCTIONS OF THE RETICULAR FORMATION

From the previous description of the vast number of connections of the reticular formation to all parts of the nervous system, it is not surprising to find that the functions are many. A few of the more important functions will be considered here.

1. **Control of skeletal muscle.** Through the reticulospinal and reticulobulbar tracts, the reticular formation can influence the activity of the alpha and gamma motor neurons. Thus the reticular formation can modulate muscle tone and reflex activity. It can also bring about reciprocal inhibition, so that, for example, when the flexor muscles contract the antagonistic extensors relax. The reticular formation, assisted by the vestibular apparatus of the inner ear and the vestibular spinal tract, plays an important role in maintaining the tone of the antigravity muscles when standing. The so-called respiratory centers of the brainstem, described by neurophysiologists in the control of the respiratory muscles, are now considered to be part of the reticular formation.

   The reticular formation is important in controlling the muscles of facial expression when associated with emotion. For example, when a person smiles or laughs in response to a joke the motor control is provided by the reticular formation on both sides of the brain. The descending tracts are separate from the corticobulbar fibers. This means that a person who has suffered a stroke that involves the corticolbulbar fibers and exhibits facial paralysis on the lower part of the face is still able to smile symmetrically.
2. **Control of somatic and visceral sensations.** The reticular formation by virtue of its central location in the cerebrospinal axis can influence all ascending pathways passing to supraspinal levels. The influence may be facilitatory or inhibitory. In particular, the reticular formation may play a leading role in the "gating mechanism" for the control of the perception of pain.

3. **Control of the autonomic nervous system.** Higher control of the autonomic nervous system, from the cerebral cortex, hypothalamus, and other subcortical nuclei, can be exerted by the reticulobulbar and reticulospinal tracts, which descend to the sympathetic outflow and the parasympathetic craniosacral outflow.
4. **Control of the endocrine nervous system.** The reticular formation either directly or indirectly through the hypothalamic nuclei can influence the synthesis or release of releasing or release-inhibiting factors and thus control the activity of the hypophysis cerebri.
5. **Influence on the biological clocks.** The reticular formation by means of its multiple afferent and efferent pathways to the hypothalamus probably influences the biological rhythms.
6. **Reticular activating system.** Multiple ascending pathways carrying sensory information to higher centers are channeled through the reticular formation, which in turn projects the information to different parts of the cerebral cortex, causing a sleeping person to waken. In fact it is now believed that the state of consciousness is dependent on the continuous projection to the cortex of sensory information. Different degrees of wakefulness seem to depend on the degree of activity of the reticular formation.

From the above description it must be apparent that the network of neurons in the cerebrospinal axis, almost totally ignored in the past, is now being shown to influence practically all activities of the body.

Clinical Notes

Loss of Consciousness

Pathological lesions of the reticular formation can cause loss of consciousness and even coma. It has been suggested that the loss of consciousness that occurs in epilepsy may be due to inhibition of the activity of the reticular formation in the upper part of the diencephalon.

REVIEW QUESTIONS

Directions: Each of the incomplete statements in this section is followed by completions of the statement. Select the ONE lettered completion that is BEST in each case.

1. The reticular formation is:
   (a) incapable of influencing the activities of the alpha motor neurons in the spinal cord
   (b) an interrupted network that extends from the midbrain down to the spinal cord.
   (c) composed of neurons with short dendritic processes.
   (d) involved in the reception of afferent fibers from most sensory pathways entering the central nervous system
   (e) its descending fibers extend into the peripheral spinal nerves
2. The reticular formation:
   (a) can influence the reception of pain
   (b) has no affect on the level of consciousness
   (c) cannot influence the hypothalamic nuclei
   (d) cannot indirectly control the activity of the hypophysis cerebri
   (e) cannot influence the biological clock
3. The reticular formation is:
   (a) a network that can be divided into four longitudinal columns
   (b) involved with reticulobulbar fibers that are connected to the sensory nuclei of the cranial nerves.
   (c) not connected to the cerebral cortex
   (d) composed of neurons with unbranching dendritic processes
   (e) important in controlling the muscles of facial expression when associated with emotion

ANSWERS AND EXPLANATIONS

1. D. A. The reticular formation can influence the alpha motor neurons in the spinal cord. B. The reticular formation is a continuous network that extends downward from the cerebrum to the different levels of the entire length of the spinal cord. C. The reticular formation consists of neurons with long dendritic processes. E. The descending fibers of the reticular formation synapse on neurons at lower levels of the central nervous system but do not extend out into the peripheral nervous system.
2. A. B. The reticular formation can affect the level of consciousness. C. The reticular formation can influence the hypothalamic nuclei. D. The reticular formation can indirectly control the activity of the hypophysis cerebri through the hypothalamic nuclei. E. The reticular formation can influence the biological clock.
3. E. A. The reticular formation is a network that is divided into three longitudinal columns. B. The reticulobulbar fibers are connected to the motor nuclei of the cranial nerves. C. The reticular formation is connected to the cerebral cortex. D. The neurons of the reticular formation have long branching dendritic processes.

CHAPTER 11

Diencephalon: The Hypothalamus

CHAPTER OUTLINE

SUGGESTED PLAN FOR REVIEW OF CHAPTER 11

1. The hypothalamus, although small in size, is a very important part of the central nervous system. It controls the autonomic nervous system and the endocrine system and thus indirectly controls body homeostasis.
2. Understand the location and precise boundaries of the hypothalamus.
3. In general terms learn the names and positions of the various nuclei of the hypothalamus.
4. Have an understanding of the main afferent and efferent connections of the hypothalamus.
5. Learn in detail the hypothalamohypophyseal tract and the hypophyseal portal system. These are very important.
6. Learn the functions of the hypothalamus and be able to list some of the common clinical problems that may arise should dysfunction occur.

INTRODUCTION

The diencephalon forms the central core of the cerebrum, while the remainder of the cerebrum forms the laterally placed cerebral hemispheres. The diencephalon consists of the third ventricle and the structures that form its boundaries. It extends posteriorly to the point where the third ventricle becomes continuous with the cerebellar aqueduct and anteriorly as far as the interventricular foramina (Fig. 11-1). The diencephalon can be divided, for purposes of description, into four major parts: (1) the thalamus, (2) the subthalamus, (3) the epithalamus, and (4) the hypothalamus.

The purpose of this chapter is to describe the hypothalamus, its connections, and its functions; the remaining parts of the diencephalon will be described elsewhere.

HYPOTHALAMUS

The hypothalamus is that part of the diencephalon that extends from the region of the optic chiasma to the caudal border of the mammillary bodies. It lies below the thalamus and forms the floor and the inferior part of the lateral walls of the third ventricle (Fig. 11-1). Anterior to the hypothalamus is an area that for functional reasons is often included in the hypothalamus. Because it extends forward from the optic chiasma to the lamina terminalis and the anterior commissure, it is referred to as the **preoptic area**. Caudally, the hypothalamus merges into the tegmentum of the midbrain. The lateral boundary of the hypothalamus is formed by the internal capsule.

When observed from below, the hypothalamus is seen to be related to the following structures, from anterior to posterior: (1) the optic chiasma, (2) the tuber cinereum and the infundibulum, and (3) the mammillary bodies.

Anatomically, the hypothalamus is a relatively small area of the brain that is strategically well placed close to the limbic system, the thalamus, the ascending and descending tracts, and the hypophysis. Physiologically there is hardly any activity in the body that is not influenced by the hypothalamus.

HYPOTHALAMIC NUCLEI

Microscopically, the hypothalamus is composed of small nerve cells that are arranged in groups or nuclei, many of which are not clearly segregated from one another. For pur-

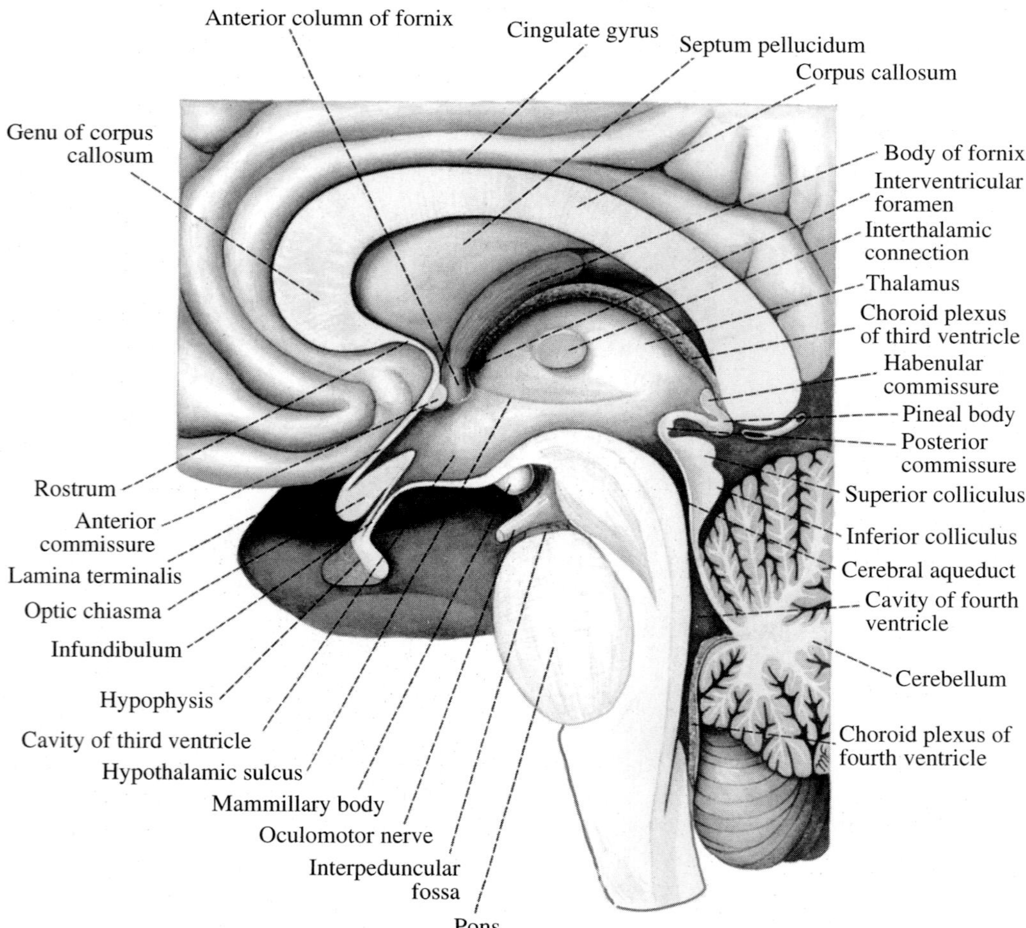

Figure 11–1 Sagittal section of the brain showing the medial surface of the diencephalon.

poses of description, the nuclei are divided by an imaginary parasagittal plane into medial and lateral zones. Lying within the plane are the columns of the fornix and the mammillothalamic tract, which serve as markers (Fig. 11-2).

Medial Zone

In the medial zone, the following hypothalamic nuclei can be recognized, from anterior to posterior: (1) part of the **preoptic nucleus**; (2) the **anterior nucleus**, which merges with the preoptic nucleus; (3) part of the **suprachiasmatic nucleus**; (4) the **paraventricular nucleus**; (5) the **dorsomedial nucleus**; (6) the **ventromedial nucleus**; (7) the **infundibular (arcuate) nucleus**; and (8) the **posterior nucleus**.

Lateral Zone

In the lateral zone, the following hypothalamic nuclei can be recognized, from anterior to posterior: (1) part of the **preoptic nucleus**, (2) part of the **suprachiasmatic nucleus**, (3) the

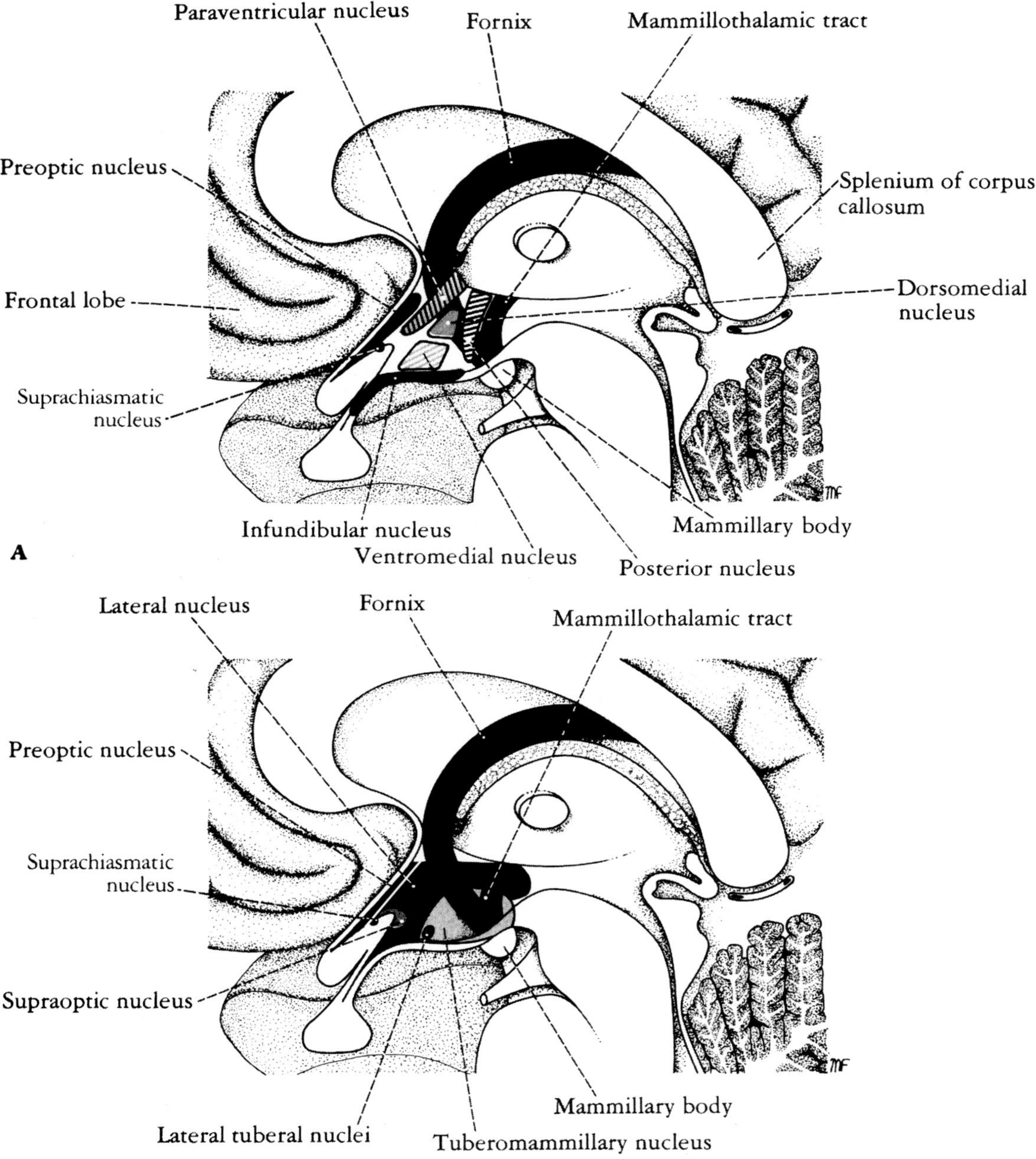

Figure 11–2 Sagittal section of the brain, showing the hypothalamic nuclei. **A**. Medial zone nuclei lying medial to the plane of the fornix and the mammillothalamic tract. **B**. Lateral zone nuclei lying lateral to the plane of the fornix and the mammillothalamic tract.

supraoptic nucleus, (4) the **lateral nucleus**, (5) the **tuberomamillary nucleus**, and (6) the **lateral tuberal nuclei**.

Some of the nuclei, for example, the preoptic nucleus, the suprachiasmatic nucleus, and the mammillary nuclei, overlap both zones. It should be emphasized that most of the hypothalamic nuclei have ill-defined boundaries.

AFFERENT CONNECTIONS OF THE HYPOTHALAMUS

The hypothalamus receives many afferent fibers from the viscera, the olfactory mucous membrane, the cerebral cortex, and the limbic system. The afferent connections are numerous and complex, and only the main pathways (Fig. 11-3) are described here:

1. **Somatic and Visceral** afferents reach the hypothalamus through collateral branches of the lemniscal afferent fibers and through the reticular formation.
2. **Visual afferents** leave the optic chiasma and pass to the suprachiasmatic nucleus.
3. **Olfaction** travels through the medial forebrain bundle.
4. **Auditory afferents** have not been identified but since auditory stimuli can influence the activities of the hypothalamus they must exist.
5. **Corticohypothalamic fibers** arise from the frontal lobe of the cerebral cortex and pass directly to the hypothalamus.
6. **Hippocampohypothalamic fibers** pass from the hippocampus through the fornix to the mammillary body. Many neurophysiologists regard the hypothalamus as the main output pathway of the limbic system.
7. **Amygdalohypothalamic fibers** pass from the amygdaloid complex to the hypothalamus through the stria terminalis and by a route that passes inferior to the lentiform nucleus.
8. **Thalamohypothalamic fibers** arise from the dorsomedial and midline thalamic nuclei.
9. **Tegmental fibers** arise from the midbrain.

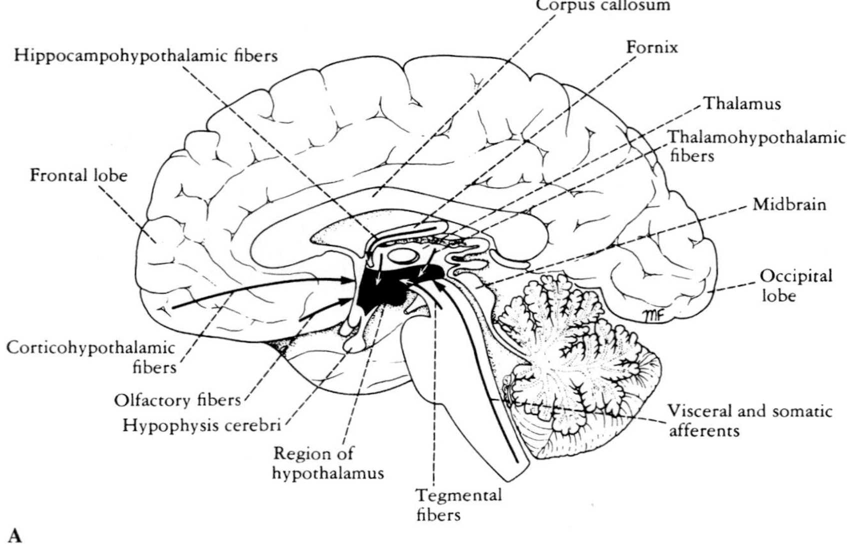

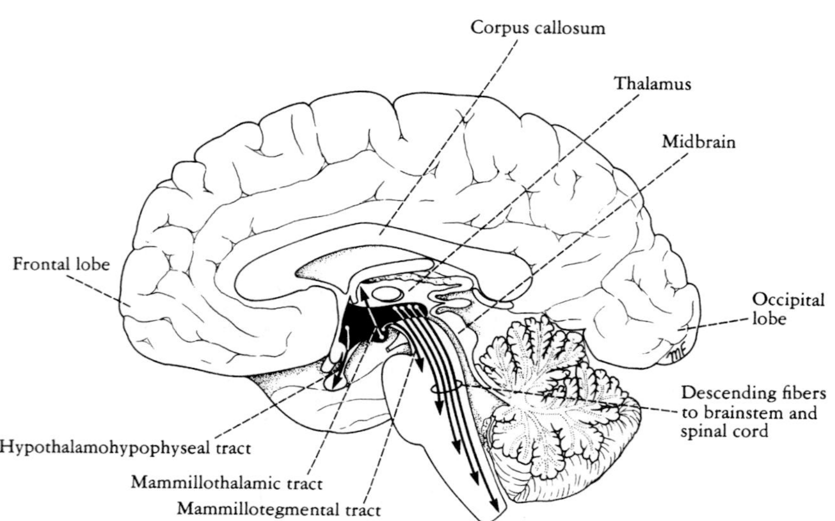

Figure 11–3 **A.** Main afferent pathways entering the hypothalamus. **B.** Main efferent pathways leaving the hypothalamus.

The main afferent connections of the hypothalamus are summarized in Table 11-1.

EFFERENT CONNECTIONS OF THE HYPOTHALAMUS

The efferent connections of the hypothalamus are also numerous and complex, and only the main pathways (Fig. 11-3) are described here:

1. **Descending fibers to the brainstem and spinal cord** influence the peripheral neurons of the autonomic nervous system. They descend through a series of neurons in the reticular formation. The hypothalamus is connected to the parasympathetic nuclei of the oculomotor, facial, glossopharyngeal, and vagus nerves in the brainstem, In a similar manner, the reticulospinal fibers connect the hypothalamus with sympathetic cells of origin in the lateral gray horns of the first thoracic segment to the second lumbar segment of the spinal cord and the sacral parasympathetic outflow at the level of the second, third, and fourth sacral segments of the spinal cord.
2. The **mammillotegmental tract** arises in the mammillary body and terminates in the anterior nucleus of the thalamus. Here the pathway is relayed to the cingulate gyrus.
3. The **mammillotegmental tract** arises from the mammillary body and terminates in the cells of the reticular formation in the tegmentum of the midbrain.
4. Multiple pathways to the **limbic system.**

The main efferent connections of the hypothalamus are summarized in Table 11-1.

CONNECTIONS OF THE HYPOTHALAMUS WITH THE HYPOPHYSIS CEREBRI

The hypothalamus is connected to the hypophysis cerebri (pituitary gland) by two pathways: (1) nerve fibers that travel from the supraoptic and paraventricular nuclei to the posterior lobe of the hypophysis, and (2) long and short portal blood vessels that connect sinusoids in the median eminence and infundibulum with capillary plexuses in the anterior lobe of the hypophysis (Fig. 11-4). These pathways enable the hypothalamus to influence the activities of the endocrine glands.

Hypothalamohypophyseal Tract

The hormones **vasopressin** and **oxytocin** are synthesized in the nerve cells of the supraoptic and paraventricular nuclei. The hormones are passed along the axons together with carrier proteins called **neurophysins** and released at the axon terminals (Fig. 11-4). Here the hormones are absorbed into the bloodstream in the capillaries of the posterior lobe of the hypophysis. The hormone vasopressin (antidiuretic hormone) is produced mainly in the nerve cells of the supraoptic nucleus. Its function is to cause vasoconstriction. It also has an important antidiuretic function,

Table 11–1 Summary of the Main Afferent and Efferent Connections of the Hypothalamus

Pathway	Origin	Destination
Afferent		
Medial and lateral lemnisci, reticular formation	Viscera and somatic structures	Hypothalamic nuclei
Medial forebrain bundle	Olfactory mucous membrane	Hypothalamic nuclei
Corticohypothalamic fibers	Frontal lobe of cerebral cortex	Hypothalamic nuclei
Hippocampohypothalamic fibers, possibly main output pathway of limbic system	Hippocampus	Nuclei of mammillary body
Amygdalohypothalamic fibers	Amygdaloid complex	Hypothalamic nuclei
Thalamohypothalamic fibers	Dorsomedial and midline nuclei of thalamus	Hypothalamic nuclei
Tegmental fibers	Tegmentum of midbrain	Hypothalamic nuclei
Efferent		
Mammillothalamic tract	Nuclei of mammillary body	Anterior nucleus of thalamus, relayed to cingulate gyrus
Mammillotegmental tract	Nuclei of mammillary body	Reticular formation in tegmentum of midbrain
Descending fibers in reticular formation to brainstem and spinal cord	Preoptic, anterior, posterior, and lateral nuclei of hypothalamus	Craniosacral parasympathetic and thoracolumbar sympathetic outflows

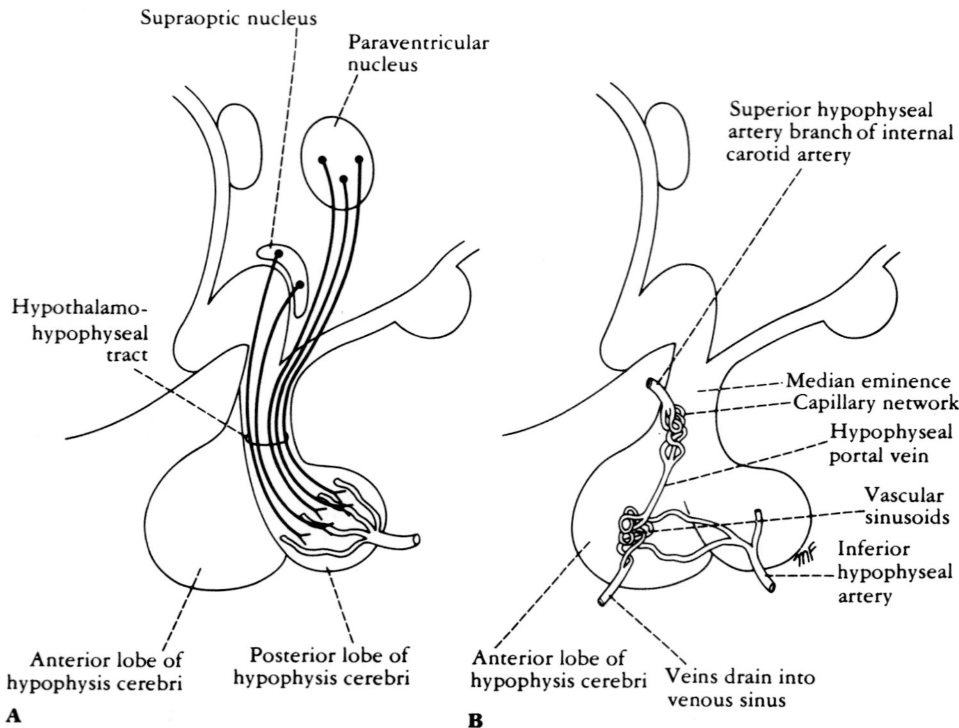

Figure 11–4 **A.** Hypothalamohypophyseal tract. **B.** Hypophyseal portal system.

causing an increased absorption of water in the distal convoluted tubules and collecting tubules of the kidney. The other hormone is oxytocin, which is mainly produced in the paraventricular nucleus. Oxytocin stimulates the contraction of the smooth muscle of the uterus and causes contraction of the myoepithelial cells that surround the alveoli and ducts of the breasts.

The supraoptic nucleus, which produces vasopressin, acts as an **osmoreceptor**. Should the osmotic pressure of the blood circulating through the nucleus be too high, the nerve cells increase their production of vasopressin and the antidiuretic effect of this hormone will increase the reabsorption of water from the kidney. By this means, the osmotic pressure of the blood will return to normal limits.

Hypophyseal Portal System

The hypophyseal portal system is formed on each side from the superior hypophyseal artery, which is a branch of the internal carotid artery (Fig. 11-4). The artery enters the median eminence and divides into tufts of capillaries. These capillaries drain into long and short descending vessels that end in the anterior lobe of the hypophysis by dividing into vascular sinusoids that pass between the secretory cells of the anterior lobe.

The portal system carries **releasing hormones** and **release-inhibiting hormones**, which are produced in the neurons of the hypothalamus, to the secretory cells of the anterior lobe of the hypophysis. The releasing hormones stimulate the production and release of **adrenocorticotropic hormone** (ACTH), **follicle-stimulating hormone** (FSH), **luteinizing hormone** (LH), **thyrotropic hormone** or **thyroid-stimulating hormone** (TSH), and **growth hormone** (GH). The release of inhibiting hormones inhibits the release of **melanocyte-stimulating hormone** (MSH) and **luteotropic hormone** (LTH). LTH (also known as the **lactogenic hormone** or **prolactin**) stimulates the corpus luteum to secrete progesterone and the mammary gland to produce milk. The growth hormone inhibitory hormone (somatostatin) inhibits the release of GH.

A summary of the hypothalamic releasing and inhibitory hormones and their effects on the anterior lobe of the pituitary is provided in Table 11-2.

The neurons of the hypothalamus that are responsible for the production of the releasing hormones and the release-inhibiting hormones are influenced by the afferent fibers passing to the hypothalamus. They also are influenced by the level of the hormone produced by the target organ controlled by the hypophysis. Should the level of thyroxin in the blood, for example, fall, then the releasing factor for the thyrotropic hormone would be produced in increased quantities.

Table 11-3 summarizes the presumed nuclear origin of the pituitary releasing and inhibitory hormones in the hypothalamus.

Table 11–2 Summary of the Hypothalamic Releasing and Inhibitory Hormones and Their Effects on the Anterior Lobe of the Pituitary

Hypothalamic Regulatory Hormone	Anterior Pituitary Hormone	Functional Result
Growth hormone–releasing hormone (GHRH)	Growth hormone (GH)	Stimulates linear growth in epiphyseal cartilages
Growth hormone–inhibiting hormone (GHIH) or somatostatin	Growth hormone (GH) (reduced production)	Reduces linear growth in epiphyseal cartilages
Prolactin-releasing hormone (PRH)	Prolactin (luteotropic hormone, LTH)	Stimulates lactogenesis
Prolactin-inhibiting hormone (PIH), dopamine	Prolactin (luteotropic hormone, LTH) (reduced production)	Reduces lactogenesis
Corticotropin-releasing hormone (CRH)	Adrenocorticotropic hormone (ACTH)	Stimulates adrenal gland to produce corticosteroids and sex hormones
Thyrotropin-releasing hormone (TRH)	Thyroid-stimulating hormone (TSH)	Stimulates thyroid gland to produce thyroxine
Luteinizing hormone—releasing hormone (LHRH), ? follicle-stimulating–releasing hormone (FRH)	Luteinizing hormone (LH) and follicle-stimulating hormone (FSH)	Ovary, stimulates follicles and production of estrogen and progesterone

Table 11–3 Summary of the Presumed Nuclear Origin of the Pituitary Releasing and Inhibitory Hormones in the Hypothalamus

Hypothalamic Regulatory Hormone	Presumed Nuclear Origin
Growth hormone–releasing hormone (GHRH)	Infundibular or arcuate nucleus
Growth hormone–inhibiting hormone (GHIH) or somatostatin	Suprachiasmatic nucleus
Prolactin-releasing hormone (PRH)	?
Prolactin-inhibiting hormone (PIH)	?
Corticotropin-releasing hormone (CRH)	Paraventricular nuclei
Thyrotropin-releasing hormone (TRH)	Paraventricular and dorsomedial nuclei and adjacent areas
Luteinizing hormone–releasing hormone (LHRH)	Preoptic and anterior nuclei

FUNCTIONS OF THE HYPOTHALAMUS

Autonomic Control

The hypothalamus has a controlling influence on the autonomic nervous system and integrates the autonomic and neuroendocrine systems, thus preserving body homeostasis. The hypothalamus should be regarded as a higher nervous center for the control of lower autonomic centers in the brainstem and spinal cord.

Electrical stimulation of the hypothalamus in animal experiments shows that the anterior hypothalamic area and the preoptic area influence parasympathetic responses; these include lowering of the blood pressure, slowing of the heart rate, contraction of the bladder, increased motility of the gastrointestinal tract, increased acidity of the gastric juice, salivation, and pupillary constriction.

Stimulation of the posterior and lateral nuclei causes sympathetic responses, which include elevation of blood pressure, acceleration of the heart rate, cessation of peristalsis in the gastrointestinal tract, pupillary dilation, and hyperglycemia.

Endocrine Control

The nerve cells of the hypothalamic nuclei, by producing the releasing factors or release-inhibiting factors (Table 11-2), control the hormone production of the anterior lobe of the pituitary gland. The anterior lobe hormones include GH, prolactin (LTH), ACTH, TSH, LH, and FSH. Some of these hormones act directly on body tissues, while others, such as ACTH, act through an endocrine organ, which in turn produces additional hormones that influence the activities of general body tissues. It should be pointed out that each stage is controlled by negative and positive feedback mechanisms.

Neurosecretion. The secretion of vasopressin and oxytocin by the supraoptic and paraventricular nuclei is discussed on page 129.

Temperature Regulation

The anterior portion of the hypothalamus controls those mechanisms that dissipate heat loss. Experimental stimulation of this area causes dilation of skin blood vessels and sweating, which lower the body temperature. Stimulation of the posterior portion of the hypothalamus results in vasoconstriction of the skin blood vessels and inhibition of sweating; there also may be shivering, in which the skeletal muscles produce heat.

Regulation of Food and Water Intake

Stimulation of the lateral region of the hypothalamus initiates eating and increases food intake. This lateral region is

Table 11–4 Summarizing the Functions of the Main Hypothalamic Nuclei

Hypothalamic Nucleus	Presumed Function
Supraoptic nucleus	Vasopressin (antidiuretic hormone)
Paraventricular nucleus	Oxytocin
Preoptic and anterior nuclei	Parasympathetic control
Posterior and lateral nuclei	Sympathetic control
Anterior hypothalamic nuclei	Temperature regulation (response to heat)
Posterior hypothalamic nuclei	Temperature regulation (response to cold)
Lateral hypothalamic nuclei	Hunger center
Medial hypothalamic nuclei	Satiety center
Lateral hypothalamic nuclei	Thirst center
Suprachiasmatic nucleus	Circadian rhythms

sometimes referred to as the **hunger center**. Stimulation of the medial region of the hypothalamus inhibits eating and reduces food intake. This area is referred to as the **satiety center**.

Experimental stimulation of other areas in the lateral region of the hypothalamus causes an immediate increase in water intake; this area is referred to as the **thirst center**. The hypothalamus also exerts control on the osmolarity of the blood through the secretion of vasopressin by the posterior lobe of the hypophysis and its influence on the distal convoluted tubules and collecting tubules of the kidneys.

Emotion and Behavior

Emotion and behavior are a function of the hypothalamus, the limbic system, and the prefrontal cortex. The hypothalamus is the integrator of afferent information received from the other areas of the nervous system and brings about the physical expression of emotion; it can produce an increase in the heart rate, elevate the blood pressure, cause dryness of the mouth, flushing or pallor of the skin, and sweating, and can often produce a massive peristaltic activity of the gastrointestinal tract.

Control of Circadian Rhythms

The hypothalamus controls many circadian rhythms, including body temperature, adrenocortical activity, eosinophil count, and renal secretion. Sleeping and wakefulness, although dependent on the activities of the thalamus, the limbic system, and the reticular activating system, are also controlled by the hypothalamus. Lesions of the anterior part of the hypothalamus seriously interfere with the rhythm of sleeping and waking. The suprachiasmatic nucleus, which receives afferent fibers from the retina, appears to play an important role in controlling the biological rhythms. Nerve impulses generated in response to variations in the intensity of light are transmitted via this nucleus to influence the activities of many of the hypothalamic nuclei.

Table 11-4 summarizes the functions of the main hypothalamic nuclei.

Clinical Notes

Hypothalamic Lesions

The most common abnormalities associated with hypothalamic lesions include severe obesity and wasting, genital hypoplasia, hyperthermia and hypothermia, diabetes insipidus, disturbances of sleep, and emotional disorders.

REVIEW QUESTIONS

Directions: Each of the numbered items in this section is followed by answers that are positively phrased. Select the ONE lettered answer that is an EXCEPTION.

1. The following statements concerning the position of the hypothalamus are correct **except:**
   (a) The hypothalamus lies in the center of the limbic system.
   (b) The hypothalamus lies below the thalamus in the tectum of the midbrain.
   (c) The lateral boundary of the hypothalamus is formed by the internal capsule.
   (d) The hypothalamus extends forward as far as the optic chiasma.
   (e) The hypothalamus extends posteriorly as far as the caudal border of the mammillary bodies.
2. The following statements concerning the nuclei of the hypothalamus are correct **except:**
   (a) The margins of the different nuclei cannot be seen with the naked eye.
   (b) The suprachiasmatic nucleus overlaps both the medial and lateral groups of nuclei.
   (c) The columns of the fornix and the mammillothalamic tract divide the nuclei of the hypothalamus into medial and lateral groups.
   (d) The medial nuclei of the hypothalamus are related medially to the cavity of the third ventricle.
   (e) The preoptic nucleus is confined to the lateral zone of nuclei.

3. The following statements concerning the afferent fibers of the hypothalamus are correct **except:**
   (a) The limbic system sends fibers to the hypothalamus.
   (b) The pineal gland sends afferent fibers to the hypothalamus.
   (c) Tegmental fibers arise from the midbrain.
   (d) Visceral and somatic afferent fibers reach the hypothalamus through collateral branches of the lemniscal afferent fibers.
   (e) The stria terminalis serves to conduct fibers from the amygdaloid complex to the hypothalamus.
4. The following statements concerning the functions of the hypothalamus are correct **except:**
   (a) The anterior hypothalamic area and the preoptic area can influence the parasympathetic part of the autonomic system.
   (b) The posterior and lateral nuclei of the hypothalamus can influence the activity of the sympathetic part of the autonomic system.
   (c) Stimulation of the anterior nuclei of the hypothalamus can lower the body temperature.
   (d) The medial nuclei of the hypothalamus can influence the intake of food.
   (e) The hypothalamus preserves the body homeostasis.
5. The following statements concerning the hypothalamus are correct **except:**
   (a) The hypothalamus integrates the functions of the autonomic and endocrine systems.
   (b) The visceral afferents to the hypothalamus reach their destination via the medial longitudinal bundle.
   (c) The nerve cells of the hypothalamus produce releasing factors that control the production of various pituitary hormones.
   (d) The mammillary bodies lie posterior to the tuber cinereum on the inferior aspect of the hypothalamus.
   (e) The hypothalamus, although small, plays a very important role in controlling bodily functions.
6. The following statements concerning the hypophyseal portal system are correct **except:**
   (a) The portal system carries releasing hormones and release-inhibiting hormones to the secretory cells of the anterior lobe of the pituitary gland.
   (b) The blood vessels begin superiorly in the median eminence and end below in the posterior lobe of the hypophysis.
   (c) The afferent fibers entering the hypothalamus can influence the production of releasing hormones by the nerve cells.
   (d) The portal system is fed by arteries that are branches of the internal carotid artery.
   (e) The portal system ends by dividing into vascular sinusoids that pass between the secretory cells of the pituitary gland.
7. The following statements concerning the hypothalamohypophyseal tract are correct **except:**
   (a) Vasopressin stimulates the distal convoluted tubules and collecting tubules of the kidney, causing an increased absorption of water from the urine.
   (b) The hormones travel in the axoplasm of the neurons in the tract with neurophysins.
   (c) The nerve cells of the lateral hypothalamic nuclei produce the hormone vasopressin.
   (d) Oxytocin stimulates the contraction of the smooth muscle of the uterus.
   (e) On reaching the axon terminals, the hormones are absorbed into the bloodstream in the capillaries of the posterior lobe of the hypophysis.
8. The following statements concerning efferent connections of the hypothalamus are correct **except:**
   (a) The mammillotegmental tract connects the mammillary body to the reticular formation in the midbrain.
   (b) The parasympathetic nucleus of the oculomotor nerve receives descending fibers from the hypothalamus.
   (c) The anterior nucleus of the thalamus receives fibers from the mammillary body.
   (d) The supraoptic nucleus sends fibers to the cerebellar cortex.
   (e) The reticulospinal fibers connect the hypothalamus to the parasympathetic outflow at the level of the second, third, and fourth sacral segments of the spinal cord.
9. The following nuclei of the hypothalamus are confined to the lateral zone **except:**
   (a) The supraoptic nucleus
   (b) The lateral nucleus
   (c) The lateral tuberal nuclei
   (d) The tuberomamillary nucleus
   (e) The paraventricular nucleus
10. The following statements concerning the hypothalamus are correct **except:**
   (a) The neurons of the hypothalamus are insensitive to the blood level of the hormone produced by the target endocrine organ controlled by the hypophysis.
   (b) The portal system carries releasing hormones that stimulate the production and release of ACTH and FSH.
   (c) The portal system carries inhibiting hormones that inhibit the release of MSH.
   (d) The growth inhibitory hormone inhibits the release of growth hormone.
   (e) Stimulation of the medial region of the hypothalamus inhibits eating and reduces food intake.

Directions: Read the case history then answer the question. You will be required to select ONE BEST lettered answer.

While crossing a road, a 28-year-old man was hit by a car and sustained severe head injuries. Following a slow recovery he was finally released from the hospital without any neurological deficits. Three months later he complained to his physician of frequency of micturition and passing large quantities of pale urine. He also noticed that he was always thirsty and drank large quantities of water. Diabetes insipidus had developed secondary to the trauma.

11. Which of the following does **not** explain his condition?
    (a) The condition could have been caused by trauma to the posterior lobe of the hypophysis.
    (b) The condition could have been caused by trauma to the supraoptic nucleus of the hypothalamus.
    (c) The passing of large quantities of pale urine can be explained by the reduced production of vasopressin by the hypothalamus.
    (d) The increased water consumption was secondary to the voiding of large quantities of urine.
    (e) When there are lesions of the posterior lobe of the hypophysis, the vasopressin is unable to enter the bloodstream.

ANSWERS AND EXPLANATIONS

1. B. The hypothalamus is situated in the diencephalon and does not lie in the midbrain.
2. E. The preoptic nucleus is situated partly in the medial zone and partly in the lateral zone.
3. B. The pineal gland sends no afferent fibers to the hypothalamus.
4. D. Stimulation of the lateral nuclei of the hypothalamus can initiate eating and increase food intake.
5. B. The visceral afferents of the hypothalamus reach their destination through collateral branches of the lemnisci and through the reticular formation.
6. B. The blood vessels begin above in the median eminence and end below in the anterior lobe of the hypophysis.
7. C. The hormone vasopressin is produced by the nerve cells of the supraoptic and paraventricular nuclei of the hypothalamus.
8. D. The supraoptic nucleus does not send fibers to the cerebellar cortex.
9. E. The paraventricular nucleus is confined to the medial zone of the hypothalamus.
10. A. The neurons of the hypothalamus are sensitive to the blood level of the hormone produced by the target endocrine organ controlled by the hypophysis.
11. E. In patients with lesions of the posterior lobe of the hypophysis, some vasopressin produced by the neurons of the supraoptic nucleus usually escapes directly into the bloodstream.

CHAPTER 12

Diencephalon: The Thalamus

CHAPTER OUTLINE

SUGGESTED PLAN FOR REVIEW OF CHAPTER 12

1. Realize that the thalamus is a very important relay station for the ascending sensory pathways to the cerebral cortex.
2. Using sagittal, coronal, and horizontal diagrams of the brain, accurately localize the thalamus. If possible, look at specimens of the brain in the laboratory.
3. Understand the subdivisions of the thalamus and the different nuclei.
4. Recognize the position of the ventral posterolateral nucleus of the thalamus and realize that it is the relay station for the important ascending sensory tracts.
5. Note the positions of the medial and lateral geniculate bodies and learn their functions.
6. Review the main connections of the thalamic nuclei. Note that, in contrast to all other sensory pathways, the olfactory afferent pathway reaches the cerebral cortex without synapsing in one of the thalamic nuclei.
7. Learn the functions of the thalamus.

INTRODUCTION

The thalamus is a large, ovoid mass of gray matter that forms the major part of the diencephalon. There are two thalami and one is situated on each side of the third ventricle (Fig. 12-1). The anterior end of the thalamus is narrow and rounded and forms the posterior boundary of the interventricular foramen. The posterior end is expanded to form the **pulvinar**. The inferior surface is continuous with the tegmentum of the midbrain. The medial surface of the thalamus forms part of the lateral wall of the third ventricle and is usually connected to the opposite thalamus by a band of gray matter (Fig. 12-1), the **interthalamic connection** (interthalamic adhesion).

The purpose of this chapter is to describe briefly the structure of the thalamus, its connections, and its functions.

SUBDIVISIONS OF THE THALAMUS

The thalamus is covered on its superior surface by a thin layer of white matter, called the **stratum zonale**, and on its lateral surface by another layer, the **external medullary lamina** (Fig. 12-1). The gray matter of the thalamus is divided by a vertical sheet of white matter, the **internal medullary lamina**, into medial and lateral halves (Fig. 12-1). The internal medullary lamina consists of nerve fibers that pass from one thalamic nucleus to another. Anterosuperiorly, the internal medullary lamina splits so that it is Y-shaped. The thalamus thus is subdivided into three main parts; the **anterior part** lies between the limbs of the Y, and the **medial and lateral parts** lie on the sides of the stem of the Y.

Each of the three parts of the thalamus contains a group of thalamic nuclei (Fig. 12-1). Smaller nuclear groups are situated within the internal medullary lamina, and some are located on the medial and lateral surfaces of the thalamus.

Anterior Part

This part of the thalamus contains the **anterior thalamic nuclei.** They receive the mammillothalamic tract from the mammillary nuclei. These anterior thalamic nuclei also receive reciprocal connections with the cingulate gyrus and hypothalamus. The function of the anterior thalamic nuclei is closely associated with that of the limbic system and is concerned with emotional tone and the mechanisms of recent memory.

Medial Part

This part of the thalamus contains the large **dorsomedial nucleus** and several smaller nuclei. The dorsomedial nucleus has two-way connections with the whole prefrontal cortex of the frontal lobe of the cerebral hemisphere. It also has similar connections with the hypothalamic nuclei. It is interconnected with all other groups of thalamic nuclei. The medial part of the thalamus is responsible for the integration of a large variety of sensory information, including somatic, visceral, and olfactory information, and the relation of this information to one's emotional feelings and subjective states.

Lateral Part

The nuclei are subdivided into a dorsal tier and a ventral tier (Fig. 12-1).

DORSAL TIER OF THE NUCLEI

This tier includes the **lateral dorsal nucleus,** the **lateral posterior nucleus,** and the **pulvinar**. The details of the connections of these nuclei are not clear. However, they are known to have interconnections with other thalamic nuclei and with the parietal lobe, cingulate gyrus, and occipital and temporal lobes.

VENTRAL TIER OF THE NUCLEI

This tier consists of the following in a craniocaudal sequence:

1. **Ventral anterior nucleus** (Fig. 12-1). This nucleus is connected to the reticular formation, the substantia nigra, the corpus striatum, and the premotor cortex as well as to many of the other thalamic nuclei. Since this nucleus lies on the pathway between the corpus striatum and the motor areas of the frontal cortex, it probably influences the activities of the motor cortex.
2. **Ventral lateral nucleus** (Fig. 12-1). This nucleus has connections similar to those of the ventral anterior nucleus but, in addition, has a major input from the cerebellum and a minor input from the red nucleus. Its main projections pass to the motor and premotor regions of the cerebral cortex. Here again this thalamic nucleus probably influences motor activity.
3. **Ventral posterior nucleus.** This nucleus is subdivided into the **ventral posteromedial nucleus** and the **ventral posterolateral nucleus** (Fig. 12-1). The ventral posteromedial (VPM) nucleus receives the ascending trigeminal and gustatory pathways, while the ventral posterolateral (VPL) nucleus receives the important ascending sensory tracts, the medial and spinal lemnisci.

The thalamocortical projections from these important nuclei pass through the posterior limb of the internal capsule and corona radiata to the primary somatic sensory areas of the cerebral cortex in the postcentral gyrus (areas 3, 1, and 2).

Other Nuclei of the Thalamus

These nuclei include the intralaminar nuclei, the midline nuclei, the reticular nucleus, and the medial and lateral geniculate bodies.

The **intralaminar nuclei** are small collections of nerve cells within the internal medullary lamina (Fig. 12-1). They receive afferent fibers from the reticular formation and also fibers from the spinothalamic and trigeminothalamic tracts; they send efferent fibers to other thalamic nuclei, which in turn project to the cerebral cortex, and fibers to the corpus striatum. The nuclei are believed to influence the levels of consciousness and alertness in an individual.

The **midline nuclei** consist of groups of nerve cells adjacent to the third ventricle and in the interthalamic con-

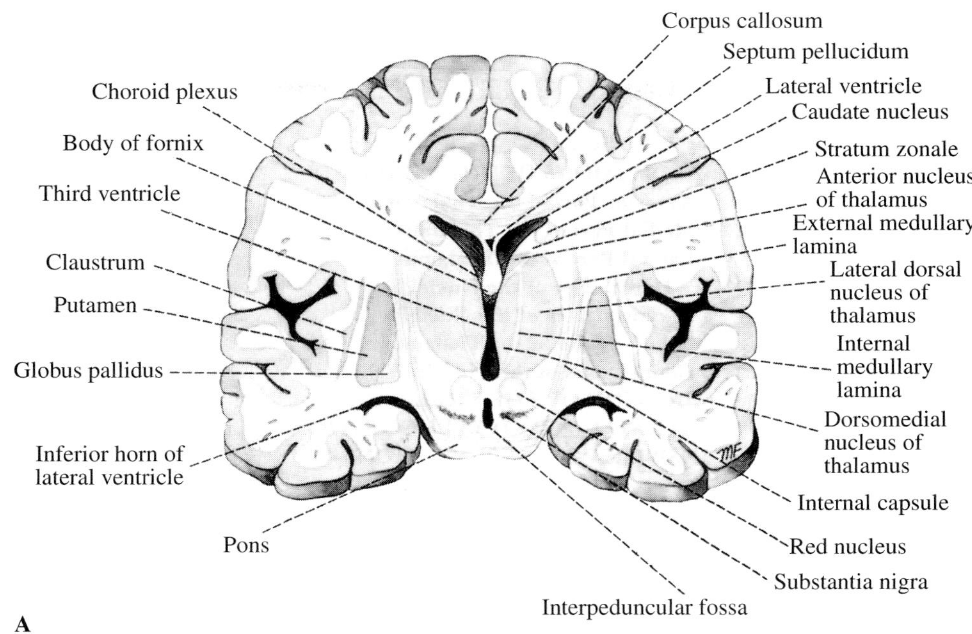

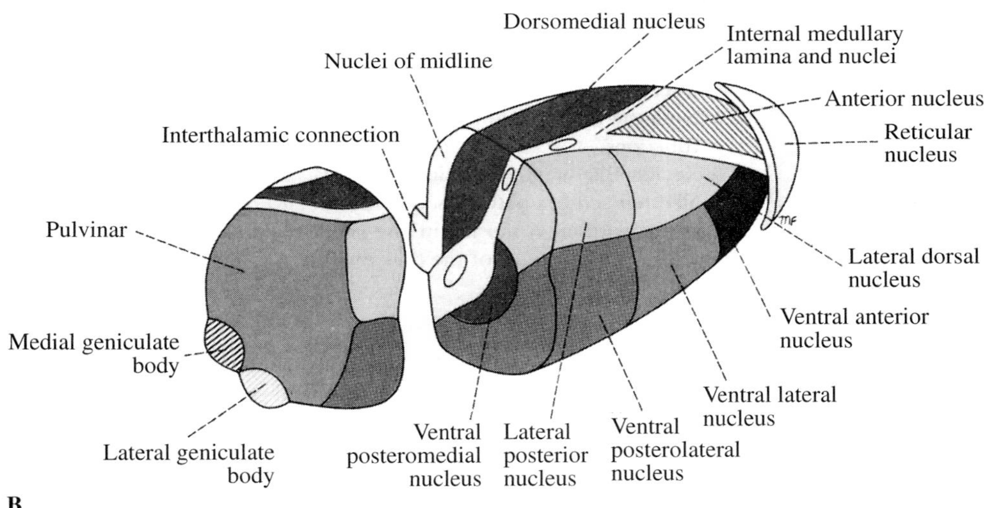

Figure 12–1 **A.** Coronal section of the cerebral hemispheres, showing the position and relations of the thalamus. **B.** The nuclei of the thalamus.

nection (Fig. 12-1). They receive afferent fibers from the reticular formation. Their precise functions are unknown.

The **reticular nucleus** is a thin layer of nerve cells sandwiched between the external medullary lamina and the posterior limb of the internal capsule (Fig. 12-1). Afferent fibers converge on this nucleus from the cerebral cortex and the reticular formation, and its output is mainly to other thalamic nuclei. The function of this nucleus is not fully understood, but it may be concerned with a mechanism by which the cerebral cortex regulates thalamic activity.

The **medial geniculate body** forms part of the auditory pathway and is a swelling on the posterior surface of the thalamus beneath the pulvinar (Fig. 12-1). Afferent fibers to the medial geniculate body form the **inferior brachium** and come from the inferior colliculus. It will be remembered that the inferior colliculus receives the termination of the fibers of the lateral lemniscus. The medial geniculate body receives auditory information from both ears but predominantly from the opposite ear.

The efferent fibers leave the medial geniculate body to form the auditory radiation, which passes to the auditory cortex of the superior temporal gyrus.

The **lateral geniculate body** forms part of the visual pathway and is a swelling on the undersurface of the pulvinar of the thalamus (Fig. 12-1). The nucleus consists of six layers of nerve cells and is the terminus of all but a few fibers of the optic tract (except the fibers passing to the pretectal nucleus). The fibers are the axons of the ganglion cell layer of the retina and come from the temporal half of the ipsilateral eye and from the nasal half of the contralateral eye, the latter fibers crossing the midline in the optic chiasma. Each lateral geniculate body, therefore, receives visual information from the opposite field of vision.

The efferent fibers leave the lateral geniculate body to form the visual radiation, which passes to the visual cortex of the occipital lobe.

Connections of the Thalamic Nuclei

The main connections of the various thalamic nuclei are summarized in Figure 12-2.

A summary of the various thalamic nuclei, their nervous connections, and their functions is provided in Table 12-1.

FUNCTIONS OF THE THALAMUS

1. The thalamus is made up of collections of nerve cells that are centrally placed in the brain and are interconnected.
2. A vast amount of sensory information (except smell) converges on the thalamus and is integrated through the interconnections between the nuclei. The resulting information pattern is distributed to other parts of the central nervous system. It is probable that olfactory information is first integrated at a lower level with taste and other sensations and is relayed to the thalamus from the amygdaloid complex and hippocampus through the mammillothalamic tract.
3. The thalamus and the cerebral cortex are closely linked. The fiber connections have been established, and it is known that following removal of the cortex the thalamus can appreciate crude sensations. However, the cerebral cortex is required for the interpretation of sensations based on past experiences.

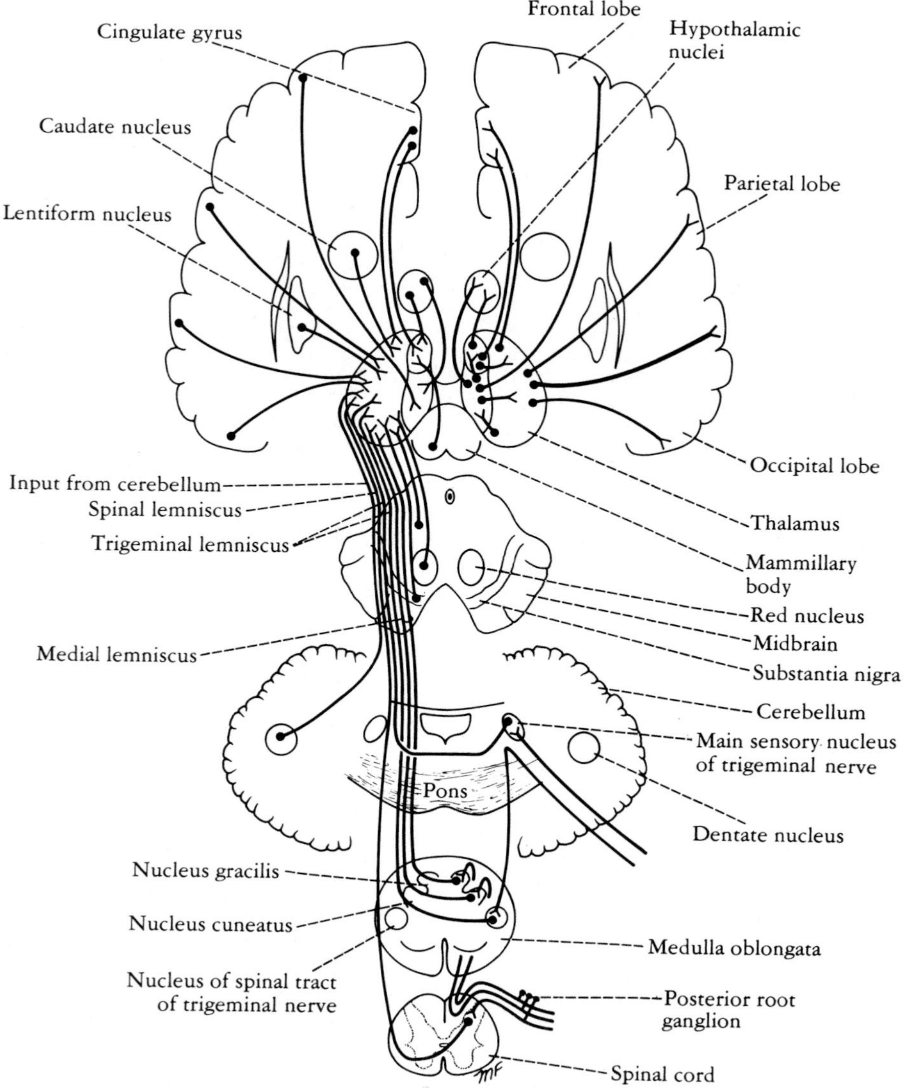

Figure 12–2 The main connections of the thalamus. The afferent fibers are shown on the left and the efferent fibers on the right.

Table 12–1 The Various Thalamic Nuclei, Their Nervous Connections, and Their Functions

Thalamic Nucleus	Afferent Neuronal Loop	Efferent Neuronal Loop	Function
Anterior	Mammillothalamic tract, cingulate gyrus, hypothalamus	Cingulate gyrus, hypothalamus	Emotional tone, mechanisms of recent memory
Dorsomedial	Prefrontal cortex, hypothalamus, other thalamic nuclei	Prefrontal cortex, hypothalamus, other thalamic nuclei	Integration of somatic, visceral, and olfactory information and relation to emotional feelings and subjective states
Lateral dorsal, lateral posterior, pulvinar	Cerebral cortex, other thalamic nuclei	Cerebral cortex, other thalamic nuclei	Unknown
Ventral anterior	Reticular formation, substantia nigra, corpus striatum, premotor cortex, other thalamic nuclei	Reticular formation, substantia nigra, corpus striatum, premotor cortex, other thalamic nuclei	Influences activity of motor cortex
Ventral lateral	As for ventral anterior nucleus but also major input from cerebellum and minor input from red nucleus		Influences motor activity of motor cortex
Ventral posteromedial (VPM)	Trigeminal lemniscus, gustatory fibers	Primary somatic sensory (areas 3, 1, 2) cortex	Relays common sensations to consciousness
Ventral posterolateral (VPL)	Medial and spinal lemnisci	Primary somatic sensory (areas 3, 1, 2) cortex	Relays common sensations to consciousness
Intralaminar	Reticular formation, spinothalamic and trigeminothalamic tracts	To cerebral cortex via other thalamic nuclei, corpus striatum	Influences levels of consciousness and alertness
Midline	Reticular formation	Unknown	Unknown
Reticular	Cerebral cortex, reticular formation	Other thalamic nuclei	Cerebral cortex regulates thalamus
Medial geniculate body	Inferior colliculus, lateral lemniscus from both ears but predominantly contralateral ear	Auditory radiation to superior temporal gyrus	Hearing
Lateral geniculate body	Optic tract	Optic radiation to visual cortex of occipital lobe	Visual information from opposite field of vision

4. The thalamus possesses certain very important nuclei that include the ventral posteromedial nucleus, the ventral posterolateral nucleus, the medial geniculate body, and the lateral geniculate body.
5. The ventroanterior and ventrolateral nuclei of the thalamus form part of the basal nuclei circuit and thus are involved in the performance of voluntary movements. These nuclei receive input from the globus pallidus and send fibers to the prefrontal, supplemental, and premotor areas of the cerebral cortex.
6. The large dorsomedial nucleus has extensive connections with the frontal lobe cortex and hypothalamus. There is considerable evidence that this nucleus lies on the pathway that is concerned with subjective feeling states and the personality of the individual.
7. The intralaminar nuclei are closely connected with the activities of the reticular formation and they receive much of their information from this source. Their strategic position enables them to control the level of overall activity of the cerebral cortex. They are thus able to influence the levels of consciousness and alertness in an individual.

Clinical Notes

Lesions of the Thalamus

Sensory Loss

These lesions usually result from thrombosis or hemorrhage of one of the arteries supplying the thalamus. Damage to the ventral posteromedial nucleus and the ventral posterolateral nucleus will result in the loss of all forms of sensation, including light touch, tactile localization and discrimination, and muscle joint sense from the opposite side of the body.

Thalamic Pain

Thalamic pain may occur in a patient who is recovering from a thalamic infarct. Spontaneous pain that is often excessive and unpleasant occurs on the opposite side of the body. The painful sensation may be aroused by light touch or cold and may fail to respond to powerful analgesic drugs.

REVIEW QUESTIONS

Directions: Each of the numbered items or incomplete statements in this section is followed by answers or completions of the statement. Select the ONE lettered answer or completion that is BEST in each case.

1. The thalamus lies:
   (a) in the floor of the third ventricle
   (b) medial to the internal capsule
   (c) lateral to the medial geniculate body
   (d) lateral to the putamen
   (e) anterior to the caudate nucleus
2. The thalamus is:
   (a) connected to the opposite thalamus by a band of white matter that crosses the third ventricle
   (b) expanded at its anterior end to form the pulvinar
   (c) covered on its lateral surface by a layer of gray matter called the external medullary lamina
   (d) divided into anterior and posterior parts by the internal medullary lamina
   (e) a cell station for the integration of all sensations received via the afferent fibers
3. From a functional point of view, the thalamus can:
   (a) not influence the levels of consciousness and alertness
   (b) not appreciate crude sensations if the cerebral cortex is not functioning
   (c) recognize the sensation of smell as the result of receiving afferent fibers directly from the nasal mucous membrane
   (d) not relay all forms of sensation from the opposite side of the body following destruction of the ventral posteromedial and the ventral posterolateral nuclei
   (e) produce spontaneous sensations of cold following thrombosis of its arterial supply
4. Which of the following statements concerning the thalamic nuclei is **not** correct?
   (a) The anterior thalamic nuclei are involved with emotional tone.
   (b) The dorsomedial nucleus has connections with the prefrontal cortex.
   (c) The ventral posterolateral nucleus sends fibers to the postcentral gyrus through the posterior limb of the internal capsule.
   (d) The intralaminar nuclei lie within the internal medullary lamina.
   (e) The nuclei consist of groups of neurons that are well defined and can be seen with the naked eye.
5. Which of the following statements concerning the thalamus is **not** correct?
   (a) The lateral geniculate body receives fibers from the optic tract of the same side.
   (b) The medial geniculate body is connected to the auditory area of the cerebral cortex on the same side.
   (c) The ventral posterolateral nucleus receives afferent sensory information from the lateral lemniscus.
   (d) The anterior thalamic nucleus is concerned with the mechanisms of recent memory.
   (e) The midline nuclei receive afferent fibers from the reticular formation.
6. Which of the following statements concerning the thalamus is **not** correct?
   (a) The midline nuclei lie adjacent to the third ventricle.
   (b) The large dorsomedial nucleus has extensive connections with the hypothalamus.
   (c) The inferior brachium consists of afferent fibers that extend from the inferior colliculus to the medial geniculate body.
   (d) The nucleus of the lateral geniculate body has twelve layers of neurons that form the terminus of the majority of the nerve fibers from the optic tract.
   (e) The efferent fibers of the lateral geniculate body form the visual radiation.

Directions: Read the case history then answer the question. You will be required to select ONE BEST answer.

A 41-year-old woman suddenly had considerable sensory loss on the left side of the body, involving both superficial and deep sensations. Four days later she started to complain of agonizing pain down the left leg. The pain started spontaneously or was initiated by light touch. The neurologist made a diagnosis of a degenerative lesion of the right thalamus.

7. The patient's symptoms could be explained by the following neuroanatomical facts **except:**
   (a) The ventral posterolateral nucleus of the right thalamus receives afferent fibers via the medial and spinal lemnisci.
   (b) The ascending tracts to the right thalamus bring sensory information from the left side of the body.
   (c) The thalamogeniculate branch of the right posterior cerebral artery, which supplies the right thalamus, may have been blocked by a thrombus.
   (d) The severe pain in the left leg forms part of the thalamic syndrome.
   (e) Contralateral hemiparesis (involving the left leg in this patient) never occurs in patients with thalamic lesions.

ANSWERS AND EXPLANATIONS

1. B. A. The thalamus lies in the lateral wall of the third ventricle. C. The thalamus lies anterior to the medial geniculate body. D. The thalamus lies medial to the putamen of the lentiform nucleus. E. The thalamus lies medial to the caudate nucleus.
2. E. A. The thalamus is connected to the thalamus of the opposite side across the third ventricle by a band of gray matter called the interthalamic connection. B. The posterior end of the thalamus is expanded to form the pulvinar. C. The thalamus is covered on its lateral surface by a layer of white matter called the external medullary

lamina. D. The thalamus is divided into medial and lateral parts by a sheet of white matter called the internal medullary velum.

3. D. A. The thalamus influences the levels of consciousness and alertness. B. The thalamus appreciates crude sensations if the cerebral cortex is not functioning. C. The thalamus does not directly receive the sensations of smell. E. Destruction of the thalamus, caused by an arterial thrombosis, can produce spontaneous sensations of pain on the opposite side of the body.
4. E
5. C. The ventral posterolateral nucleus of the thalamus receives afferent sensory information from the medial lemniscus.
6. D. The nucleus of the lateral geniculate body is made up of six layers of nerve cells.
7. E. Contralateral hemiparesis can occur in patients with degenerative lesions of the thalamus. This complication can be explained on the basis that edema can occur in the nearby posterior limb of the internal capsule, causing damage to the important motor corticospinal fibers.

CHAPTER 13

Basal Nuclei (Basal Ganglia)

CHAPTER OUTLINE

SUGGESTED PLAN FOR REVIEW OF CHAPTER 13

1. Be able to define the term basal nuclei and know the names of its parts.
2. Understand what is meant by the term corpus striatum.
3. Be able to locate on a specimen the caudate nucleus, the lentiform nucleus, the amygdaloid nucleus, and the claustrum.
4. Understand the main connections of the basal nuclei.
5. Learn the functions of the basal nuclei relative to muscular movements.
6. Read through the common clinical syndromes associated with disease of the basal nuclei. Learn about Parkinson's disease.

INTRODUCTION

The term *basal nuclei* is applied to a collection of masses of gray matter situated within each cerebral hemisphere. They are the corpus striatum, the amygdaloid nucleus, and the claustrum. The basal nuclei play an important role in the control of posture and voluntary movement.

The purpose of this chapter is to describe briefly the basal nuclei, their connections, and their functions.

CORPUS STRIATUM

The corpus striatum is situated lateral to the thalamus. It is almost completely divided by a band of nerve fibers, the **internal capsule**, into the caudate nucleus and the lentiform nucleus (Fig. 13-1).

Caudate Nucleus

The caudate nucleus is a large C-shaped mass of gray matter that is closely related to the lateral ventricle and lies lateral to the thalamus (Fig. 13-1). The lateral surface of the nucleus is related to the internal capsule, which separates it from the lentiform nucleus. For purposes of description, it can be divided into a head, a body, and a tail.

The **head** of the caudate nucleus is large and rounded and forms the lateral wall of the anterior horn of the lateral ventricle (Figs. 13-1 and 13-2). The head is continuous inferiorly with the putamen of the lentiform nucleus.* Just superiorly to this point of union, strands of gray matter pass through the internal capsule, giving the region a striated appearance, hence the term **corpus striatum**.

*The caudate nucleus and the putamen are sometimes referred to as the neostriatum or striatum.

The **body** of the caudate nucleus is long and narrow and is continuous with the head in the region of the interventricular foramen. The body of the caudate nucleus forms part of the floor of the body of the lateral ventricle (Fig. 13-1).

The **tail** of the caudate nucleus is long and slender and is continuous with the body in the region of the posterior end of the thalamus (Fig. 13-2). It follows the contour of the lateral ventricle and continues forward in the roof of the inferior horn of the lateral ventricle. It terminates anteriorly in the **amygdaloid nucleus** (Fig. 13-1).

Lentiform Nucleus

The lentiform nucleus is a wedge-shaped mass of gray matter, whose broad convex base is directed laterally and its blade medially (Fig. 13-2). It is buried deep in the white matter of the cerebral hemisphere and is related medially to the internal capsule, which separates it from the caudate nucleus and the thalamus. The lentiform nucleus is related laterally to a thin sheet of white matter, the **external capsule**, that separates it from a thin sheet of gray matter, called the **claustrum**. The claustrum, in turn, separates the external capsule from the subcortical white matter of the insula. A vertical plate of white matter divides the nucleus into a larger, darker lateral portion, the **putamen,** and an inner lighter portion, the **globus pallidus** (Fig. 13-2). Inferiorly at its anterior end, the putamen is continuous with the head of the caudate nucleus.

AMYGDALOID NUCLEUS

The amygdaloid nucleus is situated in the temporal lobe close to the uncus (Fig. 13-1). The amygdaloid nucleus is considered to be part of the limbic system and is described in Chapter 15.

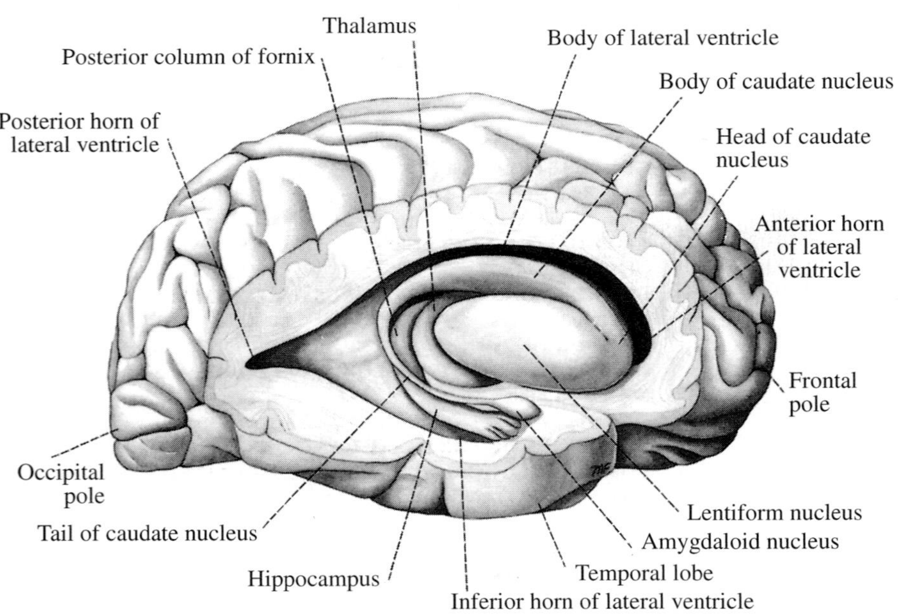

Figure 13–1 Lateral view of the right cerebral hemisphere showing the lentiform nucleus, the caudate nucleus, the thalamus, and the hippocampus.

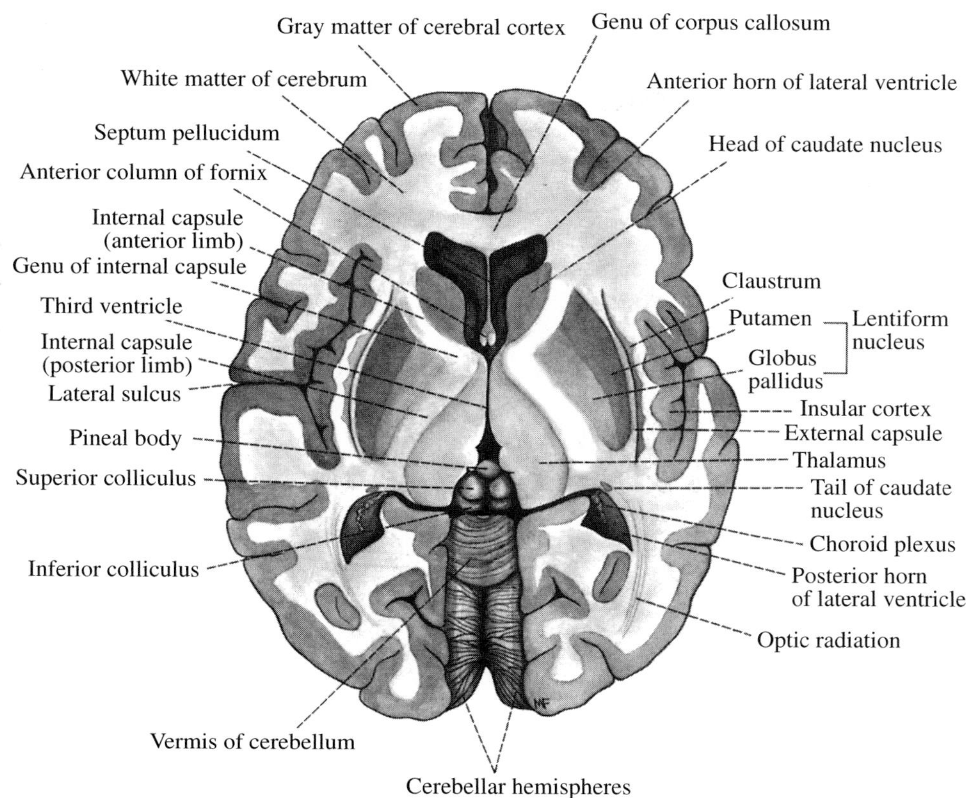

Figure 13–2 Horizontal section of the cerebrum as seen from above, showing the relationship between the lentiform nucleus, the caudate nucleus, the thalamus, and the internal capsule.

CLAUSTRUM

The claustrum is a thin sheet of gray matter that is separated from the lateral surface of the lentiform nucleus by the external capsule (Fig. 13-2). Lateral to the claustrum is the subcortical white matter of the insula. The function of the claustrum is unknown.

CONNECTIONS OF THE CORPUS STRIATUM

Afferent Fibers

CORTICOSTRIATE FIBERS

All parts of the cerebral cortex send axons to the caudate nucleus and the putamen (Fig. 13-3). Each part of the cerebral cortex projects to a specific part of the caudate-putamen complex. Most of the projections are from the cortex of the same side. The largest input is from the sensory-motor cortex. Glutamate is the neurotransmitter of the corticostriate fibers.

THALAMOSTRIATE FIBERS

Intralaminar nuclei of the thalamus send large numbers of axons to the caudate nucleus and the putamen (Fig. 13-3).

NIGROSTRIATE FIBERS

Cells in the substantia nigra send axons to the caudate nucleus and the putamen and liberate dopamine at their terminals as the neurotransmitter. It is believed that these fibers are inhibitory in function (Fig. 13-3).

BRAINSTEM STRIATAL FIBERS

Ascending fibers from the brainstem end in the caudate nucleus and putamen and liberate serotonin at their terminals at the neurotransmitter. It is thought that these fibers are inhibitory in function.

Efferent Fibers

STRIATOPALLIDAL FIBERS

These fibers pass from the caudate nucleus and putamen to the globus pallidus (Fig. 13-3). They have gamma-aminobutyric acid (GABA) as their neurotransmitter.

STRIATONIGRAL FIBERS

Fibers pass from the caudate nucleus and putamen to the substantia nigra (Fig. 13-3). Some of the fibers use GABA as the neurotransmitter, while others use substance P.

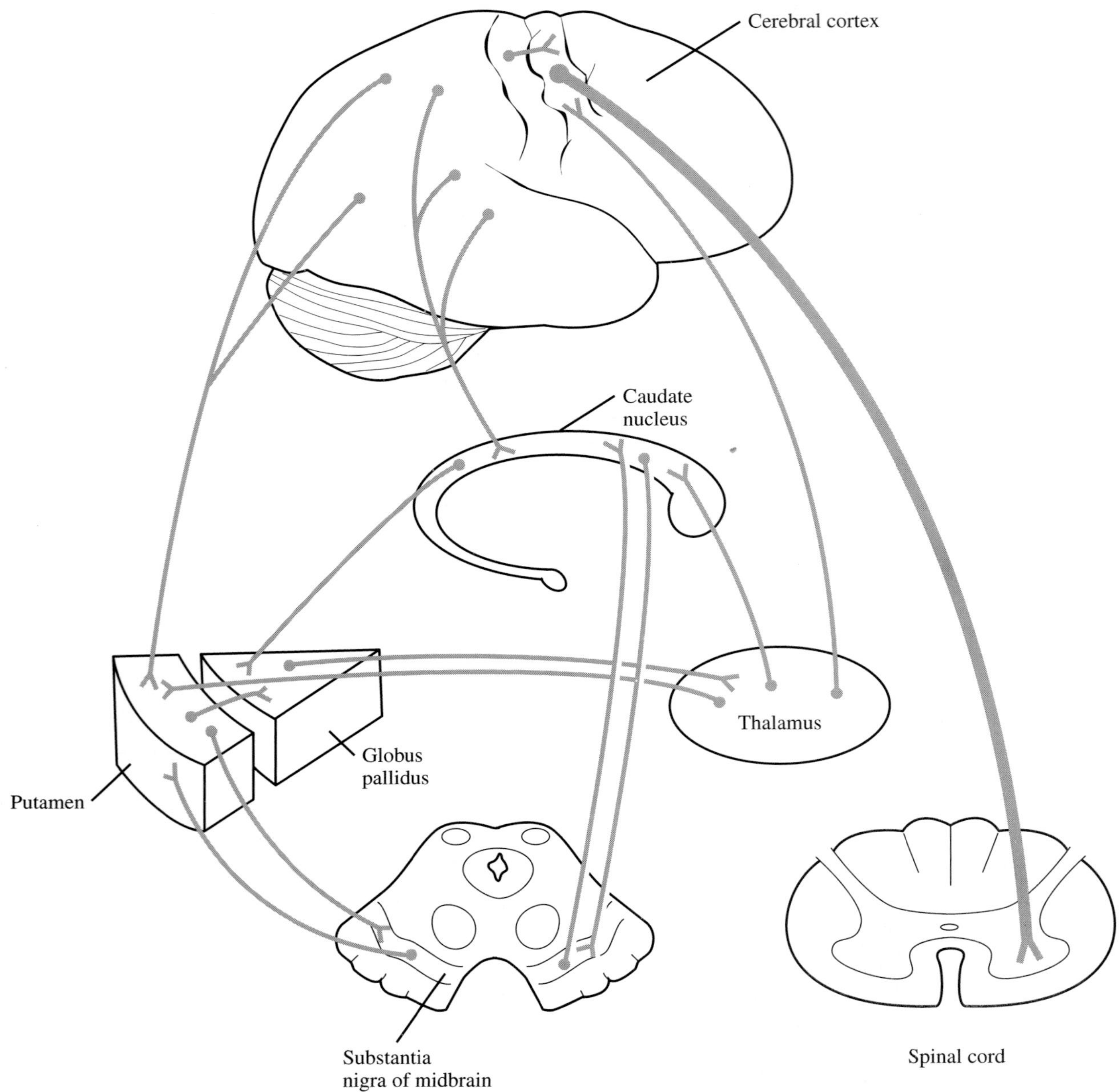

Figure 13–3 Some of the main connections between the cerebral cortex, the basal nuclei, the thalamic nuclei, the brainstem, and the spinal cord.

CONNECTIONS OF THE GLOBUS PALLIDUS

Afferent Fibers

STRIATOPALLIDAL FIBERS

These fibers pass from the caudate nucleus and putamen to the globus pallidus. As noted previously, these fibers have GABA as their neurotransmitter.

Efferent Fibers

PALLIDOFUGAL FIBERS

These fibers can be divided into four groups: (1) the ansa lenticularis, (2) the fasciculus lenticularis, (3) the pallidotegmental fibers, and (4) the pallidosubthalamic fibers.

Figure 13-4 shows the basal nuclei pathways and the known neurotransmitters.

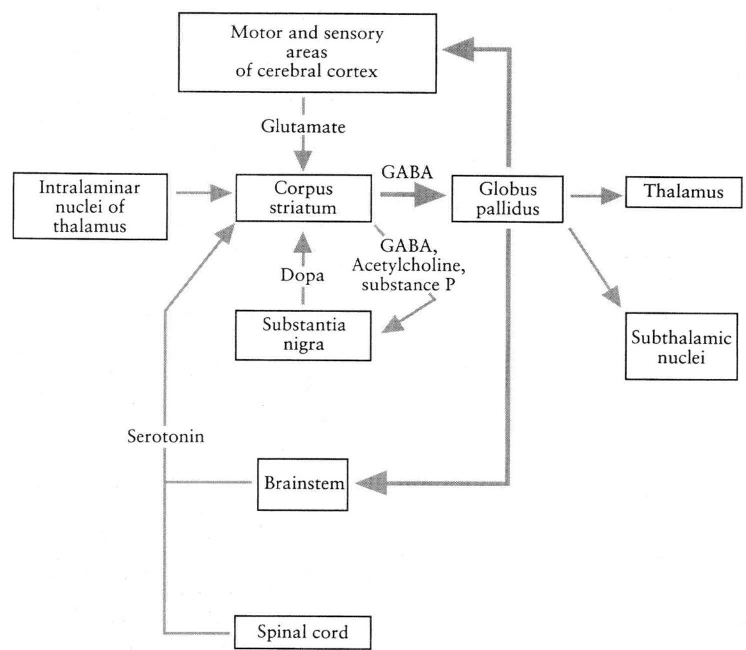

Figure 13–4 Basal nuclei pathways, showing the known neurotransmitters.

FUNCTIONS OF THE BASAL NUCLEI

The basal nuclei are joined together and connected with many different regions of the nervous system by a very complex number of neurons.

Basically, the corpus striatum receives afferent information from most of the cerebral cortex, the thalamus, the subthalamus, and the brainstem, including the substantia nigra. The information is integrated within the corpus striatum and the outflow passes back to the areas listed above. This circular pathway is believed to function as follows.

The activity of the basal nuclei is initiated by information received from the sensory cortex, the thalamus, and the brainstem. The outflow from the basal nuclei is channeled through the globus pallidus, which then influences the activities of the motor areas of the cerebral cortex or other motor centers in the brainstem. Thus the basal nuclei can control muscular movements by influencing the cerebral cortex rather than through direct descending pathways to the brainstem and spinal cord. In this way the basal nuclei assist in the regulation of voluntary movement and the learning of motor skills.

Destruction of the motor cerebral cortex prevents the individual from performing fine discrete movements of the hands and feet on the opposite side of the body. However, the individual is still capable of performing gross crude movements. If destruction of the corpus striatum then occurs, paralysis of the remaining movements of the opposite side of the body takes place.

It has been shown that the basal nuclei not only influence the execution of a particular movement of say the limbs, but also play a role in the preparation of the movements. This may be achieved by controlling the axial and girdle movements of the body and the positioning of the proximal parts of the limbs. The activity in certain neurons of the globus pallidus increases before active movements take place in the distal limb muscles. This important preparatory function enables the trunk and limbs to be placed in appropriate positions before the primary motor part of the cerebral cortex activates discrete movements in the hands and feet.

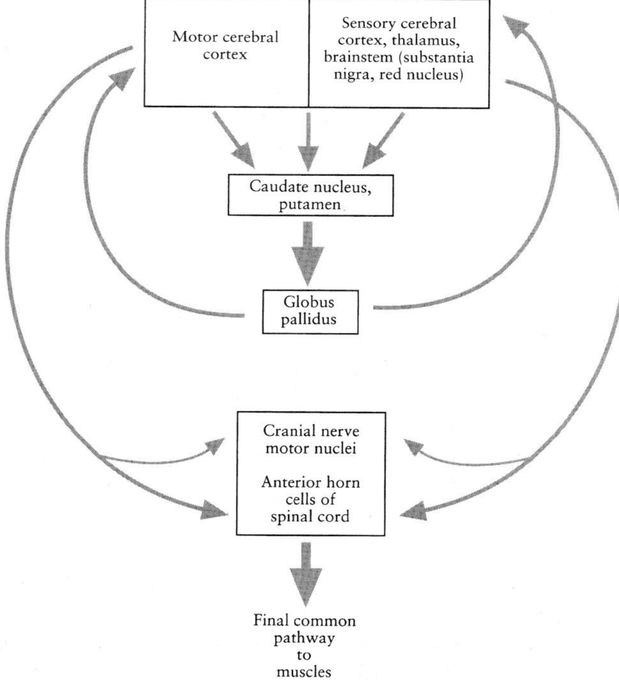

Figure 13–5 Diagram showing the main functional connections of the basal nuclei and how they may influence muscle activity.

Figure 13-5 shows the main functional connections of the basal nuclei and how they may influence muscle activity.

Clinical Notes

Chorea

In this syndrome the patient exhibits quick, jerky, irregular movements that are nonrepetitive. Swift grimaces and sudden movements of the head or limbs are good examples. In **Huntington's chorea** there is a degeneration of the GABA-secreting, substance P-secreting, and acetylcholine-secreting neurons of the striatonigral-inhibiting pathway. This results in the dopamine-secreting neurons of the substantia nigra becoming overactive so that the nigrostriatal pathway inhibits the caudate nucleus and the putamen. This inhibition produces the abnormal movements seen in this disease.

Athetosis

This consists of slow, sinuous, writhing movements that most commonly involve the distal segments of the limbs. Degeneration of the globus pallidus occurs with a breakdown of the circuitry involving the basal nuclei and the cerebral cortex.

Hemiballismus

This form of involuntary movement is confined to one side of the body. It usually involves the proximal extremity musculature, and the limb suddenly flies about in all directions out of control. The lesion occurs in the opposite subthalamic nucleus where normal smooth movements of different parts of the body are integrated.

Parkinson's Disease

This disease is associated with neuronal degeneration in the substantia nigra and to a lesser extent in the globus pallidus, putamen, and caudate nucleus. The degeneration of the inhibitory nigrostriate fibers results in a reduction in the release of the neurotransmitter dopamine within the corpus striatum. This leads to hypersensitivity of the dopamine receptors in the postsynaptic neurons in the corpus striatum, which become overactive. The signs and symptoms of the disease include tremor, cogwheel rigidity, and bradykinesis.

REVIEW QUESTIONS

Directions: Each of the numbered items in this section is followed by answers that are positively phrased. Select the ONE lettered answer that is an EXCEPTION.

1. The following statements concerning the position of the basal nuclei (ganglia) are correct **except:**
   (a) The lentiform nucleus is related medially to the internal capsule.
   (b) The putamen lies medial to the globus pallidus.
   (c) The head of the caudate nucleus lies medial to the internal capsule.
   (d) The head of the caudate nucleus is connected to the putamen.
   (e) The amygdaloid nucleus is situated in the temporal lobe of the cerebral hemisphere.
2. The following statements concerning the basal nuclei are correct **except:**
   (a) The insula forms part of the basal nuclei.
   (b) The corpus striatum is made up of the caudate nucleus and the lentiform nucleus.
   (c) The pulvinar of the thalamus is not part of the basal nuclei.
   (d) The neostriatum is formed by the caudate nucleus and the putamen.
   (e) The basal nuclei are formed of masses of gray matter buried deep in the white matter of the cerebral hemispheres.
3. The following statements concerning the caudate nucleus are correct **except:**
   (a) It is C-shaped.
   (b) It lies lateral to the thalamus.
   (c) It has a head, a body, and a tail.
   (d) The body lies in the roof of the lateral ventricle.
   (e) The tail terminates anteriorly in the amygdaloid nucleus.
4. The following statements concerning the afferent corticostriate fibers to the corpus callosum are correct **except:**
   (a) All parts of the cerebral cortex send fibers to the corpus striatum.
   (b) Glutamate is the neurotransmitter of the corticostriate fibers.
   (c) Most of the corticostriate fibers come from the cortex of the same side.
   (d) The largest input is from the sensory-motor cortex.
   (e) Each part of the cerebral cortex does not project to a specific part of the caudate-putamen complex.
5. The following statements concerning the nigrostriate fibers are correct **except:**
   (a) The fibers liberate dopamine at their terminals.
   (b) Parkinson's disease is caused by degeneration of the nigrostriate fibers.
   (c) The fibers exert an inhibitory effect on the putamen.
   (d) The caudate nucleus receives no fibers from the substantia nigra.
   (e) The nigrostriate fibers originate from cells in the substantia nigra.
6. The following statements concerning the efferent fibers of the corpus striatum are correct **except:**
   (a) None of the efferent fibers descend directly to the motor nuclei of the cranial nerves or the anterior horn cells of the spinal cord.
   (b) The efferent fibers have no effect on posture.
   (c) The striatopallidal fibers have GABA as their neurotransmitter.

(d) The striatonigral fibers pass from the caudate nucleus and putamen to the neurons in the substantia nigra.
(e) Some of the striatonigral fibers use GABA as the neurotransmitter, while others use substance P.

7. The following statements concerning the functions of the basal nuclei (ganglia) are correct **except:**
(a) The corpus striatum integrates all information received from different parts of the nervous system.
(b) The outflow of the basal nuclei is channeled through the globus pallidus, which then influences the activities of the motor areas of the cerebral cortex.
(c) The basal nuclei are capable of producing gross crude movements in the absence of the motor areas of the cerebral cortex.
(d) The basal nuclei influence muscle movements on the opposite side of the body.
(e) The globus pallidus has no influence on controlling the axial and girdle movements of the body.

Directions: Each of the numbered items in this section is followed by lettered answers. Select the ONE lettered answer that is BEST in each case.

For questions 8-12, study Figure 13-6, showing a horizontal section of the cerebrum.

8. Identify structure number 1.
(a) Head of the caudate nucleus
(b) Thalamus
(c) Putamen
(d) Globus pallidus
(e) Internal Capsule

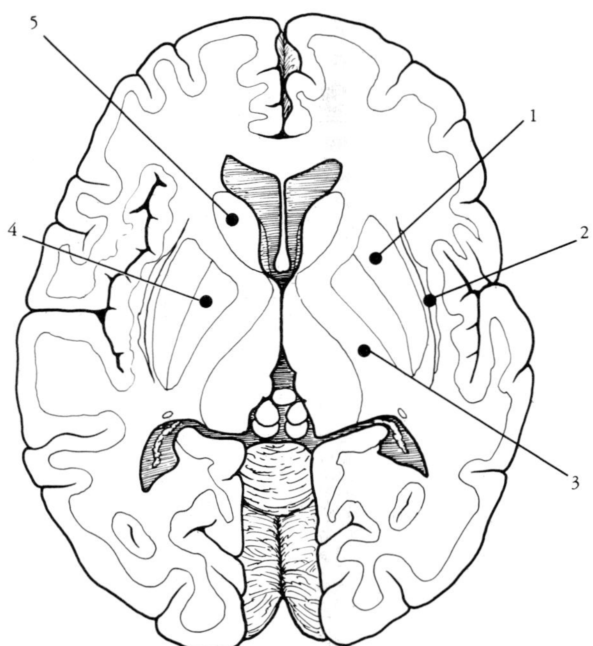

Figure 13–6 Diagram of horizontal section of the cerebrum.

9. Identify structure number 2.
(a) External capsule
(b) Internal capsule
(c) Body of lateral ventricle
(d) Insula
(e) Claustrum

10. Identify structure number 3.
(a) External capsule
(b) Thalamus
(c) Optic radiation
(d) Internal capsule
(e) Choroid plexus

11. Identify structure number 4.
(a) Putamen
(b) Thalamus
(c) Globus pallidus
(d) Caudate nucleus
(e) Claustrum

12. Identify structure number 5.
(a) Anterior horn of lateral ventricle
(b) Head of caudate nucleus
(c) Septum pellucidum
(d) Putamen
(e) Thalamus

Directions: Read the case history then answer the question. You will be required to select ONE BEST answer.

A 71-year-old man was seen by his physician because of tremor of the left arm. The patient also noticed that the muscles of his limbs sometimes felt stiff. Examination revealed that the patient rarely smiled and spoke with a weak voice. At rest, the fingers of the left hand alternately contracted and relaxed and there was a fine tremor of the wrist and elbow. There was no sensory or motor loss. A diagnosis of Parkinson's disease was made.

13. The following statements concerning this patient are correct **except:**
(a) The stiffness of the muscles of the limbs, the unsmiling face, and the weak voice are due to loss of influence of the basal nuclei on the motor areas of the cerebral cortex and the motor areas in the brainstem.
(b) The absence of sensory and motor losses is due to the fact that the ascending sensory pathways and the main descending motor tracts are unaffected by this disease.
(c) Neuronal degeneration is probably present in the substantia nigra and to a lesser extent in the globus pallidus, putamen, and caudate nucleus.
(d) The release of dopamine within the corpus striatum is reduced.
(e) The dopamine receptors in the postsynaptic neurons in the striatum are unchanged in Parkinson's disease.

ANSWERS AND EXPLANATIONS

1. B. The putamen lies lateral to the globus pallidus.
2. A. The insula is part of the cerebral cortex at the bottom of the lateral sulcus and forms no part of the basal nuclei.
3. D. The body of the caudate nucleus lies in the floor of the lateral ventricle.
4. E. Each part of the cerebral cortex projects to a specific part of the caudate-putamen complex.
5. D. The caudate nucleus receives nigrostriate fibers.
6. B. The basal nuclei (ganglia) exert control on posture and voluntary movements. Posture depends on muscle tone, and the activity of the anterior horn cells of the spinal cord are indirectly influenced by the activities of the basal nuclei.
7. E. The globus pallidus plays a role in controlling the axial and girdle movements of the body and the positioning of the proximal parts of the limbs.
8. C
9. E
10. D
11. C
12. B
13. E. In Parkinson's disease the dopamine receptors in the corpus striatum become hypersensitive and overactive.

CHAPTER 14

Cerebral Cortex

CHAPTER OUTLINE

SUGGESTED PLAN FOR REVIEW OF CHAPTER 14

1. Learn the structure of the cerebral cortex including the names and characteristic features of the different layers. Know the differences between the granular and agranular types of cortex. Note that the cerebral cortex varies in structure in different areas, whereas the cortex of the cerebellum is identical in structure in all areas.
2. Understand that the cerebral cortex is organized into vertical units of functional activity.
3. The section on the functional localization of the cerebral cortex must be carefully read and learned. Each area of the cortex discussed in this chapter must be understood and committed to memory.
4. It is essential to understand how the primary motor area and the premotor area control the movements of the contralateral side of the body. It is also important to understand how these areas on one side of the cerebral cortex control bilateral movements of the muscles of the upper part of the face, the tongue and the mandible, and the larynx and the pharynx.
5. The results of lesions of each of the cortical areas must be understood and learned. This material provides the examiners with a great many examples from which to construct suitable questions.
6. Understand what is meant by cerebral dominance.

INTRODUCTION

The cerebral cortex is the highest level of the central nervous system and always functions in association with the lower centers. It receives vast amounts of information and responds in a precise manner by bringing about appropriate changes. Many of the responses are influenced by inherited programs, while others are colored by programs learned during the individual's life and stored in the cerebral cortex.

The cerebral cortex is composed of gray matter and forms a complete covering of the cerebral hemisphere. The surface area of the cortex has been increased by throwing it into **convolutions,** or **gyri,** separated by **fissures or sulci**.

STRUCTURE OF THE CEREBRAL CORTEX

Nerve Cells

The following types of nerve cells are present in the cerebral cortex: (1) pyramidal cells, (2) stellate cells, (3) fusiform cells, (4) horizontal cells of Cajal, and (5) cells of Martinotti (Fig. 14-1).

The **pyramidal cells** measure 10 to 50 μm long. However, there are giant pyramidal cells, also known as **Betz cells**, whose cell bodies measure as much as 120 μm; these are found in the motor precentral gyrus of the frontal lobe. From the apex of each cell a dendrite extends upward toward the pia, giving off collateral branches. The axon arises from the base of the cell body and the majority enter the white matter of the cerebral hemisphere.

The **stellate cells** are polygonal and have multiple branching dendrites and a short axon, which terminates on a nearby neuron (Fig. 14-1).

The **fusiform cells** have their long axis vertical to the surface and are concentrated mainly in the deepest cortical layers (Fig. 14-1). Dendrites arise from each pole of the cell body. The axon arises from the inferior part of the cell body and enters the white matter.

The **horizontal cells of Cajal** are fusiform, horizontally oriented cells found in the most superficial layers of the cortex (Fig. 14-1). A dendrite emerges from each end of the cell

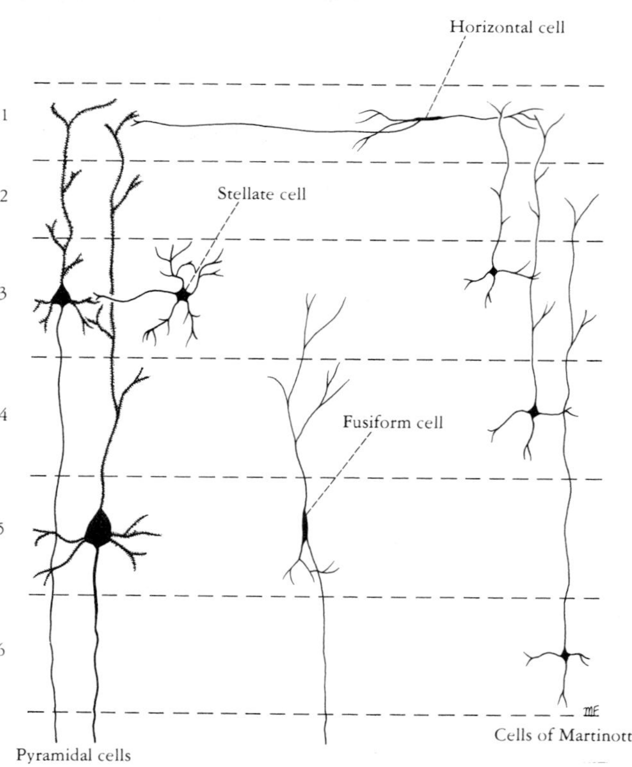

Figure 14–1 Neurons present in the cerebral cortex.

and an axon runs parallel to the surface of the cortex, making contact with the dendrites of pyramidal cells.

The **cells of Martinotti** are small, multipolar cells that are present throughout the layers of the cortex (Fig. 14-1).

Nerve Fibers

The nerve fibers of the cerebral cortex are arranged both radially and tangentially (Fig. 14-2). The **radial fibers** run at right angles to the cortical surface (Fig. 14-3). They include the afferent entering projection, association, and commissural fibers that terminate within the cortex, and the axons of pyramidal, stellate, and fusiform cells, which leave the cortex to become projection, association, and commissural fibers of the white matter of the cerebral hemisphere. The **tangential fibers** run parallel to the cortical surface and are collateral and terminal branches of afferent fibers. They also include the axons of horizontal and stellate cells and collateral branches of pyramidal and fusiform cells.

Layers

The names and characteristic features of the layers (Figs. 14-1 and 14-3) are as follows:

1. **Molecular layer (plexiform layer).** This is the most superficial layer; it consists of a dense network of tangentially oriented nerve fibers derived from the apical dendrites of the pyramidal cells and fusiform cells, the axons of the stellate cells, and the cells of Martinotti. Afferent fibers originating from the thalamus and from association and commissural fibers are also present. Scattered among these nerve fibers are the horizontal cells of Cajal.

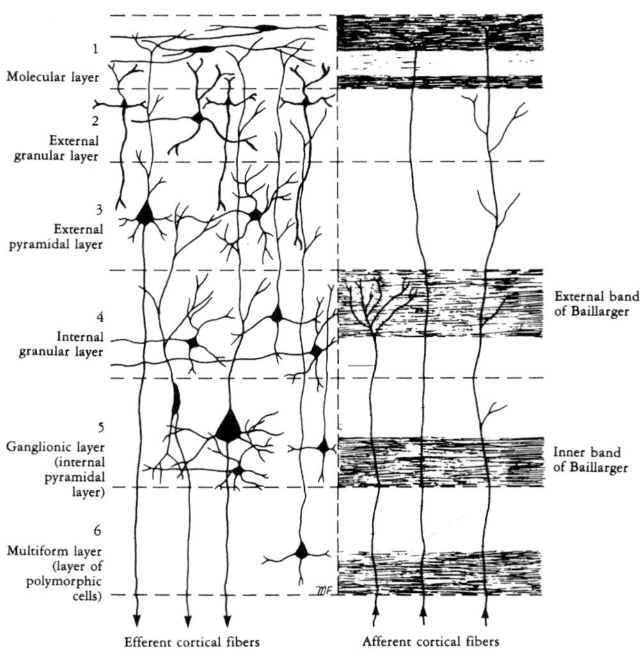

Figure 14–3 Layers of the cerebral cortex, showing neurons on the left and the nerve fibers on the right.

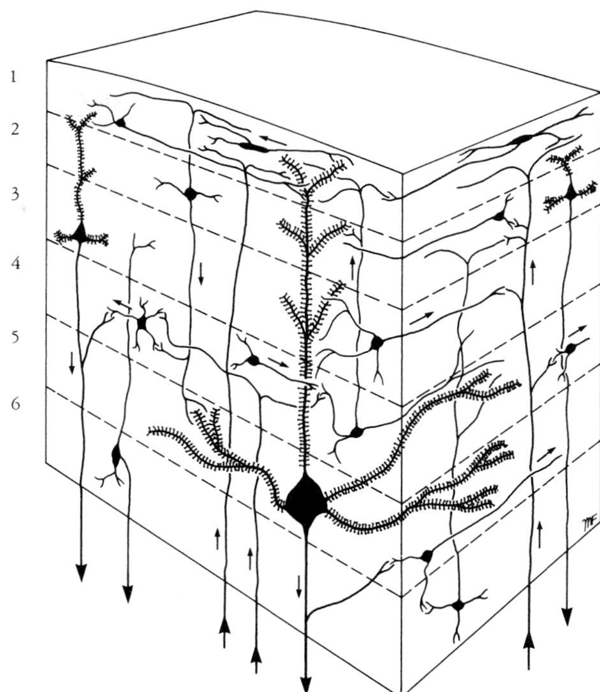

Figure 14–2 Neuronal connections of the cerebral cortex.

2. **External granular layer.** This layer contains numerous small pyramidal cells and stellate cells (Figs. 14-1 and 14-3). The dendrites of these cells terminate in the molecular layer, and the axons enter deeper layers, where they terminate or pass on to enter the white matter of the cerebral hemisphere.
3. **External pyramidal layer.** This layer is composed of pyramidal cells, whose cell body size increases from the superficial to the deeper borders of the layer (Figs. 14-1 and 14-3). The apical dendrites pass into the molecular layer and the axons enter the white matter.
4. **Internal granular layer.** This layer is composed of closely packed stellate cells (Figs. 14-1 and 14-3). There is a high concentration of horizontally arranged fibers known collectively as the **external band of Baillarger**.
5. **Ganglionic layer (internal pyramidal layer).** This layer contains very large and medium-sized pyramidal cells (Figs. 14-1 and 14-3). Scattered among the pyramidal cells are stellate cells and cells of Martinotti. In addition, there are a large number of horizontally arranged fibers that form the **inner band of Baillarger**. In the motor cortex of the precentral gyrus, the pyramidal cells of this layer are very large and are known as Betz cells. These cells account for about 3 percent of the projection fibers of the **corticospinal** or **pyramidal tract**.
6. **Multiform layer (layer of polymorphic cells).** The majority of the cells are fusiform but many of the cells are triangular or ovoid (Figs. 14-1 and 14-3). The cells of Martinotti are also conspicuous in this layer. Many nerve fibers that enter or leave the underlying white matter are present.

VARIATIONS IN CORTICAL STRUCTURE

Most areas of the cerebral cortex possess six layers and these are referred to as **homotypical**. Those areas of the cortex that have less than six layers are referred to as heterotypical. Two heterotypical areas will be described, the granular and the agranular type.

In the **granular type**, the granular layers are well developed and contain densely packed stellate cells. Thus, layers 2 and 4 are well developed, so that layers 2 through 5 merge into a single layer of predominantly granular cells. It is these cells that receive thalamocortical fibers. The granular type of cortex is found in the postcentral gyrus, in the superior temporal gyrus, and in parts of the hippocampal gyrus.

In the **agranular type** of cortex, the granular layers are poorly developed, so that layers 2 and 4 are practically absent. The pyramidal cells in layers 3 and 5 are densely packed and are very large. The agranular type of cortex is found in the precentral gyrus and other areas in the frontal lobe. These areas give rise to large numbers of efferent fibers that are associated with motor function.

MECHANISMS OF THE CEREBRAL CORTEX

The cerebral cortex is organized into vertical units of functional activity (Fig. 14-2). Such a functional unit possesses afferent fibers, internuncial neurons, and efferent fibers. An afferent fiber may synapse directly with an efferent neuron or may involve vertical chains of internuncial neurons. A single vertical chain of neurons may be involved or the wave of excitation may spread to adjacent vertical chains through short axon granular cells. The horizontal cells of Cajal permit activation of vertical units that lie some distance away from the incoming afferent fibers.

FUNCTIONAL LOCALIZATION OF THE CEREBRAL CORTEX

The simple division of cortical areas into motor and sensory is erroneous. The precentral and postcentral areas, for example, are both sensory and motor, the former predominantly motor and the latter predominantly sensory. Much of our understanding of the functional localization of the cerebral cortex is derived from clinicopathological studies in humans and electrophysiological and ablation studies in animals.

A summary of some of the main anatomical connections of the cerebral cortex is provided in Table 14-1.

Frontal Lobe

The **precentral area** is situated in the precentral gyrus and includes the anterior wall of the central sulcus and the posterior parts of the superior, middle, and inferior frontal gyri; it extends over the superomedial border of the hemisphere into the paracentral lobule (Fig. 14-4). Histologically, the characteristic feature of this area is the almost complete absence of the granular layers and the prominence of the pyramidal nerve cells. The giant pyramidal cells of Betz are concentrated in the superior part of the precentral gyrus and the paracentral lobule. The great majority of the corticospinal and corticobulbar fibers originate from the small pyramidal cells in this area. It has been estimated that the number of Betz cells present is between 25,000 and 30,000

Table 14–1 Summary of Some of the Main Anatomical Connections of the Cerebral Cortex

Function	Origin	Cortical Area	Destination
Sensory			
Somatosensory (most contralateral side of body; oral on same side; pharynx, larynx, perineum bilateral)	Ventral lateral and ventral medial nuclei of thalamus	Primary somesthetic area (Brodmann's areas 3, 1, 2), postcentral gyrus	Secondary somesthetic area, primary motor area
Vision	Lateral geniculate body	Primary visual area (Brodmann's area 17)	Secondary visual area (Brodmann's areas 18, 19)
Auditory	Medial geniculate body	Primary auditory area (Brodmann's areas 41, 42)	Secondary auditory area (Brodmann's area 22)
Taste	Nucleus solitarius	Postcentral gyrus (Brodmann's area 43)	
Smell	Olfactory bulb	Primary olfactory area, periamygdaloid and prepiriform areas	Secondary olfactory area (Brodmann's area 28)
Motor			
Fine movements (most contralateral side of body; extraocular muscles, upper face, tongue, mandible, larynx bilateral)	Thalamus from cerebellum, basal nuclei, somatosensory area, premotor area	Primary motor area (Brodmann's area 4)	Motor nuclei of brainstem and anterior horn cells of spinal cord, corpus striatum

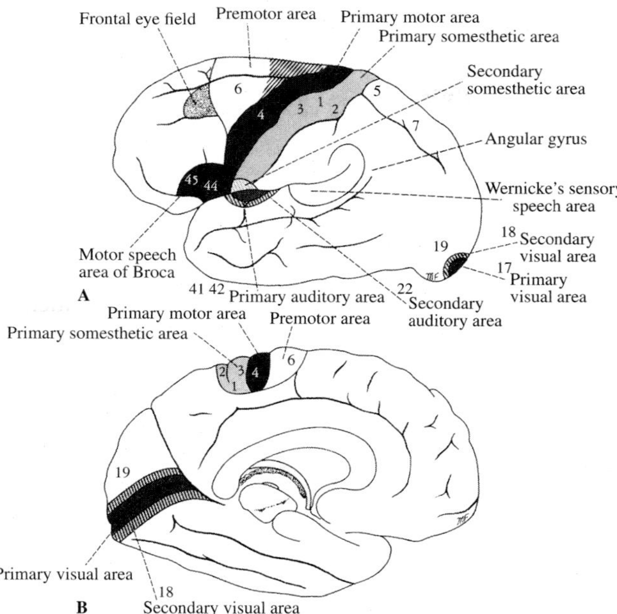

Figure 14–4 Functional localization of the cerebral cortex. **A.** Lateral view of left cerebral hemisphere. **B.** Medial view of left cerebral hemisphere.

and accounts for only about 3 percent of the corticospinal fibers. The postcentral gyrus and the secondary somatosensory areas, as well as the occipital and temporal lobes, give origin to descending tracts also; they control the sensory input to the nervous system and are not involved in muscular movement.

The precentral area can be divided into posterior and anterior regions. The posterior region—referred to as the **motor area, primary motor area,** or Brodmann's area 4—occupies the precentral gyrus extending over the superior border into the paracentral lobule (Fig. 14-4). The anterior area is known as the **premotor area, secondary motor area**, or Brodmann's area 6 and parts of areas 8, 44, and 45. It occupies the anterior part of the precentral gyrus and the posterior parts of the superior, middle, and inferior frontal gyri.

PRIMARY MOTOR AREA

The primary motor area, when electrically stimulated, produces isolated movements on the opposite side of the body and contraction of muscle groups concerned with the performance of a specific movement. Although isolated ipsilateral movements do not occur, bilateral movements of the extraocular muscles, the muscles of the upper part of the face, the tongue and the mandible, and the larynx and the pharynx do occur.

The movement areas of the body are represented in an inverted form in the precentral gyrus. Starting from below and passing superiorly are structures involved in swallowing and the tongue, jaw, lips, larynx, eyelid, and brow. The next area is an extensive region for movements of the fingers, especially the thumb, hand, wrist, elbow, shoulder, and trunk. The movements of the hip, knee, and ankle are represented in the highest areas of the precentral gyrus and of the toes on the medial surface of the cerebral hemisphere in the paracentral lobule. The anal and vesical sphincters are also controlled in the paracentral lobule. The area of cortex controlling a particular movement is proportional to the skill involved in performing the movement.

The function of the primary motor area is to carry out the individual movements of different parts of the body. To assist in this function, it receives numerous afferent fibers from the premotor area, the sensory cortex, the thalamus, the cerebellum, and the basal nuclei. The primary motor cortex is not responsible for the design of the pattern of movement but is the final station for the conversion of the design into the execution of the movement.

CLINICAL NOTES

LESIONS OF THE PRIMARY MOTOR AREA

Lesions of this area in one hemisphere result in paralysis of the contralateral extremities, the finer and more skilled movements suffering most.

The **jacksonian epileptic seizure** is due to an irritative lesion of the primary motor area (area 4). The convulsion begins in the part of the body represented in the primary motor area that is being irritated. The convulsive movement may be restricted to one part of the body, such as the face or the foot, or it may spread to involve many regions.

SECONDARY MOTOR AREA

Electrical stimulation of the secondary motor area (premotor area) produces muscular movements similar to those obtained by stimulation of the primary motor area; however, stronger stimulation is necessary to produce the same degree of movement.

The premotor area receives numerous inputs from the sensory cortex, the thalamus, and the basal nuclei. The function of the premotor area is to store programs of motor activity assembled as the result of past experience. The premotor area thus programs the activity of the primary motor area. It is particularly involved in the control of coarse postural movements through its connections with the basal nuclei.

Clinical Notes

Lesions of the Secondary Motor Area

These lesions produce difficulty in the performance of skilled movements, with little loss of strength.

Muscle Spasticity Caused by Lesions of the Primary and Secondary Motor Areas

A discrete lesion of the primary motor cortex (area 4) results in little change in the muscle tone. However, larger lesions involving the primary and secondary motor areas (areas 4 and 6), which are the most common, result in muscle spasm. The explanation for this is that the primary motor cortex gives origin to corticospinal and corticonuclear tracts and the secondary motor cortex gives origin to extrapyramidal tracts that pass to the basal nuclei and the reticular formation. The corticospinal and corticonuclear tracts tend to increase muscle tone, but the extrapyramidal fibers transmit inhibitory impulses that lower muscle tone. Destruction of the secondary motor area removes the inhibitory influence and, consequently, the muscles are spastic.

SUPPLEMENTARY MOTOR AREA

The supplementary motor area is situated in the medial frontal gyrus on the medial surface of the hemisphere and anterior to the paracentral lobule. Stimulation of this area results in movements of the contralateral limbs, but a stronger stimulus is necessary than when the primary motor area is stimulated. Removal of the supplementary motor area produces no permanent loss of movement.

FRONTAL EYE FIELD

The frontal eye field (Fig. 14-4) extends forward from the facial area of the precentral gyrus into the middle frontal gyrus (parts of Brodmann's areas 6, 8, and 9). Electrical stimulation of this region causes conjugate movements of the eyes, especially toward the opposite side. The nerve fibers from this area are thought to pass to the superior colliculus of the midbrain. The superior colliculus is connected to the nuclei of the extraocular muscles by the reticular formation. The frontal eye field controls voluntary scanning movements of the eye and is independent of visual stimuli. The involuntary following of moving objects by the eyes involves the visual area of the occipital cortex to which the frontal eye field is connected by association fibers.

Clinical Notes

Lesions of the Frontal Eye Field

Destructive lesions of the frontal eye field of one hemisphere cause the two eyes to deviate to the side of the lesion and an inability to turn the eyes to the opposite side. The involuntary tracking movement of the eyes when following moving objects is unaffected, since the lesion does not involve the visual cortex in the occipital lobe.

Irritative lesions of the frontal eye field of one hemisphere cause the two eyes to deviate periodically to the opposite side of the lesion.

MOTOR SPEECH AREA OF BROCA

The motor speech area of Broca (Fig. 14-4) is located in the inferior frontal gyrus between the anterior and ascending rami and the ascending and posterior rami of the lateral fissure (Brodmann's areas 44 and 45). In the majority of individuals, this area is important in the left or dominant hemisphere and ablation will result in paralysis of speech. In those individuals where the right hemisphere is dominant, the area on the right side is of importance. The ablation of this region in the nondominant hemisphere has no effect on speech.

Broca's speech area brings about the formation of words by its connections with the adjacent primary motor area, and the muscles of the larynx, mouth, tongue, soft palate, and the respiratory muscles are appropriately stimulated.

Clinical Notes

Lesions of the Motor Speech Area of Broca

Destructive lesions in the left inferior frontal gyrus result in the loss of ability to produce speech, i.e., **expressive aphasia**. Patients, however, retain the ability to think the words they wish to say, they can write the words, and they can understand their meaning when they see or hear them.

Lesions of the Sensory Speech Area of Wernicke

Destructive lesions restricted to Wernicke's speech area in the dominant hemisphere produce a loss of ability to understand the spoken and written word, i.e., **receptive aphasia**. Since Broca's area is unaffected, speech is unimpaired and patients can produce fluent speech. However, they are unaware of the meaning of the words they use, and they may use incorrect words or even nonexistent words. Patients are also unaware of their mistakes.

Lesions of the Motor and Sensory Speech Areas

Destructive lesions involving both Broca's and Wernicke's speech areas result in the loss of the production of speech and the loss of the understanding of the spoken and written word, i.e., **global aphasia**.

Lesions of the Dominant Angular Gyrus

Destructive lesions in the angular gyrus in the posterior parietal lobe (often considered a part of Wernicke's area) divide the pathway between the visual association area and the anterior part of Wernicke's area. This results in an inability to read (**alexia**) or write (**agraphia**).

PREFRONTAL CORTEX

The prefrontal cortex is an extensive area that lies anterior to the precentral area. It includes the greater parts of the superior, middle, and inferior frontal gyri, the orbital gyri, most of the medial frontal gyrus, and the anterior half of the cingulate gyrus (Brodmann's areas 9, 10, 11, and 12). Large numbers of afferent and efferent pathways connect the prefrontal area with other areas of the cerebral cortex, the thalamus, the hypothalamus, and the corpus striatum. The frontopontine fibers also connect this area to the cerebellum through the pontine nuclei. The commissural fibers of the forceps minor and genu of the corpus callosum unite these areas in both cerebral hemispheres.

The prefrontal area is concerned with the individual's personality. It also exerts its influence in determining the initiative and judgment of an individual.

Clinical Notes

Lesions of the Prefrontal Cortex

Destruction of the prefrontal region does not produce any marked loss of intelligence. It is an area of the cortex that is capable of associating experiences that are necessary for the production of abstract ideas, judgment, emotional feeling, and personality. Tumors or traumatic destruction of the prefrontal cortex results in the person's losing initiative and judgment. Emotional changes that occur include a tendency to euphoria. The patient no longer conforms to the accepted mode of social behavior and becomes careless of dress and appearance.

PARIETAL LOBE

Primary Somesthetic Area

The primary somesthetic area (Fig. 14-4) occupies the postcentral gyrus on the lateral surface of the hemisphere and the posterior part of the paracentral lobule on the medial surface (Brodmann's areas 3, 1, and 2). The primary somesthetic area of the cerebral cortex receives projection fibers from the ventral posterolateral and ventral posteromedial nuclei of the thalamus. The opposite half of the body is represented as inverted. The pharyngeal region, tongue, and jaws are represented in the most inferior part of the postcentral gyrus; this is followed by the face, fingers, hand, arm, trunk, and thigh. The leg and the foot areas are found on the medial surface of the hemisphere in the posterior part of the paracentral lobule. The anal and genital regions are also found in this latter area. The apportioning of the cortex for a particular part of the body is related to its functional importance. The face, lips, thumb, and index finger have particularly large areas assigned to them.

Although the majority of the sensations reach the cortex from the contralateral side of the body, some from the oral region go to the same side, and those from the pharynx, larynx, and perineum go to both sides.

Secondary Somesthetic Area

The secondary somesthetic area (Fig. 14-4) is in the superior lip of the posterior limb of the lateral fissure. The face area lies most anterior and the leg area is posterior. The body is bilaterally represented, with the contralateral side dominant. The detailed connections of this area are unknown, but the spinothalamic tracts are believed to be associated with it. The functional significance of this area is not known.

Clinical Notes

Lesions of the Sensory Cortex

The sensory cortex is necessary for the appreciation of spatial recognition, recognition of relative intensity, and recognition of similarity and difference.

Lesions of the primary somesthetic area of the cortex result in contralateral sensory disturbances, which are most severe in the distal parts of the limbs. Crude painful, tactile, and thermal stimuli often return, but this is believed to be due to the function of the thalamus. The patient remains unable to judge degrees of warmth, unable to localize tactile stimuli accurately, and unable to judge weights of objects.

Lesions of the secondary somesthetic area of the cortex do not cause recognizable sensory defects.

SOMESTHETIC ASSOCIATION AREA

The somesthetic association area (Fig. 14-4) occupies the superior parietal lobule extending onto the medial surface of the hemisphere (Brodmann's areas 5 and 7). This area has many connections with other sensory areas of the cortex. Its main function is to receive and integrate different sensory modalities. For example, it enables one to recognize objects placed in the hand without the help of vision. In other words, it not only receives information concerning the size and shape of an object but also relates this to past sensory experiences, so that the information can be interpreted and recognition occurs.

OCCIPITAL LOBE

Primary Visual Area

The primary visual area (Brodmann's area 17) is situated in the walls of the posterior part of the calcarine sulcus and occasionally extends around the occipital pole onto the lateral surface of the hemisphere (Fig. 14-4).

The visual cortex receives afferent fibers from the lateral geniculate body. The fibers first pass forward in the white matter of the temporal lobe and then turn back to the primary visual cortex in the occipital lobe. The visual cortex receives fibers from the temporal half of the ipsilateral retina and the nasal half of the contralateral retina. The right half of the field of vision, therefore, is represented in the visual cortex of the left cerebral hemisphere and vice versa. It is also important to note that the superior retinal quadrants (inferior field of vision) pass to the superior wall of the calcarine sulcus, while the inferior retinal quadrants (superior field of vision) pass to the inferior wall of the calcarine sulcus.

The macula lutea, which is the central area of the retina and the area for most perfect vision, is represented on the cortex in the posterior part of area 17 and accounts for one-third of the visual cortex. The peripheral parts of the retina in the region of the orra serrata are represented in the anterior part of area 17.

Clinical Notes

Lesions of the Primary Visual Area

Lesions involving the walls of the posterior part of one calcarine sulcus result in a loss of sight in the opposite visual field (**crossed homonymous hemianopia**). It is interesting to note that the central part of the visual field, when tested, apparently is normal. This so-called macular sparing is probably due to the patient's shifting the eyes very slightly while the visual fields are being examined. The following clinical defects should be understood. Lesions of the upper half of one primary visual area, i.e., the area above the calcarine sulcus, result in **inferior quadrantic hemianopia**, whereas lesions involving one visual area below the calcarine sulcus result in **superior quadrantic hemianopia**. Lesions of the occipital pole produce central scotomas. The most common causes of these lesions are vascular disorders, tumors, and injuries from gunshot wounds.

SECONDARY VISUAL AREA

The secondary visual area (Brodmann's areas 18 and 19) surrounds the primary visual area on the medial and lateral surfaces of the hemisphere (Fig. 14-4). This area receives afferent fibers from area 17 and other cortical areas, as well as from the thalamus. The function of the secondary visual area is to relate the visual information received by the primary visual area to past visual experiences, thus enabling the individual to recognize and appreciate what he or she is seeing.

The **occipital eye field** is thought to exist in the secondary visual area in humans. Stimulation produces conjugate deviation of the eyes, especially to the opposite side. The function of this eye field is believed to be reflex and associated with movements of the eye when it is following an object. The occipital eye fields of both hemispheres are connected by nervous pathways and also are thought to be connected to the superior colliculus. The frontal eye field, on the other hand, controls voluntary scanning movements of the eye and is independent of visual stimuli.

CLINICAL NOTES

LESIONS OF THE SECONDARY VISUAL AREA

Lesions of the secondary visual area result in a loss of ability to recognize objects seen in the opposite field of vision. The reason for this is that the area of cortex that stores past visual experiences has been lost.

TEMPORAL LOBE

Primary Auditory Area

The primary auditory area (Brodmann's areas 41 and 42) includes the gyrus of Heschl and is situated in the inferior wall of the lateral sulcus (Fig. 14-4).

Projection fibers to the auditory area arise principally in the medial geniculate body and form the **auditory radiation of the internal capsule**. The medial geniculate body receives fibers mainly from the organ of Corti of the opposite side as well as some fibers from the same side.

CLINICAL NOTES

LESIONS OF THE PRIMARY AUDITORY AREA

Because the primary auditory area in the inferior wall of the lateral sulcus receives nerve fibers from both cochleae, a lesion of one cortical area will produce slight bilateral loss of hearing, but the loss will be greatest in the opposite ear. The main defect noted is a loss of ability to locate the source of the sound. Bilateral destruction of the primary auditory areas causes complete deafness.

SECONDARY AUDITORY AREA

The secondary auditory area (auditory association cortex) is situated posterior to the primary auditory area (Fig. 14-4) in the lateral sulcus and in the superior temporal gyrus (Brodmann's area 22). This area is thought to be necessary for the interpretation of sounds.

CLINICAL NOTES

LESIONS OF THE SECONDARY AUDITORY AREA

Lesions of the cortex posterior to the primary auditory area in the lateral sulcus and in the superior temporal gyrus result in an inability to interpret sounds, and the patient may experience **word deafness (acoustic verbal agnosia).**

SENSORY SPEECH AREA OF WERNICKE

The sensory speech area of Wernicke (Fig. 14-4) is localized in the left dominant hemisphere, mainly in the superior temporal gyrus, with extensions around the posterior end of the lateral sulcus into the parietal region. Wernicke's area is connected to Broca's area by a bundle of nerve fibers called the **arcuate fasciculus**. It receives fibers from the visual cortex in the occipital lobe and the auditory cortex in the superior temporal gyrus. Wernicke's area permits the understanding of written and spoken language and allows a person to read a sentence, understand it, and say it out loud.

Since Wernicke's area represents the site on the cerebral cortex where somatic, visual and auditory association areas all come together, it should be regarded as an area of very great importance.

OTHER CORTICAL AREAS

Taste Area

The taste area is probably situated at the lower end of the postcentral gyrus in the superior wall of the lateral sulcus or in the adjoining area of the insula (Brodmann's area 43). Ascending fibers from the nucleus solitarius ascend to the ventral posterior nucleus of the thalamus, where they synapse on neurons that send fibers to the cortex.

Vestibular Area

The vestibular area is situated near the lower end of the postcentral gyrus and lies opposite the auditory area in the superior temporal gyrus. This area is concerned with the appreciation of the positions and movements of the head in space. Through its nerve connections, the movements of the eyes and the muscles of the trunk and limbs are influenced in the maintenance of posture.

Insula

This area of the cortex that is buried within the lateral sulcus is important for planning or coordinating the articulatory movements for speech.

ASSOCIATION CORTEX

The primary sensory areas and the primary motor areas form only a small part of the total cortical surface area. The remaining areas are referred to as association cortex. They have multiple inputs and outputs and are very much concerned with behavior, discrimination, and interpretation of sensory experiences. Three main association areas are recognized: prefrontal, anterior temporal, and posterior parietal.

The prefrontal cortex is discussed on page 154. The anterior temporal cortex is thought to play a role in the storage of previous sensory experiences. Stimulation may cause the individual to recall objects seen or music heard in the past. In the posterior parietal cortex the sensory input of touch, pressure, and proprioception is integrated into concepts of size, form, and texture. This ability is known as stereognosis. An appreciation of the body image is also assembled in the posterior parietal cortex. An individual is able to develop a body scheme that he or she is able to appreciate consciously. The right side of the body is represented in the left hemisphere and the left side of the body in the right hemisphere.

CLINICAL NOTES

LESIONS OF THE SOMESTHETIC ASSOCIATION AREA

Lesions of the superior parietal lobule interfere with the patient's ability to combine touch, pressure, and proprioceptive impulses, so that he or she is unable to appreciate texture, size, and form. This loss of integration of sensory impulses is called **astereognosis.** For example, with the eyes closed, the individual would be unable to recognize a key placed in his or her hand.

Destruction of the posterior part of the parietal lobe, which integrates somatic and visual sensations, will interfere with the appreciation of the body image on the opposite side of the body. The individual may fail to recognize the opposite side of the body as his or her own. The individual may fail to wash it or dress it or to shave that side of the face.

CEREBRAL DOMINANCE

An anatomical examination of the two cerebral hemispheres shows that the cortical gyri and fissures are almost identical. Moreover, nervous pathways projecting to the cortex do so largely contralaterally and equally to identical cortical areas. In addition, the cerebral commissures, especially the corpus callosum and the anterior commissure, provide a pathway for information that is received in one hemisphere to be transferred to the other. Nevertheless, we know that certain nervous activity is predominantly performed by one of the two cerebral hemispheres. Handedness, perception of language, and speech are functional areas of behavior that are in most individuals controlled by the dominant hemisphere. On the other hand, spatial perception and recognition of faces and music are interpreted by the nondominant hemisphere.

More than 90 percent of the adult population is right-handed and is therefore left hemisphere dominant. About 96 percent of the adult population is left hemisphere dominant for speech. During childhood, one hemisphere slowly comes to dominate the other, and it is only after the first decade that the dominance becomes fixed. This would explain why a 5-year-old child with damage to the dominant hemisphere can easily learn to become left-handed and speak well, whereas in the case of the adult this is almost impossible.

CLINICAL NOTES

ALZHEIMER'S DISEASE

Alzheimer's disease is a degenerative disease of the brain occurring in middle to late life, but an early form of the disease is now well recognized. The disease affects more than 4 million people in the United States, resulting in over 100,000 deaths per year. The risk of the disease rises sharply with advancing years.

The cause of Alzheimer's disease is unknown but there is evidence of a genetic predisposition.

Early memory loss, a disintegration of personality, complete disorientation, deterioration in speech, and restlessness are common signs. In the late stages the patient may become mute, incontinent, and bedridden and usually dies of some other disease.

Microscopically, changes eventually occur throughout the cerebral cortex. Many so-called senile plaques are found in the atrophic cortex. The plaques result from the accumulation of several proteins around deposits of Beta amyloid. In the center of each plaque is an extracellular collection of degenerating nervous tissue; surrounding the core is a rim of large abnormal neuronal processes, probably presynaptic terminals, filled with an excess of intracellular neurofibrils that are tangled and twisted, forming neurofibrillary tangles. The neurofibrillary tangles are aggregations of the microtubular protein tau. There is a marked loss of choline acetyltransferase, the biosynthetic enzyme for acetylcholine, in the areas of the cortex in which the senile plaques occur. This is thought to be due to loss of the ascending projection fibers rather than a loss of cortical cells. As these cellular changes occur, the affected neurons die.

As yet, there is no clinical test for making the definite diagnosis of Alzheimer's disease. Reliance is placed on taking a careful history, and carrying out numerous neurological, and psychiatric examinations spaced out over time. In this way other causes of dementia can be excluded.

REVIEW QUESTIONS

Directions: Each of the numbered items or incomplete statements in this section is followed by answers or by completions of the statement. Select the ONE lettered answer or completion that is BEST in each case.

1. The cerebral cortex is
   (a) absent from the bottom of each cerebral sulcus
   (b) composed of a mixture of gray and white matter
   (c) not connected by axons to the caudate nucleus
   (d) organized into vertical functional units
   (e) made up of four layers of nerve cells
2. The microscopic structure of the cerebral cortex shows
   (a) a granular type of cortex in the postcentral gyrus
   (b) that the horizontal cells of Cajal are restricted to the deep layers
   (c) Betz cells present in very large numbers in the visual cortex
   (d) the cells of Martinotti are confined to the superficial layers
   (e) the bands of Baillarger run vertically
3. The cerebral cortex has
   (a) entering projection, association, and commissural fibers running tangentially to the surface beneath the pia mater
   (b) large pyramidal cells in the ganglionic layer of the precentral gyrus
   (c) horizontal cells of Cajal which restrict the activity of incoming afferent fibers
   (d) no nervous connection with the putamen
   (e) very shallow sulci in the prefrontal areas
4. Concerning the cerebral cortex:
   (a) The precentral gyrus is entirely motor in function
   (b) A homotypical cortex possesses four layers of cortex
   (c) In the agranular type of cortex, the pyramidal cells in layers 3 and 5 are densely packed
   (d) Clinicopathological studies are of little value in determining the functional localization of the cerebral cortex
   (e) Ablation studies of the cerebral cortex in animals have contributed very little to our understanding of the function of the different parts of the cerebral cortex
5. Concerning the precentral area:
   (a) It is located in the precentral gyrus and the anterior wall of the central sulcus and the posterior parts of the superior, middle, and inferior frontal gyri
   (b) The granular layers are conspicuous
   (c) The giant Betz cells are concentrated in the inferior part of the precentral gyrus
   (d) The majority of the corticospinal fibers arise from the large pyramidal cells in this area
   (e) Brodmann's area 4 occupies the anterior part of this area
6. Concerning the primary motor area:
   (a) It controls the contraction of groups of muscles
   (b) It is concerned with the performance of specific movements on the opposite side of the body
   (c) The movement areas of the body are represented in an inverted form in the precentral gyrus
   (d) There is an extensive area representing the movements of the thumb and fingers.
   (e) All of the above are correct
7. The insula of the cerebrum is located in which area?
   (a) Medial to the corpus striatum
   (b) In the longitudinal fissure
   (c) In the parietal lobe
   (d) Deep in the lateral fissure between the parietal and temporal lobes
   (e) Between the temporal and occipital lobes.
8. During brain surgery under local anesthesia, a surgeon exposes the left postcentral gyrus 7 cm lateral to the midline, stimulates this area with an electrode, and asks the patient what he feels. The patient might reply:
   (a) that he feels pain in his left leg
   (b) that he feels as if something is touching his right index finger
   (c) that he hears a ringing noise
   (d) that he sees flashes of light in both eyes
   (e) The patient would not reply because he would lose consciousness

9. Lesions of the posterior part of the parietal lobe (area 7) of the right hemisphere may result in:
   (a) Paralysis of the left side of the face
   (b) Anesthesia of the left arm
   (c) Receptive aphasia
   (d) Paralysis of the right leg
   (e) Inability to recognize objects in the left visual half-fields
10. The olfactory association cortex includes the:
   (a) Parahippocampal gyrus
   (b) Superior temporal gyrus
   (c) Hypothalamus
   (d) Paracentral gyrus
   (e) Cuneus
11. The corticospinal tracts originate from:
   (a) Cells of Martinotti
   (b) Pyramidal cells
   (c) Horizontal cells
   (d) Stellate cells
   (e) Golgi type II cells
12. The cerebral cortex is an essential component of the pathway included in:
   (a) Pupillary light reflex
   (b) Consensual light reflex
   (c) Corneal reflex
   (d) Gag reflex
   (e) Accommodation reflex
13. Stimulation of the middle frontal cortex (area 8) of the cerebral cortex would most likely produce:
   (a) Contraction of the muscles of the contralateral leg
   (b) Visual agnosia
   (c) Auditory hallucinations
   (d) Conjugate eye movements
   (e) Fasciculations in the muscles of the ipsilateral hand
14. Motor seizures limited to the right arm with no loss of consciousness are often due to lesions of which cortical area?
   (a) Wernicke's area in the left hemisphere
   (b) Striate cortex in the right hemisphere (area 17)
   (c) Precentral gyrus in the left hemisphere (area 4)
   (d) Broca's area in the left hemisphere
   (e) Posterior parietal cortex in the right hemisphere (area 7)
15. Which of the following connects Wernicke's area in the temporal lobe to Broca's area in the frontal lobe?
   (a) Inferior longitudinal fasciculus
   (b) Corpus callosum
   (c) Arcuate fasciculus
   (d) Corona radiata
   (e) Cingulum
16. Which of the following regions of the body has the largest representation in cortical area 4?
   (a) Trunk muscles
   (b) Muscles of the forearm
   (c) Muscles of mastication
   (d) Muscles of the thumb
   (e) Muscles of the foot
17. Representation of the body parts (somatotopic representation) is found in the:
   (a) postcentral gyrus
   (b) angular gyrus
   (c) primary visual area
   (d) Wernicke's area
   (e) hippocampal gyrus
18. Area 17 in the cerebral cortex is located in the:
   (a) precentral gyrus
   (b) superior temporal gyrus
   (c) parahippocampal gyrus
   (d) occipital lobe
   (e) inferior temporal gyrus
19. Area 4 in the cerebral cortex is located in the:
   (a) middle temporal gyrus
   (b) insula
   (c) occipital lobe
   (d) precentral gyrus
   (e) cingulate gyrus
20. Area 41 in the cerebral cortex is located in the:
   (a) superior temporal gyrus
   (b) superior parietal lobule
   (c) middle temporal gyrus
   (d) postcentral gyrus
   (e) precentral gyrus
21. Areas 3, 1, and 2 in the cerebral cortex are located in the:
   (a) precentral gyrus
   (b) postcentral gyrus
   (c) superior temporal gyrus
   (d) occipital lobe
   (e) middle frontal gyrus
22. Area 19 in the cerebral cortex is located in:
   (a) parietal lobe
   (b) occipital lobe
   (c) frontal lobe
   (d) cingulate gyrus
   (e) parahippocampal gyrus
23. The association fibers of the cerebrum:
   (a) cross from one hemisphere to the other
   (b) remain in the same hemisphere but pass from place to place within the hemisphere
   (c) project from motor areas of the cortex to the tegmentum of the midbrain
   (d) conduct impulses from the spinal cord to the sensory areas of the cortex
   (e) run from the deep layers of the cerebral cortex to the superficial layers

For questions 24-28 study Figure 14-5, showing an axial (horizontal) CT scan of the brain.

24. Identify structure number 1
   (a) frontal lobe
   (b) choroid plexus
   (c) anterior horn of the lateral ventricle
   (d) thalamus
   (e) lentiform nucleus
25. Identify structure number 2
   (a) frontal lobe
   (b) parietal lobe
   (c) temporal lobe
   (d) occipital lobe
   (e) cerebellum

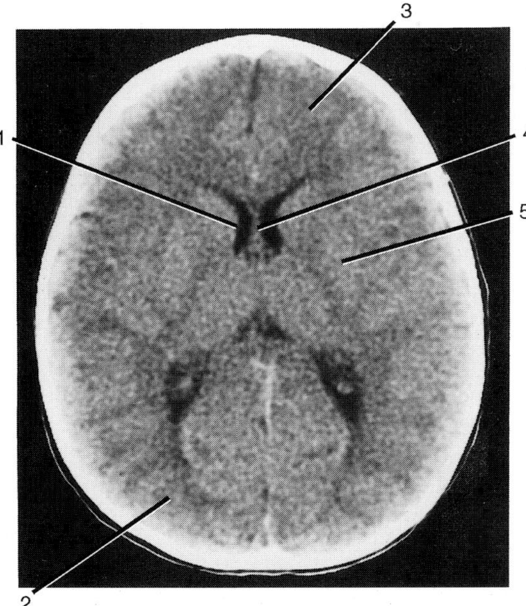

Figure 14–5 Axial (horizontal) CT scan of the brain.

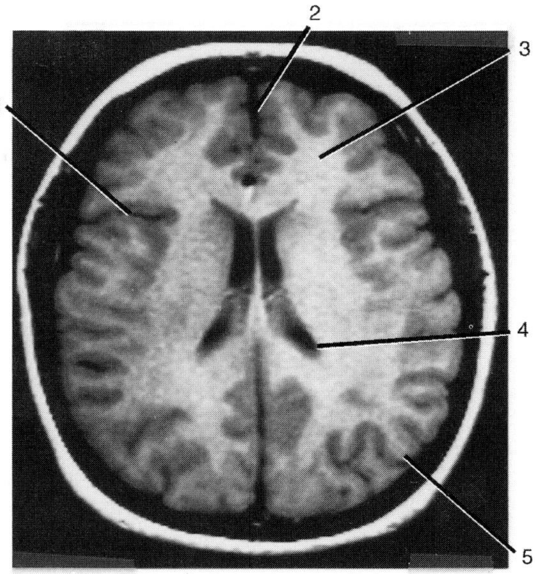

Figure 14–6 Axial (horizontal) MRI scan of the brain.

26. Identify structure number 3
    (a) corpus callosum
    (b) parietal lobe
    (c) lentiform nucleus
    (d) frontal lobe
    (e) temporal lobe
27. Identify structure number 4
    (a) body of the fornix
    (b) septum pellucidum
    (c) genu of the corpus callosum
    (d) rostrum
    (e) choroid plexus
28. Identify the structure number 5
    (a) caudate nucleus
    (b) internal capsule
    (c) lentiform nucleus
    (d) claustrum
    (e) optic radiation

For questions 29-33 study Figure 14-6, showing an axial (horizontal) MRI scan of the brain.

29. Identify structure number 1
    (a) lateral sulcus
    (b) parieto-occipital sulcus
    (c) central sulcus
    (d) longitudinal fissure
    (e) gray matter of occipital lobe
30. Identify structure number 2
    (a) precentral sulcus
    (b) superior frontal sulcus
    (c) lateral sulcus
    (d) longitudinal fissure
    (e) crista galli
31. Identify structure number 3
    (a) white matter of parietal lobe
    (b) gray matter of frontal lobe
    (c) white matter of frontal lobe
    (d) orbital plate of the frontal bone
    (e) forceps major
32. Identify structure number 4
    (a) anterior horn of the lateral ventricle
    (b) body of the lateral ventricle
    (c) inferior horn of the lateral ventricle
    (d) posterior horn of the lateral ventricle
    (e) fourth ventricle
33. Identify structure number 5
    (a) gray matter of parietal lobe
    (b) gray matter of occipital lobe
    (c) forceps minor
    (d) cortex of cerebellar hemisphere
    (e) transverse venous sinus

For questions 34-40 study Figure 14-7, showing a lateral view of the left cerebral hemisphere.

34. Identify the functional area number 1
    (a) primary motor area
    (b) secondary motor area
    (c) secondary auditory area
    (d) secondary somesthetic area
    (e) frontal eye field
35. Identify the functional area number 2
    (a) primary somesthetic area
    (b) secondary somesthetic area
    (c) primary auditory area
    (d) secondary auditory area
    (e) primary motor area

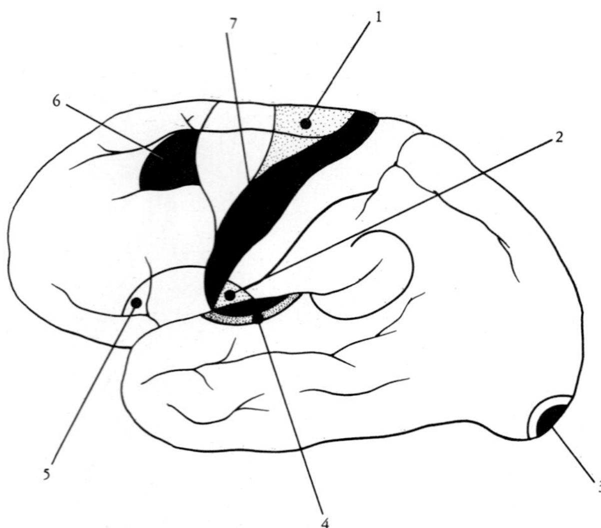

Figure 14–7 Lateral view of the left cerebral hemisphere.

36. Identify the functional area number 3
    (a) primary auditory area
    (b) secondary auditory area
    (c) primary visual area
    (d) secondary visual area
    (e) Wernicke's sensory speech area
37. Identify the functional area number 4
    (a) primary motor area
    (b) primary auditory area
    (c) primary speech area
    (d) primary visual area
    (e) secondary auditory area
38. Identify the functional area number 5
    (a) secondary somesthetic area
    (b) motor speech area
    (c) primary motor area
    (d) secondary motor area
    (e) frontal eye field
39. Identify the functional area number 6
    (a) premotor area
    (b) motor speech area
    (c) primary motor area
    (d) frontal eye field
    (e) primary auditory area
40. Identify the functional area number 7
    (a) primary motor area
    (b) primary somesthetic area
    (c) frontal eye field
    (d) motor speech area
    (e) secondary somesthetic area

Directions: Each of the numbered items in this section is followed by answers that are positively phrased. Select the ONE lettered answer that is an EXCEPTION.

41. The following information concerning the primary motor area is correct **except:**
    (a) Movements of the toes are represented on the medial surface of the cerebral hemisphere
    (b) The anal and urethral sphincters are represented on the paracentral lobule
    (c) The primary motor area receives afferent fibers from the thalamus
    (d) The primary motor area is responsible for the design of the pattern of muscular movement
    (e) The area of cortex controlling a particular movement is proportional to the skill involved in performing the movement
42. The following facts regarding the visual cortex are correct **except:**
    (a) Areas 18 and 19 are visual association areas
    (b) Primary area 17 surrounds the calcarine sulcus
    (c) It is called the striate cortex because of the bands of Baillarger
    (d) Inferior retinal quadrants are projected onto the superior visual cortex
    (e) Because of the large number of stellate cells, the cortex is called granular
43. The prefrontal cortex receives projection fibers from the following structures of the nervous system **except:**
    (a) Thalamus
    (b) Putamen
    (c) Caudate nucleus
    (d) Hypothalamus
    (e) Substantia nigra
44. In the maintenance of normal posture, the alpha motor neurons may receive direct and/or indirect nervous input from the following **except** the:
    (a) Labyrinth and neck muscles
    (b) Cerebral cortex
    (c) Cerebellum
    (d) Muscles and joints
    (e) Nucleus solitarius
45. The precentral gyrus receives inputs either directly or indirectly from the following areas of the nervous system when voluntary movements are performed **except** the:
    (a) Limbic system
    (b) Ascending tracts in the medial lemniscus
    (c) Stria medullaris
    (d) Eyes
    (e) Cerebellum
46. The following facts concerning the hand area on the motor cortex are correct **except:**
    (a) It may be involved in jacksonian epilepsy
    (b) It is larger than the chest area
    (c) It is on the lateral surface of the cerebral hemisphere
    (d) It is one of the smallest areas on the precentral gyrus
    (e) It contains Betz cells and other pyramidal cells

Directions: Read the case history then answer the question. A 57-year-old woman was examined by a neurologist for a suspected brain tumor. With the patient's eyes closed, a spoon was placed in her right hand and she was asked to recognize the object. After moving the spoon around in her hand, she was unable to recognize it. However, on opening her eyes the patient was embarrassed and immediately recognized what was in her hand.

47. This patient was demonstrating astereognosis. In this condition the following facts could be correct **except:**
    (a) This patient has a lesion involving the left parietal lobe
    (b) The tumor involves the left superior parietal lobule
    (c) This area of the cerebral cortex is known as the somesthetic association area
    (d) It is unnecessary for the patient to move the spoon around in her right hand in order to recognize the object
    (e) The association area is where the sensations of touch, pressure, and proprioception are integrated

ANSWERS AND EXPLANATIONS

1. D. (A) The cerebral cortex covers the entire cerebral hemisphere and there are no exceptions. (B) The cerebral cortex is composed entirely of gray matter. (C) The cerebral cortex does send axons to the caudate nucleus. (E) Most areas of the cerebral cortex are made up of six layers; however there are some important exceptions (see p. 154).
2. A. (B) The horizontal cells of Cajal are found in the most superficial layers of the cortex. (C) Betz cells are found in the motor precentral gyrus of the frontal lobe. (D) The cells of Martinotti are present throughout the layers of the cerebral cortex. (E) The bands of Baillarger run horizontally.
3. B. (A) Entering projection, association, and commissural fibers run at right angles to the cortical surface and are known as known as radial fibers. (C) The horizontal cells of Cajal permit activation of functional units some distance away from the incoming afferent fibers. (D) The cerebral cortex sends many axons to the putamen. (E) The sulci in the prefrontal area are similar in depth to other regions of the cortex.
4. C. (A). The precentral gyrus has both motor and sensory functions but the motor function predominates. (B). A homotypical cortex possesses six layers. (D). Clinicopathological studies have been of great value in determining the functional significance of different areas of the cerebral cortex. (E). Experimental ablation studies in animals have provided a great deal of important information regarding cerebral cortical function
5. A. (B). The granular layers are inconspicuous. (C). The giant cells of Betz are concentrated in the superior part of the precentral gyrus. (D). The majority of the corticospinal fibers arise from the small pyramidal cells. (E). Brodmann's area 4 is the primary motor area and occupies the posterior part of the precentral gyrus.
6. E
7. D
8. B. Stimulation of the left postcentral gyrus 7 cm lateral to the midline would excite the cortical area for the right index finger.
9. E
10. A
11. B
12. E. For further details, see page 193.
13. D
14. C
15. C
16. D
17. A
18. D
19. D
20. A
21. B
22. B
23. B
24. C
25. D
26. D
27. B
28. C
29. A
30. D
31. C
32. D
33. B
34. B
35. B
36. C
37. E
38. B
39. D
40. A
41. D. The primary motor area is not responsible for the design of the pattern of muscular movement but is the final station for the conversion of the design into the execution of the movement.
42. D. The inferior retinal quadrants are projected onto the inferior visual cortex.
43. E
44. E
45. C
46. D
47. D. When testing for the presence of astereognosis, it is essential that the patient be allowed to finger the object so that the sensations of touch, pressure, and proprioception are appreciated and integrated in the superior parietal lobule.

CHAPTER 15

Limbic System

CHAPTER OUTLINE

SUGGESTED PLAN FOR REVIEW OF CHAPTER 15

1. Understand that the limbic system consists of a group of structures clustered around the hypothalamus. Learn the names of these structures and know their positions.
2. Understand what is meant by such terms as alveus, fimbria, and dentate gyrus.
3. Learn the position of the parts of the fornix; they are commonly asked in spot examinations when brain specimens are used.
4. Understand how the different parts of the limbic system are connected to the remainder of the nervous system.
5. Learn the functions of the limbic system.

INTRODUCTION

The word limbic means border or margin and the term limbic system includes a group of structures that lie in the border zone between the cerebral cortex and the hypothalamus. The limbic system is involved with many other structures beyond the border zone in the control of emotion, behavior, and drive; it also appears to be important to memory.

Anatomically the limbic structures include the subcallosal, cingulate, and parahippocampal gyri, the hippocampal formation, amygdaloid nucleus, mammillary bodies, and the anterior thalamic nucleus (Fig. 15-1). The alveus, the fimbria, the fornix, the mammillothalamic tract, and the stria terminalis constitute the connecting pathways of this system.

HIPPOCAMPAL FORMATION

The hippocampal formation consists of the hippocampus, the dentate gyrus, and the parahippocampal gyrus.

The **hippocampus** is a curved elevation of gray matter that extends throughout the entire length of the floor of the inferior horn of the lateral ventricle. It is named hippocampus because it resembles a "sea horse" in coronal section. Its anterior end is expanded to form the **pes hippocampus**. The convex ventricular surface is covered with ependyma, beneath which lies a thin layer of white matter called the **alveus**. The alveus consists of nerve fibers that have originated in the hippocampus and these converge medially to form a bundle called the **fimbria**. The fimbria in turn becomes continuous with the crus of the fornix. The hippocampus terminates posteriorly beneath the splenium of the corpus callosum.

The **dentate gyrus** is a narrow, notched band of gray matter that lies between the fimbria of the hippocampus and the parahippocampal gyrus (Fig. 15-1).

The **parahippocampal gyrus** is continuous with the hippocampus along the medial edge of the temporal lobe.

AMYGDALOID NUCLEUS

The amygdaloid nucleus (body) resembles an almond and is situated close to the tip of the inferior horn of the lateral ventricle (Fig. 15-1). It is fused with the tip of the tail of the caudate nucleus, which has passed anteriorly in the roof of the inferior horn of the lateral ventricle. The stria terminalis emerges from its posterior aspect.

CONNECTING PATHWAYS OF THE LIMBIC SYSTEM

These pathways are the alveus, the fimbria, the fornix, the mammillothalamic tract, and the stria terminalis.

The **alveus** consists of nerve fibers that originate in the hippocampal cortex. The fibers converge on the medial border of the hippocampus to form a bundle called the **fimbria**.

The fimbria now leaves the posterior end of the hippocampus as the **crus of the fornix**. This curves posteriorly and superiorly beneath the splenium of the corpus callosum and around the posterior surface of the thalamus. The two crura now converge to form the **body of the fornix**. The body of the fornix splits anteriorly into two anterior **columns of the fornix**. Each column then joins the mammillary body.

The **mammillothalamic tract** provides important connections between the mammillary body and the anterior nuclear group of the thalamus.

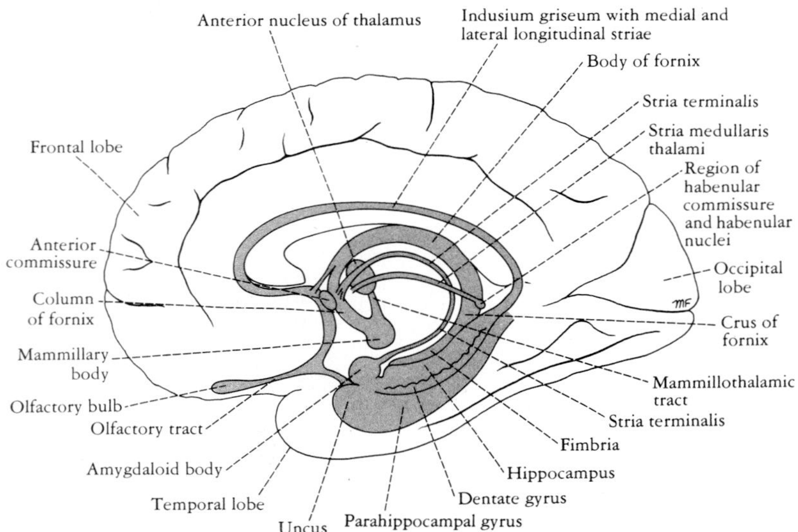

Figure 15–1 The medial surface of the right cerebral hemisphere showing the parts of the limbic system.

The **stria terminalis** emerges from the posterior aspect of the amygdaloid nucleus and follows the curve of the caudate nucleus and comes to lie in the floor of the body of the lateral ventricle.

STRUCTURE OF THE HIPPOCAMPUS

The cortical structure of the parahippocampal gyrus is six-layered. As the cortex is traced into the hippocampus, there is a gradual transition from a six- to a three-layered arrangement. These three layers are the superficial molecular layer, consisting of nerve fibers and scattered small neurons; the **pyramidal layer**, consisting of many large pyramidal-shaped neurons; and the inner **polymorphic layer**, which is similar in structure to the polymorphic layer of the cortex seen elsewhere.

Afferent Connections

Afferent connections of the hippocampus can be divided into six groups (Fig. 15-2).

1. Fibers arising in the cingulate gyrus pass to the hippocampus.
2. Fibers arising from the septal nuclei (nuclei lying within the midline close to the anterior commissure) pass posterior in the fornix to the hippocampus.
3. Fibers arising from one hippocampus pass across the midline to the opposite hippocampus in the fornix.
4. Fibers arising from the indusium griseum (vestigial layer of gray matter on the superior surface of the corpus callosum, Fig. 15-2) pass posteriorly to the hippocampus.
5. Fibers from the entorhinal area or olfactory association cortex pass to the hippocampus.
6. Fibers arising from the dentate and parahippocampal gyri travel to the hippocampus.

Efferent Connections

Axons of the large pyramidal cells of the hippocampus form the alveus and the fimbria and continue as the fornix. The fibers within the fornix are distributed to the following regions (Fig. 15-2):

1. Fibers pass to the anterior commissure to enter the mammillary body, where they end in the medial nucleus.
2. Fibers pass to the anterior commissure to end in the anterior nuclei of the thalamus.
3. Fibers pass to the anterior commissure to enter the tegmentum of the midbrain.
4. Fibers pass to the anterior commissure to end in the septal nuclei, the lateral preoptic area, and the anterior part of the hypothalamus.
5. Fibers join the habenular nuclei.

Consideration of the above complex anatomical pathways indicates that the structures comprising the limbic system are not only interconnected, but also send projection fibers to many different parts of the nervous system. Physiologists now recognize the importance of the hypothalamus as being the major output pathway of the limbic system. The hypothalamus, by means of its connections through the reticular formation with the outflow of the autonomic nervous system, and its control of the endocrine system, is able to influence many aspects of emotional behavior.

FUNCTIONS OF THE LIMBIC SYSTEM

There is considerable evidence to indicate that the limbic system is concerned with emotional behavior, particularly the reactions of fear and anger and the emotions associated with sexual behavior. There also is evidence that the hippocampus is concerned with recent memory. Memory for remote past events usually is unaffected by lesions of this structure.

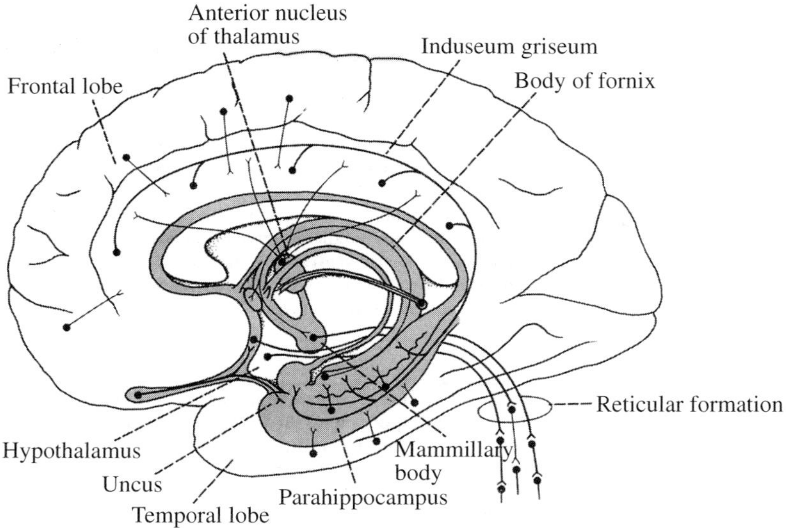

Figure 15–2 Diagram showing some afferent and efferent connections of the limbic system.

CLINICAL NOTES

MALFUNCTION OF THE LIMBIC SYSTEM

This malfunction is involved in psychiatric disorders, including schizophrenia, depression, and senile dementia. Antipsychotic drugs block limbic dopamine receptors.

REVIEW QUESTIONS

Directions: Each of the incomplete statements in this section is followed by completions of the statement. Select the ONE lettered completion that is BEST in each case.

1. The limbic system is:
   (a) phylogenetically among the youngest parts of the brain
   (b) in the form of a ring that surrounds the upper end of the brain stem
   (c) the terminus of nerve fibers that arise from the nucleus gracilis and nucleus cuneatus
   (d) not concerned with emotions, such as the reactions to fear and anger
   (e) functionally uninvolved in sexual behavior
2. The limbic system:
   (a) exerts control over the autonomic system
   (b) outflow does not involve the hypothalamus
   (c) possesses nerve fibers that arise from the cingulate gyrus but do not pass to the hippocampus
   (d) has efferent connections that do not pass from the hippocampus through the fornix
   (e) is not capable of producing changes in blood pressure or respiration

ANSWERS AND EXPLANATIONS

1. B. (A) The limbic structures are phylogenetically among the oldest of the brain. (C) No nerve fibers pass to the limbic system from the nucleus gracilis and nucleus cuneatus. (D) The limbic system is concerned with emotions, such as the reactions of fear and anger. (E) Sexual behavior is definitely affected by the limbic system.
2. A. (B) The hypothalamus is considered to be part of the outflow of the limbic system. (C) Nerve fibers arise from the cingulate gyrus and pass to the hippocampus. (D) The hippocampus sends efferent nerve fibers through the fornix. (E) The limbic system is capable of producing changes in blood pressure and respiration.

CHAPTER 16

Blood Supply of the Brain

CHAPTER OUTLINE

SUGGESTED PLAN FOR REVIEW OF CHAPTER 16

1. The blood supply to the brain is important since many clinical problems arise as the result of arterial hemorrhage or thrombosis. It follows, therefore, that examination questions in this area are common.
2. Be able to make simple diagrams of (a) the circle of Willis and (b) the arterial supply to the cortex on the lateral and medial surfaces of the cerebral hemispheres.
3. Know the blood supply to the internal capsule. This important structure contains the major ascending and descending pathways to the cerebral cortex and it is commonly disrupted as the result of arterial hemorrhage or thrombosis (stroke).
4. Understand the venous drainage of the brain; the details need not be committed to memory.

INTRODUCTION

The normal cerebral blood flow averages 50 to 60 ml/100 g of brain per minute. Positron emission tomography (PET) is now used to measure regional cerebral blood flow. The main arterial inflow is provided by four arteries: two internal carotids and two vertebrals. The two vertebral arteries unite to form the basilar artery, and the basilar artery and the carotids unite to form an important arterial circle, the circle of Willis. The hemispheres are supplied by branches from this circle. The blood is drained by thin-walled valveless cerebral veins into the cranial venous sinuses. The cerebral blood flow is related to the metabolic activity of the nerve tissue and is mainly regulated locally by the concentrations of carbon dioxide, oxygen, and hydrogen ions. Unconsciousness occurs in 5-10 seconds after the cessation of cerebral blood flow and irreversible brain damage rapidly follows.

ARTERIES OF THE BRAIN

The brain is supplied by the two internal carotid and the two vertebral arteries. The four arteries lie within the subarachnoid space and their branches anastomose on the inferior surface of the brain to form the **circle of Willis**.

Internal Carotid Artery

The internal carotid artery begins at the bifurcation of the common carotid artery. It ascends the neck and enters the skull by passing through the carotid canal of the temporal bone. After horizontally running forward through the cavernous sinus, it emerges on the medial side of the anterior clinoid process by perforating the dura mater. It now enters the subarachnoid space and divides into the **anterior** and **middle cerebral arteries** (Fig. 16-1).

BRANCHES OF THE CEREBRAL PORTION

1. The **ophthalmic artery** arises as the internal carotid artery emerges from the cavernous sinus.
2. The **posterior communicating artery** is a small vessel that arises from the internal carotid artery close to its terminal bifurcation (Fig. 16-1). It runs posteriorly above the oculomotor nerve to join the posterior cerebral artery, thus forming part of the circle of Willis.
3. The **choroidal artery**, a small branch, originates from the internal carotid artery close to the terminal bifurcation. The choroidal artery enters the choroid plexus of the inferior horn of the lateral ventricle. It gives off small branches to the crus cerebri, the lateral geniculate body, the optic tract, and the internal capsule.
4. The **anterior cerebral artery** is the smaller terminal branch of the internal carotid artery (Fig. 16-1). It runs forward and medially to enter the longitudinal fissure between the cerebral hemispheres. Here, it is joined to the anterior cerebral artery of the opposite side by the **anterior communicating artery**. It curves backward over the corpus callosum and, finally, anastomoses with the posterior cerebral artery (Fig. 16-1). The **cortical branches**

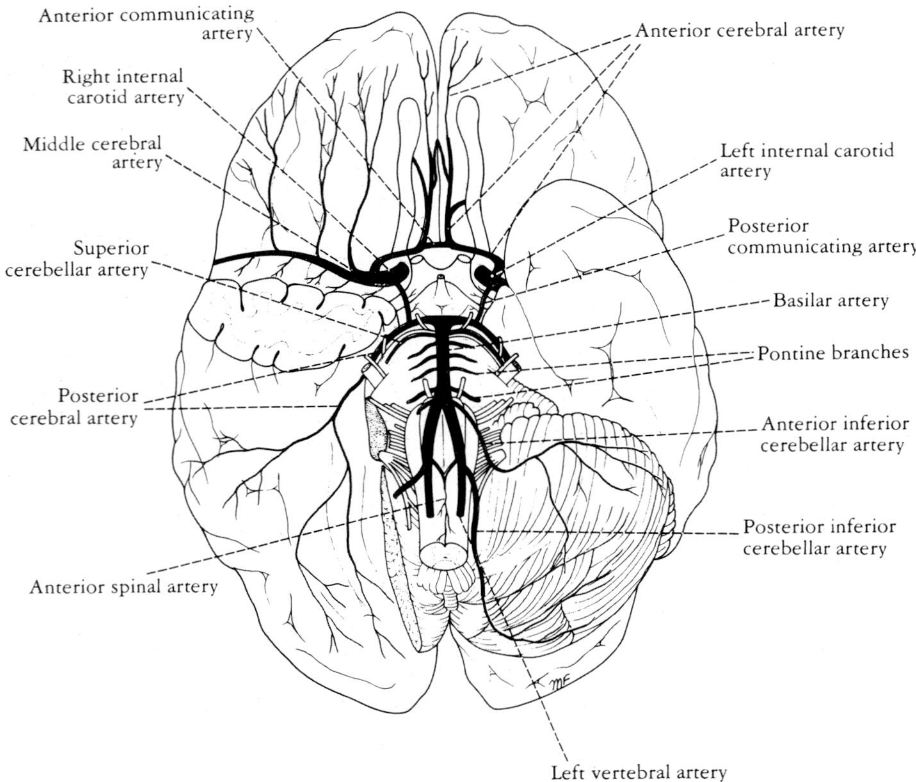

Figure 16–1 Arteries of the inferior surface of the brain. Note the formation of the circle of Willis.

supply all the medial surface of the cerebral cortex as far back as the parieto-occipital sulcus (Fig. 16-2). They also supply a strip of cortex about 1 inch (2.5 cm) wide on the adjoining lateral surface. The anterior cerebral artery thus supplies the "leg area" of the precentral gyrus. A group of **central branches** pierces the anterior perforated substance and helps to supply parts of the lentiform and caudate nuclei and the internal capsule.

5. The **middle cerebral artery**, the largest branch of the internal carotid, runs laterally in the lateral cerebral sulcus (Fig. 16-1). **Cortical branches** supply the entire lateral surface of the hemisphere, except for the narrow strip supplied by the anterior cerebral artery, the occipital pole, and the inferolateral surface of the hemisphere, which are supplied by the posterior cerebral artery (Fig. 16-2). This artery thus supplies all the motor areas except the "leg area." **Central branches** supply the lentiform and caudate nuclei and the internal capsule.

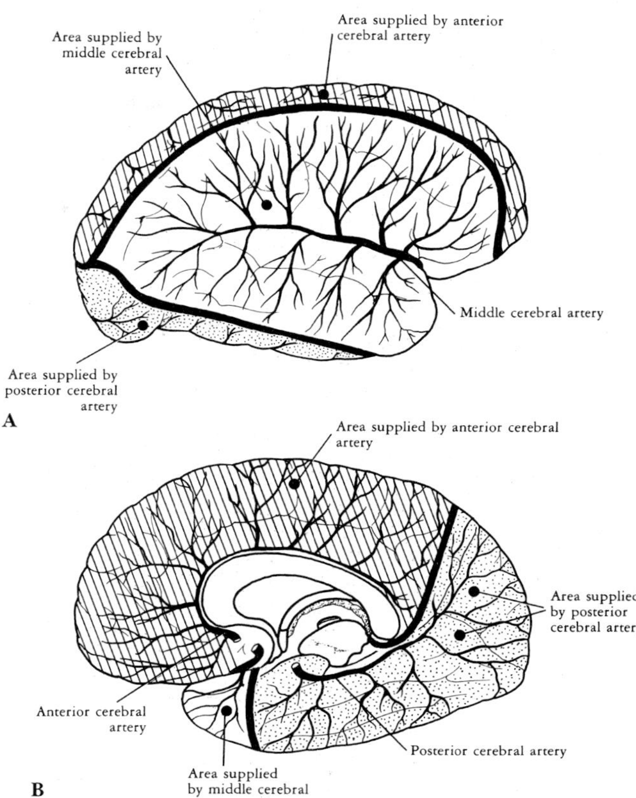

Figure 16–2 Areas of the cortex supplied by the cerebral arteries. **A.** The lateral surface of the right cerebral hemisphere. **B.** The medial surface of the right cerebral hemisphere.

Vertebral Artery

The vertebral artery, a branch of the first part of the subclavian artery, ascends the neck through the foramina in the transverse processes of the upper six cervical vertebrae. It enters the skull through the foramen magnum and pierces the meninges to enter the subarachnoid space. It then passes upward, forward, and medially on the medulla oblongata. At the lower border of the pons, it joins the vessel of the opposite side to form the **basilar artery**.

BRANCHES OF THE CRANIAL PORTION

1. The meningeal branches supply the bone and dura in the posterior cranial fossa.
2. The posterior spinal artery may arise from the vertebral artery or the posterior inferior cerebellar artery. It descends close to the posterior roots of the spinal nerves. The arteries are reinforced by radicular arteries that enter the vertebral canal through the intervertebral foramina.
3. The anterior spinal artery is formed from a contributory branch from each vertebral artery near its termination (Fig. 16-1). The single artery descends on the anterior surface of the medulla oblongata and spinal cord along the anterior median fissure. The artery is reinforced by radicular arteries that enter the vertebral canal through the intervertebral foramina.
4. The posterior inferior cerebellar artery supplies the inferior surface of the vermis, the nuclei of the cerebellum, and the undersurface of the cerebellar hemisphere; it also supplies the medulla oblongata and the choroid plexus of the fourth ventricle.
5. The medullary arteries are small branches that are distributed to the medulla oblongata.

Basilar Artery

The basilar artery, formed by the union of the two vertebral arteries (Fig. 16-1), ascends in a groove on the anterior surface of the pons and ends by dividing into the two posterior cerebral arteries.

BRANCHES

1. The **pontine arteries** are several small vessels that enter the pons (Fig. 16-1).
2. The **labyrinthine artery** accompanies the facial and the vestibulocochlear nerves into the internal acoustic meatus and supplies the internal ear.
3. The **anterior inferior cerebellar artery** supplies the anterior and inferior parts of the cerebellum. A few branches pass to the pons and the upper part of the medulla oblongata.
4. The **superior cerebellar artery** arises close to the termination of the basilar artery and supplies the superior surface of the cerebellum. It also supplies the pons and the pineal gland.
5. The **posterior cerebral artery** curves backward around the midbrain and is joined by the posterior communicating branch of the internal carotid artery (Fig. 16-1). **Cortical branches** supply the inferolateral and medial surfaces of the temporal lobe and the lateral and medial surfaces of the occipital lobe (Fig. 16-2), including the visual cortex. **Central branches** pierce the brain substance

and supply parts of the thalamus and the lentiform nucleus, and the midbrain, the pineal gland, and the medial geniculate bodies. A **choroidal branch** supplies the choroid plexuses of the lateral ventricle and third ventricle.

Circle of Willis

The circle of Willis lies in the interpeduncular fossa at the base of the brain. It is formed by the anastomosis between the two internal carotid arteries and the two vertebral arteries (Figs. 16-1 and 16-3). The anterior communicating, anterior cerebral, internal carotid, posterior communicating, posterior cerebral, and basilar arteries all contribute to the circle. The circle of Willis allows blood that enters by either internal carotid or vertebral arteries to be distributed to any part of both cerebral hemispheres. Cortical and central branches arise from the circle and supply the brain substance. Variations in the sizes of the arteries forming the circle are common and the absence of one or both posterior communicating arteries has been reported.

Although the cerebral arteries anastomose with one another at the circle of Willis and by means of branches on the surface of the cerebral hemispheres, once they enter the brain substance no further anastomoses occur.

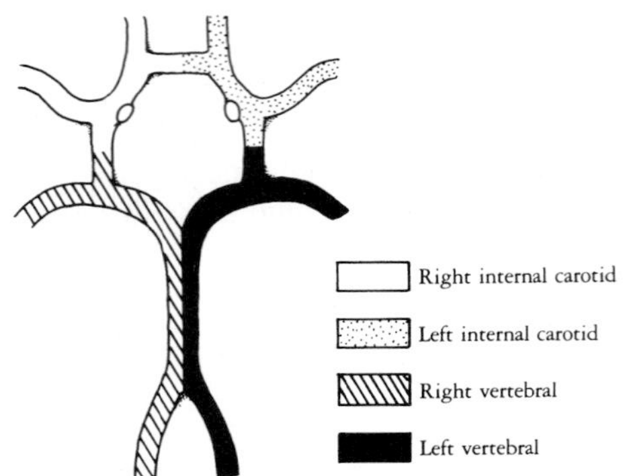

Figure 16–3 Circle of Willis showing the distribution of blood from the four main arteries.

Arteries to Specific Brain Areas

The **corpus striatum** and the **internal capsule** are supplied mainly by the medial and lateral striate central branches of the middle cerebral artery; the central branches of the anterior cerebral artery supply the remainder of these structures.

The **thalamus** is supplied mainly by branches of the posterior communicating, basilar, and posterior cerebral arteries.

The **midbrain** is supplied by the posterior cerebral, superior cerebellar, and basilar arteries.

The **pons** is supplied by the basilar and the anterior, inferior, and superior cerebellar arteries.

The **medulla oblongata** is supplied by the vertebral, anterior and posterior spinal, posterior inferior cerebellar, and basilar arteries.

The **cerebellum** is supplied by the superior cerebellar, anterior inferior cerebellar, and posterior inferior cerebellar arteries.

Nerve Supply to the Cerebral Arteries

Although the cerebral arteries are innervated by sympathetic postganglionic nerve fibers, they apparently play little or no part in the control of cerebral vascular resistance in humans. They do, however, protect the brain from hypertension during severe exercise, by causing vasoconstriction.

The most powerful vasodilator substances for cerebral blood vessels are raised carbon dioxide and hydrogen ion concentrations and reduced oxygen concentrations.

Clinical Notes

Interruption of the Cerebral Circulation

Unconsciousness occurs in 5-10 seconds if the blood flow to the brain is completely cut off. Irreversible brain damage with death of nervous tissue rapidly follows complete arrest of cerebral blood flow. It has been estimated that neuronal function ceases after about 1 minute and that irreversible changes start to occur after about 4 minutes, although this time may be longer if the patient's body has been cooled. Cardiac arrest due to coronary thrombosis is the most common cause of this condition.

Anterior Cerebral Artery Occlusion

Occlusion of the anterior cerebral artery distal to the communicating artery may produce the following signs and symptoms:

1. Contralateral hemiparesis and hemisensory loss involving mainly the leg and foot (paracentral lobule of cortex)
2. Inability to identify objects correctly, apathy, and personality changes (frontal and parietal lobes)

Middle Cerebral Artery Occlusion

Occlusion of the middle cerebral artery may produce the following signs and symptoms:

1. Contralateral hemiparesis and hemisensory loss involving mainly the face and arm (precentral and postcentral gyri)
2. Aphasia if the left hemisphere is affected (rarely if the right hemisphere is affected)
3. Contralateral homonymous hemianopia (damage to the optic radiation)
4. Anosognosia if the right hemisphere is affected (rarely if the left hemisphere is affected)

Posterior Cerebral Artery Occlusion

Occlusion of the posterior cerebral artery may produce the following signs and symptoms:

1. Contralateral homonymous hemianopia with some degree of macular sparing (damage to the calcarine cortex, macular sparing due to the occipital pole receiving collateral blood supply from the middle cerebral artery)
2. Visual agnosia (ischemia of the left occipital lobe)
3. Impairment of memory (possible damage to the medial aspect of the temporal lobe)

INTERNAL CAROTID ARTERY OCCLUSION

The occlusion of the internal carotid artery can occur without causing symptoms or signs or can cause massive cerebral ischemia depending on the degree of collateral anastomoses.

1. The symptoms and signs are those of middle cerebral artery occlusion, including contralateral hemiparesis and hemianesthesia.
2. There is partial or complete loss of sight on the same side but permanent loss is rare (emboli dislodged from the internal carotid artery reach the retina through ophthalmic artery).

VERTEBROBASILAR ARTERY OCCLUSION

The vertebral and basilar arteries supply all the parts of the central nervous system in the posterior cranial fossa, and through the posterior cerebral arteries they supply the visual cortex on both sides. The clinical signs and symptoms are extremely varied.

LATERAL AND MEDIAL MEDULLARY SYNDROMES

Blockage of the posterior inferior cerebellar artery to the lateral part of the medulla produces the **lateral medullary syndrome**. Blockage of the vertebral artery or its anterior spinal branch to the medial part of the medulla produces the **medial medullary syndrome**.

VEINS OF THE BRAIN

The veins of the brain have very thin walls and possess no valves. They emerge from the brain and lie in the subarachnoid space. They pierce the arachnoid mater and the meningeal layer of the dura and drain into the cranial venous sinuses.

External Cerebral Veins

The **superior cerebral veins** ascend over the lateral surface of the cerebral hemisphere and drain into the superior sagittal sinus.

The **superficial middle cerebral vein** drains the lateral surface of the cerebral hemisphere. It empties into the cavernous sinus.

The **deep middle cerebral vein** drains the insula and is joined by the **anterior cerebral and striate veins** to form the **basal vein**. The basal vein joins the great cerebral vein, which drains into the straight sinus.

Internal Cerebral Veins

The two internal cerebral veins are formed by the union of the **thalamostriate vein** and the **choroid vein** at the interventricular foramen. The two veins run posteriorly and unite to form the **great cerebral vein**, which empties into the straight sinus.

Veins of Specific Brain Areas

The **midbrain** is drained by veins that open into the basal or great cerebral veins.

The **pons** is drained by veins that open into the basal vein, cerebellar veins, or neighboring venous sinuses.

The **medulla oblongata** is drained by veins that open into the spinal veins and neighboring venous sinuses.

The **cerebellum** is drained by veins that empty into the great cerebral vein or adjacent venous sinuses.

REVIEW QUESTIONS

Directions: Each of the numbered items in this section is followed by answers that are positively phrased. Select the ONE lettered answer that is an EXCEPTION.

1. The following statements concerning the cerebral blood flow are correct **except:**
   (a) The blood flow is related to the local metabolic activity of the nervous system
   (b) A low oxygen tension in the cerebral blood causes vasodilation of the cerebral blood vessels
   (c) Numerous anastomoses take place between the cerebral arteries once they have gained entrance to the nervous tissue
   (d) The sympathetic nerve fibers have very little control over the diameter of the cerebral arteries
   (e) Positron emission tomography can be used to measure regional cerebral blood flow
2. The following statements concerning the interruption of cerebral blood flow are correct **except:**
   (a) Unconsciousness takes place within about 10 seconds

(b) Cooling the patient's body slows down the process of neuronal degeneration
(c) Cardiac arrest is one of the most common causes of this condition
(d) Irreversible brain damage starts to occur after the blood flow has ceased for about 4 minutes.
(e) A cerebral blood flow of 10 ml/100 g of brain per minute is considered to be normal

3. The following statements concerning the arterial supply to the brain are correct **except:**
(a) The nuclei of the cerebral hemispheres receive their nourishment by diffusion of tissue fluid from the blood vessels on the surface of the brain
(b) The main arteries that supply the brain lie within the subarachnoid space
(c) The basilar artery is formed by the union of the two vertebral arteries
(d) The cerebral arteries anastomose on the surface of the brain
(e) The entire blood supply of the cerebral cortex comes from cortical branches of the anterior, middle, and posterior cerebral arteries

4. The following statements concerning the circle of Willis are correct **except:**
(a) It lies in the interpeduncular fossa at the base of the brain
(b) It is rarely subject to anatomical variation
(c) It lies within the subarachnoid space
(d) It permits the arterial blood to flow across the midline to the opposite side of the brain
(e) It permits the arterial blood to flow forward or backward should the internal carotid or vertebral artery be occluded

5. The following statements concerning the blood supply to the internal capsule are correct **except:**
(a) It is supplied by the central branches of the middle cerebral artery
(b) It is supplied by central branches of the anterior cerebral artery
(c) It is supplied by perforating branches of the posterior cerebral artery
(d) It is a common site for cerebral hemorrhage
(e) Blockage of the arterial supply could compromise both the ascending sensory and the descending motor tracts

Directions: Each of the incomplete statements in this section is followed by completions of the statement. Select the ONE completion that is BEST in each case.

For questions 6-10 study Figure 16-4, showing the lateral surface of the right cerebral hemisphere.

6. The number 1 area of the cerebral cortex receives its arterial supply from the:
(a) anterior cerebral artery
(b) middle cerebral artery
(c) posterior cerebral artery
(d) basilar artery
(e) posterior communicating artery

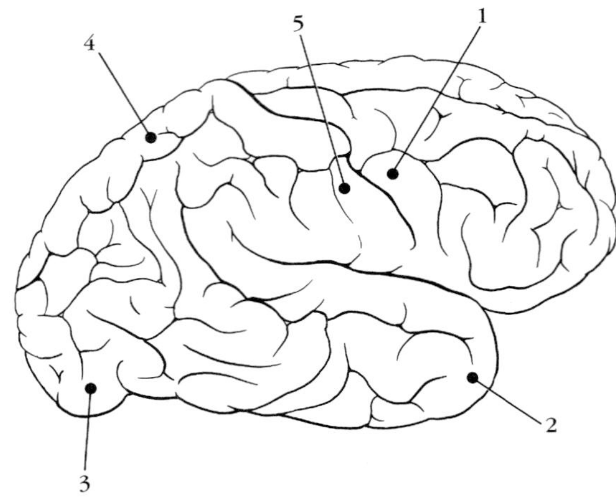

Figure 16–4 Lateral surface of the right cerebral hemisphere.

7. The number 2 area of the cerebral cortex receives its arterial supply from the:
(a) anterior communicating artery
(b) middle cerebral artery
(c) anterior cerebral artery
(d) basilar artery
(e) posterior cerebral artery

8. The number 3 area of the cerebral cortex receives its arterial supply from the:
(a) posterior cerebral artery
(b) anterior cerebral artery
(c) posterior communicating artery
(d) middle cerebral artery
(e) anterior communicating artery

9. The number 4 area of the cerebral cortex receives its arterial supply from the:
(a) middle cerebral artery
(b) basilar artery
(c) lenticulostriate artery
(d) anterior cerebral artery
(e) posterior cerebral artery

10. The number 5 area of the cerebral cortex receives its arterial supply from the:
(a) basilar artery
(b) anterior communicating artery
(c) posterior cerebral artery
(d) anterior cerebral artery
(e) middle cerebral artery

11. The pontine arteries arise from which main stem artery?
(a) Internal carotid artery
(b) External carotid artery
(c) Basilar artery
(d) Vertebral artery
(e) Posterior communicating artery

12. The posterior inferior cerebellar artery arises from which main stem artery?
(a) Basilar artery
(b) Posterior cerebral artery
(c) Anterior cerebral artery
(d) Middle cerebral artery
(e) Vertebral artery

13. The posterior communicating artery arises from which main stem artery?
    (a) Basilar artery
    (b) Vertebral artery
    (c) Internal carotid artery
    (d) External carotid artery
    (e) Anterior cerebral artery
14. The anterior communicating artery arises from which main stem artery?
    (a) Anterior cerebral artery
    (b) Middle cerebral artery
    (c) Posterior cerebral artery
    (d) Basilar artery
    (e) Internal carotid artery
15. The superior cerebellar artery arises from which main stem artery?
    (a) Basilar artery
    (b) Vertebral artery
    (c) Posterior communicating artery
    (d) Internal carotid artery
    (e) Middle cerebral artery
16. The great cerebral vein drains into which venous sinus?
    (a) Transverse sinus
    (b) Superior sagittal sinus
    (c) Straight sinus
    (d) Inferior sagittal sinus
    (e) Cavernous sinus
17. The internal cerebral vein drains into which venous sinus?
    (a) Superior sagittal sinus
    (b) Transverse sinus
    (c) Cavernous sinus
    (d) Straight sinus
    (e) Inferior sagittal sinus
18. The superior cerebral vein drains into which venous sinus?
    (a) Straight sinus
    (b) Occipital sinus
    (c) Cavernous sinus
    (d) Superior sagittal sinus
    (e) Inferior sagittal sinus
19. The superficial middle cerebral vein drains into which venous sinus?
    (a) Intercavernous sinus
    (b) Straight sinus
    (c) Inferior sagittal sinus
    (d) Cavernous sinus
    (e) Superior sagittal sinus
20. The thalamostriate vein drains into which venous sinus?
    (a) Straight sinus
    (b) Inferior sagittal sinus
    (c) Superior sagittal sinus
    (d) Cavernous sinus
    (e) Transverse sinus

For questions 21-25 study Figure 16-5, showing a lateral internal carotid arteriogram.

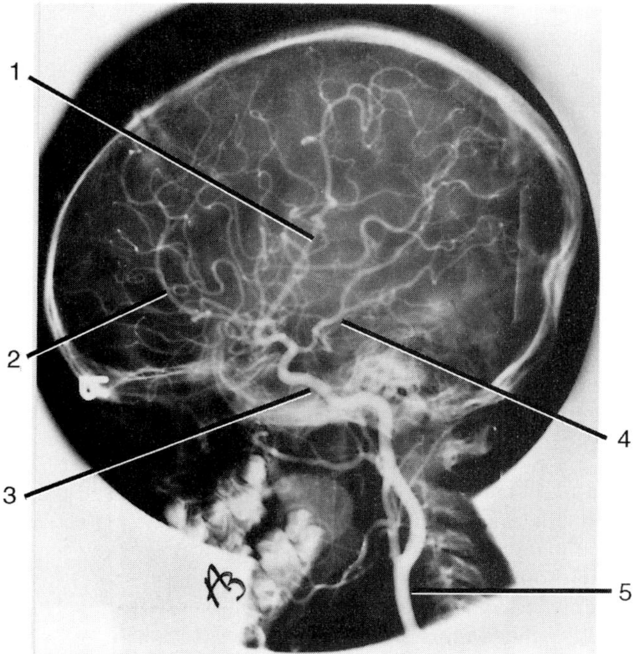

Figure 16–5 Lateral internal carotid arteriogram.

21. The number 1 artery is the:
    (a) internal carotid artery
    (b) posterior cerebral artery
    (c) anterior cerebral artery
    (d) common carotid artery
    (e) middle cerebral artery
22. The number 2 artery is the:
    (a) anterior cerebral artery
    (b) middle cerebral artery
    (c) posterior cerebral artery
    (d) internal carotid artery
    (e) common carotid artery
23. The number 3 artery is the:
    (a) basilar artery
    (b) internal carotid artery
    (c) middle cerebral artery
    (d) anterior cerebral artery
    (e) posterior cerebral artery
24. The number 4 artery is the:
    (a) posterior cerebral artery
    (b) internal carotid artery
    (c) common carotid artery
    (d) external carotid artery
    (e) middle cerebral artery
25. The number 5 artery is the:
    (a) common carotid artery
    (b) internal carotid artery
    (c) external carotid artery
    (d) anterior cerebral artery
    (e) middle cerebral artery

Directions: Read the case history then answer the question. A 71-year-old man was walking along the street when he suddenly collapsed. On admission to the emergency department of the local hospital he was found to have paralysis on the right side of his body, mainly involving the right leg. There was also some sensory loss of the right foot and ankle. The sudden onset of the right-sided hemiplegia and hemianesthesia made the diagnosis of a cerebrovascular accident most probable.

26. The following considerations in this patient are correct **except:**
    (a) The lesion may involve the left cerebral hemisphere
    (b) The right-sided hemiplegia most probably involves the left precentral gyrus
    (c) Since the signs of the paralysis are limited to the right leg and foot, the vascular defect probably involves the upper part of the precentral gyrus and the paracentral lobule
    (d) The loss of cutaneous sensation on the right foot and ankle may be due to a lesion of the left postcentral gyrus and the paracentral lobule
    (e) The left middle cerebral artery or one of its branches may be blocked by a thrombus or an embolus

ANSWERS AND EXPLANATIONS

1. C. Once a cerebral artery enters the substance of the brain, it does not anastomose with another artery.
2. E. The normal cerebral blood flow is about 50 to 60 mg/100 g of brain per minute.
3. A. The nuclei that lie deep within the cerebral hemispheres receive their arterial supply from the central branches of the cerebral arteries.
4. B. The circle of Willis is subject to frequent anatomical variations. Cerebral and communicating arteries, anterior and posterior, may be absent, reduced in size, or double.
5. C. The posterior cerebral artery does not supply the internal capsule.
6. B
7. B
8. A
9. D
10. E
11. C
12. E
13. C
14. A
15. A
16. C
17. D
18. D
19. D
20. A
21. E
22. A
23. B
24. A
25. A
26. E. The cortical branches of the anterior cerebral artery supply all the medial surface of the cerebral hemisphere as far back as the parieto-occipital sulcus. They also supply a strip of cortex about 1 inch wide on the adjoining lateral surface. The left anterior cerebral artery, and not the left middle cerebral artery, thus supplies the "right leg area" of the left precentral gyrus.

CHAPTER 17

The Cerebrospinal Fluid, the Ventricles of the Brain, and the Brain Barriers

CHAPTER OUTLINE

SUGGESTED PLAN FOR REVIEW OF CHAPTER 17

1. Know the composition and functions of the cerebrospinal fluid (CSF).
2. Be able to describe the formation, circulation, and absorption of the CSF. Know the sites where the circulation is commonly obstructed.
3. Learn the boundaries and openings of the lateral, third, and fourth ventricles. Be able to identify the structures that lie beneath the floor of the fourth ventricle.
4. Understand the subarachnoid space and know the locations of the main cisterns.
5. Learn in detail the anatomy of spinal tap; this is a common clinical procedure.
6. Know the CSF pressure and remember that it is expressed in millimeters (mm) of water and not mercury. Know what Queckenstedt's sign is.
7. Be able to define the following: (a) hydrocephalus, (b) blood-brain barrier, and (c) blood–cerebrospinal fluid barrier.
8. Learn the detailed structure of the blood-brain barrier.

INTRODUCTION

The cerebrospinal fluid is a clear, colorless liquid that fills the ventricles of the brain and bathes the external surface of the brain and spinal cord. It is formed from the choroid plexuses within the ventricles and circulates through the three openings in the roof of the fourth ventricle to reach the subarachnoid space. The fluid is produced continuously at a rate of about 0.5 ml per minute and with a total volume of about 130 ml; this corresponds to a turnover time of about 5 hours.

COMPOSITION AND PRESSURE OF CEREBROSPINAL FLUID

The CSF has a specific gravity of about 1.007. It possesses, in solution, inorganic salts similar to those in the blood plasma. The glucose content is about half that of blood and there is only a trace of protein. A few cells are present and these are lymphocytes. The normal lymphocyte count is 0 to 3 cells per cu mm. In the lateral recumbent position the cerebrospinal fluid pressure, as measured by spinal tap, is about 60 to 150 mm of water. This pressure may be easily raised by straining, coughing, or compressing the internal jugular veins in the neck.

Table 17-1 summarizes the physical characteristics and composition of the CSF.

Table 17–1 Summary of the Physical Characteristics and Composition of the Cerebrospinal Fluid

Appearance	Clear and colorless
Volume	130 ml
Rate of production	0.5 ml/min
Pressure (spinal tap with patient in lateral recumbent position)	60–150 mm of water
Composition	
Protein	15–45 mg/100 ml
Glucose	50–85 mg/100 ml
Chloride	720–750 mg/100 ml
Cells	0–3 lymphocytes/cu mm

FUNCTION OF THE CEREBROSPINAL FLUID

The CSF serves as a protective cushion between the central nervous system and the surrounding bones. Because the density of the brain is only slightly greater than that of the CSF, the latter provides mechanical buoyancy and support for the brain. The close relationship of the fluid to the nervous tissue and the blood enables it to serve as a reservoir and assist in the regulation of the contents of the skull. The CSF is an ideal physiological substrate and probably plays an active part in the nourishment of the nervous tissue; it almost certainly assists in the removal of products of neuronal metabolism. The secretions of the pineal gland possibly influence the activities of the pituitary gland by circulating through the CSF in the third ventricle (Box 17-1).

Box 17–1 Functions of the Cerebrospinal Fluid

1. Cushions and protects the central nervous system from trauma.
2. Provides mechanical buoyancy and support for the brain.
3. Serves as a reservoir and assists in the regulation of the contents of the skull.
4. Nourishes the central nervous system.
5. Removes metabolites from the central nervous system.
6. Serves as a pathway for pineal secretions to reach the pituitary gland.

FORMATION OF CEREBROSPINAL FLUID

The CSF is formed in the choroid plexuses of the lateral, third, and fourth ventricles; some originates as tissue fluid in the brain substance.

The choroid plexuses have a folded surface and consist of a core of vascular connective tissue covered with cuboidal epithelium of the ependyma. The blood of the capillaries is separated from the ventricular lumen by fenestrated endothelium, a basement membrane, and the surface epithelium. The ependymal cells of the choroid plexuses actively secrete the CSF.

CIRCULATION OF CEREBROSPINAL FLUID

The fluid passes from the lateral ventricles into the third ventricle through the interventricular foramina (Fig. 17-1). It then passes into the fourth ventricle through the cerebral aqueduct. The circulation is aided by the arterial pulsations of the choroid plexuses and the cilia on the ependymal cells lining the ventricles.

From the fourth ventricle, the fluid passes through the median aperture (**foramen of Magendie**) and the lateral foramina (**foramina of Luschka**) of the lateral recesses of the fourth ventricle and enters the subarachnoid space. The fluid then flows superiorly through the interval in the tentorium cerebelli to reach the inferior surface of the cerebrum (Fig. 17-1). It now moves superiorly over the lateral aspect of each cerebral hemisphere. Some of the CSF moves inferiorly in the subarachnoid space around the spinal cord and cauda equina. The pulsations of the cerebral and spinal arteries and the movements of the vertebral column facilitate this flow of fluid.

ABSORPTION OF CEREBROSPINAL FLUID

The CSF is absorbed into the **arachnoid villi** that project into the dural venous sinuses, especially the **superior sagittal sinus** (Fig. 17-1). The arachnoid villi are grouped together to form **arachnoid granulations**. Each arachnoid villus is a diverticulum of the subarachnoid space that pierces the dura mater.

Absorption of CSF into the venous sinuses occurs when the CSF pressure exceeds that in the sinus. Studies of the arachnoid villi indicate that fine tubules lined with endothelium permit a direct flow of fluid from the subarachnoid space into the lumen of the venous sinuses. Should the venous pressure rise and exceed the CSF pressure, compression of the villi closes the tubules and prevents the reflux of blood into the subarachnoid space.

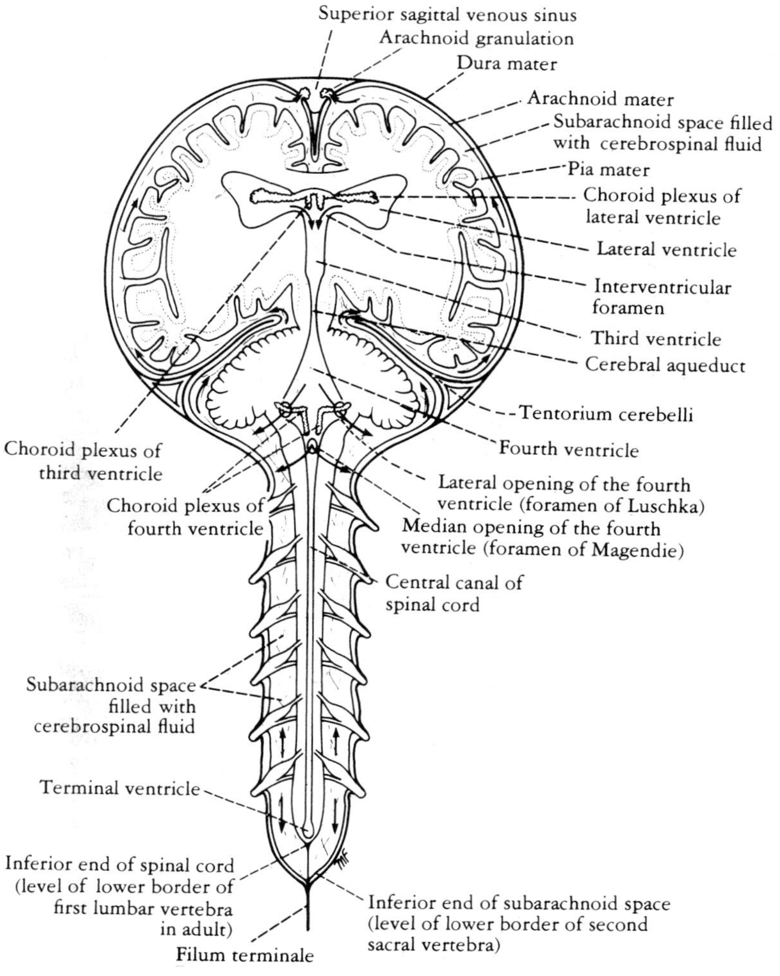

Figure 17–1 Circulation of the cerebrospinal fluid.

Some of the CSF is absorbed directly into the veins in the subarachnoid space and escapes through the perineural lymph vessels of the cranial and spinal nerves.

VENTRICULAR SYSTEM

The ventricles of the brain are the lateral ventricles, the third ventricle, and the fourth ventricle (Fig.17-1). They are developmentally derived from the cavity of the neural tube. They are lined throughout with **ependyma** and are filled with **cerebrospinal fluid**.

Lateral Ventricles

There are two lateral ventricles and one is present in each cerebral hemisphere (Fig. 17-2). Each ventricle is a roughly C-shaped cavity and includes a **body,** which occupies the parietal lobe and from which **anterior, posterior,** and **inferior horns** extend into the frontal, occipital, and temporal lobes, respectively. The lateral ventricles communicate with the cavity of the third ventricle through the **interventricular foramen** (Fig. 17-1), which lies in the medial wall of each ventricle. The **choroid plexus of the lateral ventricles** projects into each ventricle on its medial aspect.

Third Ventricle

The third ventricle is a slitlike cleft between the two thalami. It communicates anteriorly with the lateral ventricles through the interventricular foramina (of Monro) and posteriorly with the fourth ventricle through the cerebral aqueduct (of Sylvius) (Fig. 17-1). The **choroid plexuses of the third ventricle** hang from the roof.

The blood supply of the choroid plexuses of the third and lateral ventricles is derived from the choroidal branches of the internal carotid and basilar arteries. The venous blood drains into the internal cerebral veins.

Cerebral Aqueduct (Aqueduct of Sylvius)

The cerebral aqueduct, a narrow channel about 3/4 inch (1.8 cm) long, connects the third with the fourth ventricle (Fig. 17-1). It is lined with ependyma and is surrounded by a layer of gray matter called the **central gray**. The direction of flow of CSF is from the third to the fourth ventricle. There is no choroid plexus in the cerebral aqueduct.

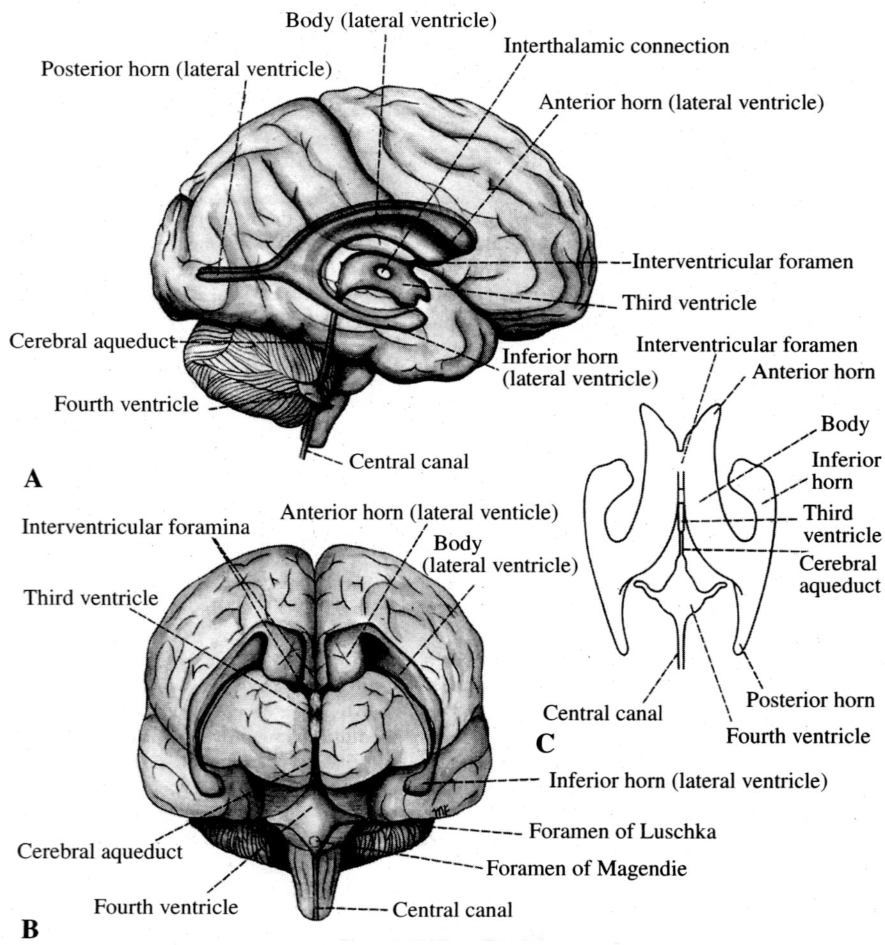

Figure 17–2 Cast of the ventricular cavities of the brain as seen from lateral view (**A**), anterior view (**B**), and superior view (**C**).

Fourth Ventricle

The fourth ventricle is a tent-shaped cavity filled with cerebrospinal fluid. It is situated anterior to the cerebellum and posterior to the pons and the superior half of the medulla oblongata (Fig. 17-2). It is continuous above with the cerebral aqueduct and below with the central canal of the spinal cord. The fourth ventricle possesses lateral boundaries, a roof, and a rhomboid-shaped floor. The lateral boundaries are formed by the **superior and inferior cerebellar peduncles**.

The roof the fourth ventricle projects into the cerebellum. It is formed by the **superior medullary velum** above and the **inferior medullary velum** below. The inferior medullary velum is pierced in the midline by a large opening, the **median aperture, the foramen of Magendie**.

The floor is formed by the posterior surface of the pons and the cranial half of the medulla oblongata (see Fig. 8-6). In the midline is the **median sulcus**. On each side of this sulcus is the **median eminence**, which is bounded laterally by the **sulcus limitans**. Lateral to the sulcus limitans there is the **vestibular area**, beneath which lie the vestibular nuclei. The **facial colliculus**, produced by the fibers of the facial nerve looping over the abducens nucleus, lies at the inferior end of the medial eminence.

Strands of nerve fibers, the **stria medullaris**, emerge from the median sulcus and pass laterally to enter the inferior cerebellar peduncle. Inferior to the stria lies the hypoglossal triangle formed by the underlying **hypoglossal nucleus** and lateral to this lies the **vagal triangle** produced by the underlying dorsal motor nucleus of the vagus.

Lateral recesses extend around the sides of the medulla and open anteriorly as the **lateral openings of the fourth ventricle**, or the **foramina of Luschka** (Fig. 17-1). It is through these two openings and the foramen of Magendie that the CSF enters the subarachnoid space.

The **choroid plexus of the fourth ventricle** is suspended from the interior half of the roof of the ventricle. The blood supply to the plexus is from the posterior inferior cerebellar arteries.

CENTRAL CANAL OF THE SPINAL CORD AND MEDULLA OBLONGATA

The central canal opens superiorly into the fourth ventricle. Inferiorly, it extends through the inferior half of the medulla oblongata and through the entire length of the spinal cord. In the conus medullaris of the spinal cord, it expands to form the **terminal ventricle**. The central canal is closed at its lower end, is filled with cerebrospinal fluid, and is lined with ependyma. The central canal is surrounded by gray matter, the **gray commissure**. There is no choroid plexus in the central canal

SUBARACHNOID SPACE

The subarachnoid space is the interval between the arachnoid mater and pia mater and envelops the brain and spinal cord (Fig. 17-1). The space is filled with CSF and contains the large blood vessels of the brain. Inferiorly, the subarachnoid space extends beyond the lower end of the spinal cord and invests the **cauda equina**. The subarachnoid space ends below at the level of the interval between the second and third sacral vertebrae.

Subarachnoid Cisterns

In certain locations around the base of the brain, the arachnoid does not closely follow the surface of the brain so that the subarachnoid space expands to form cisterns. The **cerebellomedullary cistern** lies between the cerebellum and the medulla oblongata, the **pontine cistern** lies on the anterior surface of the pons, and the **interpeduncular cistern** lies on the anterior surface of the midbrain between the crura cerebri.

Extensions of the Subarachnoid Space

A sleeve of the subarachnoid space extends around the optic nerve to the back of the eyeball. Here the arachnoid mater and pia mater fuse with the sclera. The central artery and vein of the retina cross this extension of the subarachnoid space to enter the optic nerve and they may be compressed in patients with raised CSF pressure. Small extensions of the subarachnoid space also occur around the other cranial and spinal nerves.

The subarachnoid space also extends around the arteries and veins of the brain and spinal cord at points where they penetrate the nervous tissue. The pia mater, however, quickly fuses with the outer coat of the blood vessel below the surface of the brain and spinal cord, thus closing off the subarachnoid space.

CLINICAL NOTES

SPINAL TAP

A spinal tap can be performed to withdraw a sample of CSF for microscopic or bacteriological examination or to inject drugs to combat infection or induce anesthesia. Fortunately, the spinal cord terminates inferiorly at the level of the lower border of the first lumbar vertebra in the adult. (In the infant it may reach inferiorly to the third lumbar vertebra.) The subarachnoid space extends inferiorly as far as the lower border of the second sacral vertebra.

With the patient lying on one side with the vertebral column well flexed, the space between adjoining laminae in the lumbar region is opened to a maximum. An imaginary line joining the highest points on the iliac crests passes over the fourth lumbar spine. Using a careful aseptic technique and local anesthesia, the physician passes the spinal tap needle, fitted with a stylet, into the vertebral canal above or below the fourth lumbar spine. The needle will pass through the following anatomical structures before it enters the subarachnoid space: (1) skin, (2) superficial fascia, (3) supraspinous ligament, (4) interspinous ligament, (5) ligamentum flavum, (6) areolar tissue containing the internal vertebral venous plexus, (7) dura mater, and (8) arachnoid mater. The depth to which the needle will have to pass will vary from 1 inch (2.5 cm) or less in a child to as much as 4 inches (10 cm) in an obese adult.

The CSF pressure can be measured by attaching a manometer to the needle. When the patient is in the recumbent position, the **normal pressure is about 60 to 150 mm of water**. The pressure shows oscillations corresponding to the movements of respiration and the arterial pulse.

A block of the subarachnoid space in the vertebral canal, which may be caused by a tumor of the spinal cord or the meninges, may be detected by compressing the internal jugular veins in the neck. This raises the cerebral venous pressure and inhibits the absorption of CSF in the arachnoid granulations, thus producing a rise in the manometer reading of the CSF pressure. If this rise fails to occur, the subarachnoid space is blocked and the patient is said to exhibit a positive **Queckenstedt's sign**.

Papilledema

An abnormal rise in CSF pressure, as may occur in the presence of a cerebral tumor, will compress the thin walls of the retinal vein as it crosses the extension of the subarachnoid space to enter the optic nerve. This will result in congestion of the retinal vein, bulging forward of the optic disc, and edema of the disc; the last condition is known as **papilledema**. Since both subarachnoid extensions are continuous with the intracranial subarachnoid space, both eyes will exhibit papilledema. Persistent papilledema leads to optic atrophy and blindness.

Blockage of the Circulation of Cerebrospinal Fluid

An obstruction of the interventricular foramen by a tumor will block the drainage of the lateral ventricle on that side. The continued production of cerebrospinal fluid by the choroid plexus of that ventricle will cause distention of that ventricle and atrophy of the surrounding neural tissue.

An obstruction in the cerebral aqueduct may be congenital or result from inflammation or pressure from a tumor. This causes a symmetrical distention of both lateral ventricles and distention of the third ventricle.

Obstruction of the median aperture (foramen of Magendie) in the roof of the fourth ventricle and the two lateral apertures (foramina of Luschka) in the lateral recesses of the fourth ventricle by inflammatory exudate, or by tumor growth, will produce symmetrical dilatation of both lateral ventricles and the third and fourth ventricles.

Sometimes inflammatory exudate secondary to meningitis will block the subarachnoid space and obstruct the flow of cerebrospinal fluid over the outer surface of the cerebral hemispheres. Here, again, the entire ventricular system of the brain will become distended.

Hydrocephalus

Hydrocephalus is an abnormal increase in the volume of the CSF within the skull. If the hydrocephalus is accompanied by a raised CSF pressure, then it is due to either (1) an abnormal increase in the formation of the fluid, (2) a blockage of the circulation of the fluid, or (3) a diminished absorption of the fluid. Rarely, hydrocephalus occurs with a normal CSF pressure and in these patients there is a compensatory hypoplasia or atrophy of the brain substance.

BLOOD-BRAIN BARRIER

The blood-brain barrier protects the brain from toxic compounds. In certain situations, however, it is important that the nerve cells be exposed without a barrier to the circulating blood. This enables neuronal receptors to sample the plasma directly and to respond and maintain the normal internal environment of the body within very fine limits. There is no blood-brain barrier in the pineal gland, the hypothalamus, the posterior lobe of the pituitary, the tuber cinereum, the wall of the optic recess, and the area postrema at the lower end of the fourth ventricle.

The blood-brain barrier is formed by the tight junctions between the endothelial cells of the blood capillaries. In those areas where the blood-brain barrier is absent, the capillary endothelium contains fenestrations across which proteins and small organic molecules can pass from the blood to the nervous tissue.

CLINICAL NOTES

KERNICTERUS

In the newborn child or premature infant in whom the blood-brain barrier is not fully developed, toxic substances such as bilirubin can readily enter the central nervous system and produce yellowing of the brain and kernicterus.

BRAIN TRAUMA AND THE BLOOD-BRAIN BARRIER

Injury to the brain, whether it is due to direct trauma or to inflammatory or chemical toxins, can cause a breakdown of the blood-brain barrier. This allows the free diffusion of large molecules into the nervous tissue.

DRUGS AND THE BLOOD-BRAIN BARRIER

The blood-brain barrier prevents the entrance of certain drugs into the nervous tissue. Penicillin, for example, which is toxic to nervous tissue, is largely blocked by the barrier. Other antibiotics such as chloramphenicol and the tetracyclines readily cross the barrier.

BLOOD CEREBROSPINAL-FLUID BARRIER

There is free passage of water, gases, and lipid-soluble substances from the blood to the CSF. Macromolecules such as proteins and most hexoses other than glucose are unable to enter the CSF. It has been suggested that a barrier similar to the blood-brain barrier exists in the choroid plexuses and it is probable that the tight junctions between the choroidal epithelial cells serve as the barrier.

CEREBROSPINAL FLUID-BRAIN INTERFACE

There is no physiological barrier between the CSF and the extracellular compartment of the central nervous system so that the extracellular spaces of the nervous tissue are in almost direct continuity with the subarachnoid space.

REVIEW QUESTIONS

Directions: Each of the numbered items in this section is followed by answers that are positively phrased. Select the ONE lettered answer that is an EXCEPTION.

1. The following statements concerning cerebrospinal fluid are correct **except:**
   (a) The normal glucose concentration is about half that of blood
   (b) The CSF has a specific gravity of about 1.007
   (c) The total volume of CSF is about 130 ml
   (d) The CSF is produced continuously by the choroid plexuses
   (e) The normal lymphocyte count in cerebrospinal fluid is 20 to 30 cells per cu mm
2. The following statements concerning cerebrospinal fluid are correct **except:**
   (a) The normal CSF pressure in the lateral recumbent position is about 60 to 150 mm water
   (b) Compression of the internal jugular veins lowers the CSF pressure
   (c) The CSF is found in the ventricles of the brain and in the subarachnoid space
   (d) The choroid plexuses are located in the lateral, third, and fourth ventricles
   (e) The third ventricle is joined to the fourth ventricle by the aqueduct of Sylvius
3. The following statements concerning the lateral ventricle are correct **except:**
   (a) The ventricle is C-shaped and follows the curve of the caudate nucleus
   (b) It is present in the frontal, parietal, occipital, and temporal lobes of the cerebral hemisphere
   (c) It communicates with the third ventricle through its medial wall
   (d) The choroid plexus projects into the ventricle through the lateral wall
   (e) The posterior horn arises at the junction of the body with the inferior horn
4. The following statements concerning the fourth ventricle are correct **except:**
   (a) The cerebellum is located in its roof
   (b) The foramen of Magendie is situated in the inferior medullary velum
   (c) The facial colliculus lies in the floor of the upper part of the ventricle
   (d) The foramina of Luschka allow the cerebrospinal fluid to escape into the subarachnoid space
   (e) The nucleus of the fourth cranial nerve lies beneath the floor
5. The following statements concerning the subarachnoid space are correct **except:**
   (a) The space is the interval between the arachnoid and the dura mater
   (b) It is expanded to form cisterns
   (c) The space receives CSF through three holes in the fourth ventricle
   (d) It terminates below in the adult at the level of the interval between the second and third sacral vertebrae
   (e) It surrounds the cauda equina
6. The following statements concerning the circulation of the CSF are correct **except:**
   (a) The arterial pulsations of the choroidal arteries and the cerebral arteries aid the circulation of the fluid
   (b) The fluid reaches the cerebral hemispheres by passing through the notch in the tentorium cerebelli

(c) The fluid escapes from the central canal of the spinal cord through an aperture in the roof of the terminal ventricle
(d) Some of the fluid moves inferiorly around the spinal cord in the subarachnoid space
(e) The movements of the vertebral column assist in the mixing of the CSF

7. The following statements concerning the procedure of spinal tap are correct **except:**
(a) With the patient lying on the side with the vertebral column well flexed, the space between adjoining laminae in the lumbar region is opened to a maximum
(b) The needle is inserted above or below the fourth lumbar spine
(c) The needle will pierce the supraspinous and interspinous ligaments and the ligamentum flavum before penetrating the meninges
(d) The needle is not likely to pierce the internal vertebral venous plexus
(e) An imaginary line joining the highest points of the iliac crests is used to locate the level of the fourth lumbar spine

8. The following statements concerning the CSF pressure are correct **except:**
(a) The pressure shows oscillations corresponding to the arterial pulse
(b) The pressure is lowered when the patient coughs
(c) Queckenstedt's sign may be positive if the spinal part of the subarachnoid is blocked by tumor
(d) The pressure will rise if the arachnoid villi are blocked by inflammatory exudate
(e) The pressure changes with the respiratory movements of the patient

9. The following statements concerning hydrocephalus are correct **except:**
(a) It is an abnormal increase in the volume of CSF in the skull
(b) It can be caused by a blockage of the circulation of the CSF
(c) It is never accompanied by hypoplasia of the brain
(d) It can be caused by a diminished absorption of the CSF
(e) Blockage of the cerebral aqueduct can produce hydrocephalus

10. The following statements concerning the blood-brain barrier are correct **except:**
(a) The blood-brain barrier protects the brain from toxic compounds
(b) The blood-brain barrier is absent from the hypothalamus
(c) The blood-brain barrier is incompletely formed in the newborn
(d) The blood-brain barrier is formed by the tight junctions between the endothelial cells of the blood capillaries
(e) Penicillin passes freely across the blood-brain barrier

11. The following statements concerning the CSF are correct **except:**
(a) The CSF plays no role in the transport of hormones
(b) The CSF can flow directly into the venous blood at the arachnoid granulations
(c) The CSF flows directly into the neuropil of the central nervous system from the ventricles
(d) The CSF flows directly into the neuropil through the pia mater
(e) The CSF that extends along the spinal nerves is absorbed into the perineural lymph vessels

Directions: Each of the numbered items or incomplete statements in this section is followed by answers or completions of the statement. Select the ONE lettered answer or completion that is BEST in each case.

12. Which of the following statements concerning the third ventricle is (are) correct?
(a) The optic chiasma is placed in its floor
(b) The choroid plexus is situated in the floor
(c) The cavity is lined with pia mater
(d) The cavity is restricted to an area below the interthalamic connection
(e) The hypothalamus lies in its anterior wall

13. Which of the following statements concerning the formation of the CSF is (are) correct?
(a) The choroid plexuses actively secrete cerebrospinal fluid
(b) The cells responsible for the formation of the cerebrospinal fluid are the endothelial cells of the choroidal blood capillaries
(c) The tissue fluid of the brain does not contribute to the CSF
(d) There is extensive diffusion of fluid from the cerebral veins situated in the subarachnoid space
(e) The arachnoid villi actively secrete cerebrospinal fluid

For questions 14-19 study Figure 17-3, showing the floor of the fourth ventricle.

14. Structure number 1 is the:
(a) sulcus limitans
(b) vestibular area
(c) hypoglossal triangle
(d) facial colliculus
(e) medial eminence

15. Structure number 2 is the:
(a) median sulcus
(b) sulcus limitans
(c) hypoglossal triangle
(d) facial colliculus
(e) vestibular area

16. Structure number 3 is the:
(a) hypoglossal triangle
(b) vagal triangle
(c) median sulcus
(d) facial colliculus
(e) vestibular area

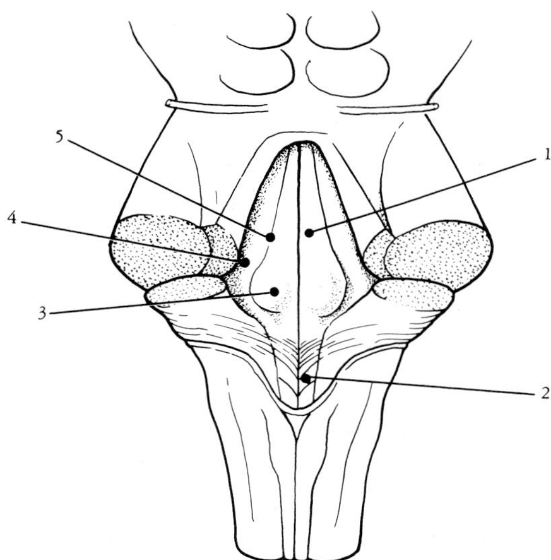

Figure 17–3 Floor of the fourth ventricle.

17. Structure number 4 is the:
    (a) facial colliculus
    (b) sulcus limitans
    (c) vestibular area
    (d) hypoglossal triangle
    (e) facial colliculus
18. Structure number 5 is the:
    (a) vestibular area
    (b) sulcus limitans
    (c) medial eminence
    (d) median sulcus
    (e) stria medullaris
19. In Figure 17-4 showing an axial (horizontal) PET scan of the brain, identify the curved white structures.
    (a) Caudate nucleus
    (b) Thalamus
    (c) Lateral ventricle
    (d) Corpus striatum
    (e) Choroid plexus

Directions: Read the case history, then answer the question. A 47-year-old man was diagnosed as having a rapidly growing intracranial tumor. One of the clinical findings on ophthalmoscopic examination was bilateral papilledema and congestion of the retinal veins.

20. The following statements concerning this patient's condition are correct **except:**
    (a) The papilledema is bilateral because the subarachnoid space extends forward around both optic nerves to the back of the eyeballs
    (b) A rise in CSF pressure compresses the retinal vein as it crosses the subarachnoid extension to enter the optic nerve
    (c) The edema of the optic disc results in the disc bulging forward
    (d) The central artery of the retina is also compressed by the rise in CSF pressure and this results in ischemia of the retina
    (e) Persistent papilledema leads to optic atrophy and blindness

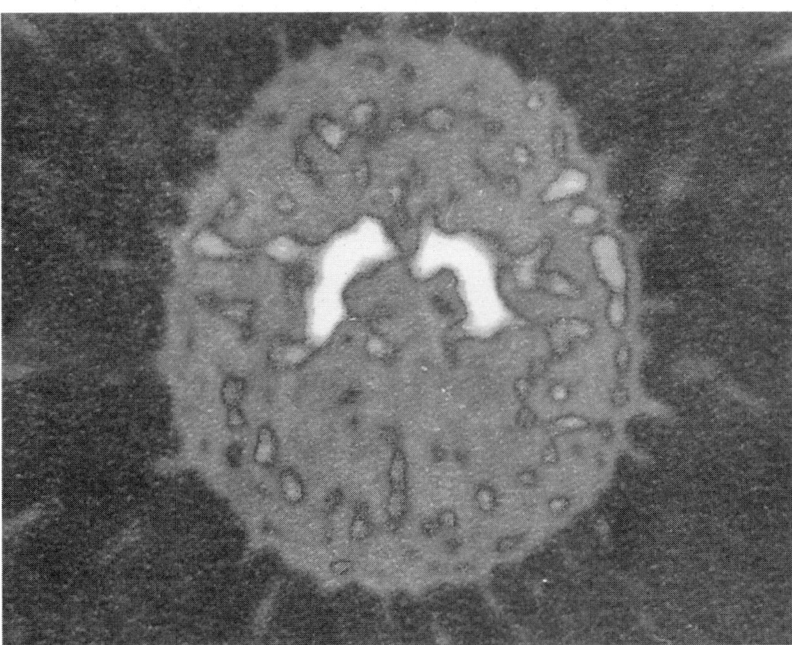

Figure 17–4 Axial (horizontal) PET scan of the brain following the injection of 18-fluoro-6-L-dopa.

ANSWERS AND EXPLANATIONS

1. E. The normal lymphocyte count of CSF is 0-3 cells per cu mm.
2. B. Compression of the internal jugular vein in the neck raises the CSF pressure because it impedes the reabsorption of the fluid into the venous sinuses
3. D. The choroid plexus projects into the lateral ventricle through the choroidal fissure on the medial wall
4. E. The nucleus of the fourth cranial nerve lies in the midbrain.
5. A. The subarachnoid space is the interval between the arachnoid mater and the pia mater.
6. C. The CSF does not escape through the roof of the terminal ventricle in the spinal cord since there is no opening.
7. D. The internal vertebral venous plexus lies embedded in areolar tissue in the epidural space within the vertebral canal. The spinal tap needle is very likely to pierce one of the veins of the plexus before it penetrates the meninges; a small drop of blood may enter the CSF, in which case the sample should be discarded.
8. B. The CSF pressure rises when the patient coughs.
9. C. Hydrocephalus can result in atrophy of the cerebral cortex.
10. E. Penicillin, which is toxic in large doses to nervous tissue, is largely blocked by the blood-brain barrier and only a small amount enters the central nervous system.
11. A. There is considerable evidence that hormones can be transported in the CSF. For example, the pineal gland probably influences the activity of the pituitary gland by the passage of substances through the CSF in the third ventricle.
12. A. B. The choroid plexus is situated in the roof of the third ventricle. C. The cavity of the ventricle is lined with ependyma. D. The interthalamic connection crosses the third ventricle so that part of the cavity lies above and part of the cavity lies below the connection. E. The hypothalamus lies in the floor of the third ventricle.
13. A. B. The choroidal ependymal cells actively secrete CSF. C. The tissue fluid of the brain substance contributes slightly to the CSF. D. The cerebral veins do not contribute to the CSF. E. The arachnoid villi are sites where the CSF enters the venous blood.
14. E
15. C
16. D
17. C
18. B
19. D. The curved white areas in Figure 17-4 show the uptake of 18-fluoro-6-L-dopa in the corpus striatum. This appearance is normal and indicates that the neurotransmitter dopamine is present in normal amounts in the corpus striatum.
20. D. The central artery of the retina has thick walls and is not compressed by a rise in CSF pressure in the subarachnoid extension around the optic nerve. Consequently, in this patient, the retina does not undergo ischemia.

CHAPTER 18

Cranial Nerves I–IV

CHAPTER OUTLINE

SUGGESTED PLAN FOR REVIEW OF CHAPTER 18

1. The cranial nerves are clinically important and testing for their integrity forms part of every physical examination. Moreover, each cranial nerve provides the examiner with many possible good questions.
2. Understand the basic information regarding the motor and sensory nuclei of the cranial nerves and note their location.
3. Learn the structure of the optic nerve and lesions of the optic pathway. The possible lesions are tricky but with patience you will understand and master them.
4. Know the various visual reflexes.
5. Because the third and fourth nerves are of small diameter and are relatively long, they frequently are damaged in head injuries. Questions are commonly directed to the defects found after injury.

INTRODUCTION

There are 12 pairs of cranial nerves, which leave the brain and pass through foramina and fissures in the skull. All the nerves are distributed in the head and neck except the tenth, which also supplies structures in the thorax and abdomen. The cranial nerves are named as follows:

1. Olfactory (I)
2. Optic (II)
3. Oculomotor (III)
4. Trochlear (IV)
5. Trigeminal (V)
6. Abducent (VI)
7. Facial (VII)
8. Vestibulocochlear (VIII)
9. Glossopharyngeal (IX)
10. Vagus (X)
11. Accessory (XI)
12. Hypoglossal (XII)

ORGANIZATION OF THE CRANIAL NERVES

The olfactory, optic, and vestibulocochlear nerves are entirely sensory. The oculomotor, trochlear, abducent, accessory, and hypoglossal nerves are entirely motor. The trigeminal, facial, glossopharyngeal, and vagus nerves are both sensory and motor nerves. The letter symbols commonly used to indicate the functional components of each cranial nerve are shown in Table 18-1. The cranial nerves have central motor and/or sensory nuclei within the brain and peripheral nerve fibers that emerge from the brain and exit from the skull to reach their effector or sensory organs.

The different components of the cranial nerves, their functions, and the openings in the skull through which the nerves leave the cranial cavity are summarized in Table 18-2.

Table 18–1 The Letter Symbols Commonly Used to Indicate the Functional Components of Each Cranial Nerve

Component	Function	Letter Symbols
Afferent nerve fibers	Sensory	
General somatic afferent	General sensations	GSA
Special somatic afferent	Hearing, balance, vision	SSA
General visceral afferent	Viscera	GVA
Special visceral afferent	Smell, taste	SVA
Efferent nerve fibers		
General somatic efferent	Somatic striated muscles	GSE
General visceral efferent	Glands and smooth muscles (parasympathetic innervation)	GVE
Special visceral efferent	Branchial arch striated muscles	SVE

MOTOR NUCLEI OF THE CRANIAL NERVES

Somatic Motor and Branchiomotor Nuclei

The somatic motor and branchiomotor nerve fibers of a cranial nerve are the axons of nerve cells situated within the brain. These nerve cell groups form motor nuclei and they innervate striated muscle. Each nerve cell with its processes is referred to as a **lower motor neuron**. Such a nerve cell is, therefore, equivalent to the motor cells found in the anterior gray columns (horns) of the spinal cord.

The motor nuclei of the cranial nerves receive impulses from the cerebral cortex through the corticonuclear fibers. These fibers originate from the pyramidal cells in the inferior part of the precentral gyrus (area 4) and from the adjacent part of the postcentral gyrus. The corticonuclear fibers descend through the **corona radiata** and the **genu of the internal capsule**. They pass through the midbrain just medial to the corticospinal fibers in the **basis pedunculi** and end by synapsing either directly on the lower motor neurons within the cranial nerve nuclei or indirectly through the **internuncial neurons**.

The majority of the corticonuclear fibers to the motor cranial nerve nuclei cross the median plane before reaching the nuclei. **Bilateral connections are present for all the cranial motor nuclei except for part of the facial nucleus that supplies the muscles of the lower part of the face and a part of the hypoglossal nucleus that supplies the genioglossus muscle.**

General Visceral Motor Nuclei

The general visceral motor nuclei form the cranial outflow of the parasympathetic portion of the autonomic nervous system. They are the **Edinger-Westphal nucleus** of the oculomotor nerve, the **superior salivatory nucleus** of the facial nerve, the **inferior salivatory nucleus** of the glossopharyngeal nerve, and the **dorsal motor nucleus** of the vagus. These nuclei receive numerous afferent fibers, including descending pathways from the hypothalamus.

SENSORY NUCLEI OF THE CRANIAL NERVES

These include somatic and visceral afferent nuclei. The sensory or afferent parts of a cranial nerve are the axons of nerve cells outside the brain and are situated in ganglia on the nerve trunks (equivalent to posterior root ganglion of a spinal nerve) or may be situated in a sensory organ such as the nose, eye, or ear. The central processes of these cells enter the brain and terminate by synapsing with cells forming the sensory nuclei. Axons from the nuclear cells now cross the midline and ascend to other sensory nuclei (e.g., the thalamus), where they synapse. The nerve cells of these nuclei send their axons to terminate in the cerebral cortex.

Table 18–2 Cranial Nerves

	Name	Components	Function	Opening in Skull
I	Olfactory	Sensory (SVA)	Smell	Openings in cribriform plate of ethmoid
II	Optic	Sensory (SSA)	Vision	Optic canal
III	Oculomotor	Motor (GSE, GVE)	Lifts upper eyelid, turns eyeball upward, downward, and medially; constricts pupil; accommodates eye	Superior orbital fissure
IV	Trochlear	Motor (GSE)	Assists in turning eyeball downward and laterally	Superior orbital fissure
V	Trigeminal*			
	Ophthalmic division	Sensory (GSA)	Cornea, skin of forehead, scalp, eyelids, and nose; also mucous membrane of paranasal sinuses and nasal cavity	Superior orbital fissure
	Maxillary division	Sensory (GSA)	Skin of face over maxilla; teeth of upper jaw; mucous membrane of nose, the maxillary sinus, and palate	Foramen rotundum
	Mandibular division	Motor (SVE)	Muscles of mastication, mylohyoid, anterior belly of digastric, tensor veli palatini, and tensor tympani	Foramen ovale
		Sensory (GSA)	Skin of cheek, skin over mandible and side of head, teeth of lower jaw and temporomandibular joint; mucous membrane of mouth and anterior part of tongue	
VI	Abducent	Motor (GSE)	Lateral rectus muscle—turns eyeball laterally	Superior orbital fissure
VII	Facial	Motor (SVE)	Muscles of face and scalp, stapedius muscle, posterior belly of digastric and stylohyoid muscles	Internal acoustic meatus, facial canal, stylomastoid foramen
		Sensory (SVA)	Taste from anterior two-thirds of tongue, floor of mouth and palate	
		Secretomotor (GVE) parasympathetic	Submandibular and sublingual salivary glands, the lacrimal gland, and glands of nose and palate	
VIII	Vestibulocochlear			
	Vestibular	Sensory (SSA)	From utricle and saccule and semicircular canals—position and movement of head	Internal acoustic meatus
	Cochlear	Sensory (SSA)	Organ of Corti—hearing	
IX	Glossopharyngeal	Motor (SVE)	Stylopharyngeus muscle—assists in swallowing	
		Secretomotor (GVE) parasympathetic	Parotid salivary gland	Jugular foramen
		Sensory (GVA, SVA, GSA)	General sensation and taste from posterior one-third of tongue, and pharynx; carotid sinus (baroreceptor) and carotid body (chemoreceptor)	
X	Vagus	Motor (GVE, SVE) Sensory (GVA, SVA, GSA)	Heart and great thoracic blood vessels; larynx, trachea, bronchi, and lungs; alimentary tract from pharynx to splenic flexure of colon; liver, kidneys, and pancreas	Jugular foramen
XI	Accessory			
	Cranial root	Motor (SVE)	Muscles of soft palate (except tensor veli palatini), pharynx (except stylopharyngeus), and larynx (except cricothyroid) in branches of vagus	Jugular foramen
	Spinal root	Motor (SVE)	Sternocleidomastoid and trapezius muscles	
XII	Hypoglossal	Motor (GSE)	Muscles of tongue (except palatoglossus) controlling its shape and movement	Hypoglossal canal

*The trigeminal nerve also carries proprioceptive impulses from the muscles of mastication and the facial and extraocular muscles.

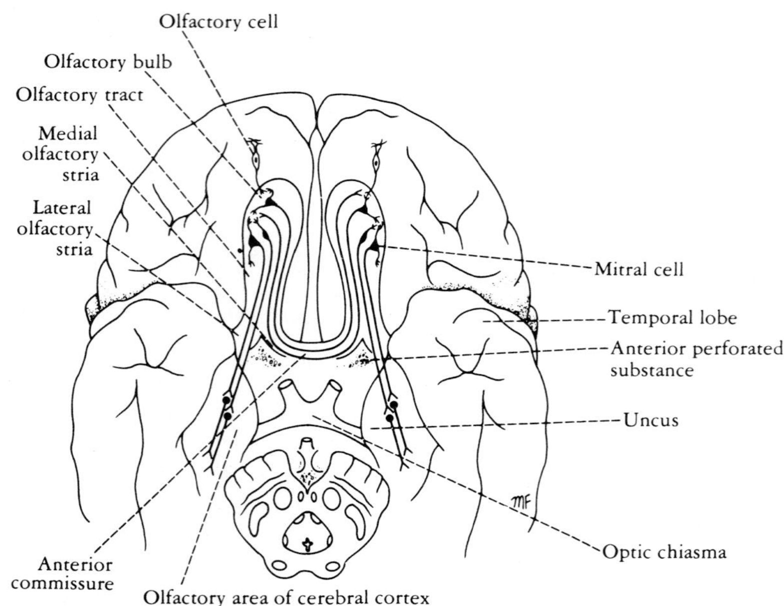

Figure 18–1 Connections between the olfactory cells and the rest of the olfactory system.

OLFACTORY NERVES (CRANIAL NERVE 1)

The olfactory nerves arise from **olfactory receptor nerve cells** in the olfactory mucous membrane located in the upper part of the nasal cavity above the level of the superior concha. Bundles of these nerve fibers pass through the openings of the cribriform plate of the ethmoid bone to enter the olfactory bulb inside the skull.

Olfactory Bulb

The incoming olfactory nerve fibers synapse with the dendrites of the **mitral cells** and form rounded areas known as **synaptic glomeruli**. Smaller nerve cells called **tufted cells** and **granular cells** also synapse with the mitral cells. The olfactory bulb, in addition, receives axons from the contralateral olfactory bulb through the olfactory tract.

Olfactory Tract

This is a narrow band of white matter that runs from the posterior end of the olfactory bulb and divides into **medial and lateral olfactory striae**. The lateral stria carries the axons to the **olfactory area of the cerebral cortex**, namely, the **periamygdaloid and prepiriform areas** (Fig. 18-1). The medial olfactory stria carries the fibers that cross the median plane in the anterior commissure to pass to the olfactory bulb of the opposite side.

The periamygdaloid and prepiriform areas of the cerebral cortex are often known as the **primary olfactory cortex**. The **entorhinal area (area 28)** of the parahippocampal gyrus, which receives numerous connections from the primary olfactory cortex, is called the **secondary olfactory cortex**. These areas of the cortex are responsible for the appreciation of olfactory sensations. Note that, in contrast to all other sensory pathways, the olfactory afferent pathway has only two neurons and reaches the cerebral cortex without synapsing in one of the thalamic nuclei. A summary of the distribution of the olfactory nerve is seen in Table 18-2, p 191.

Clinical Notes

Bilateral Anosmia

This condition can be caused by disease of the olfactory mucous membrane, such as the common cold or allergic rhinitis.

Unilateral Anosmia

Unilateral anosmia can result from disease affecting the olfactory nerves, bulb, or tract. Examples are fractures of the cribriform plate of the ethmoid, frontal lobe tumors, and meningiomas of the anterior cranial fossa.

OPTIC NERVE (CRANIAL NERVE II)

The optic nerve is composed of axons from the **ganglion cell layer** of the retina. The nerve emerges from the back of the eyeball and leaves the orbital cavity of the skull through the optic canal. It unites with the optic nerve of the opposite side to form the **optic chiasma** (Fig. 18-2).

In the chiasma, the fibers from the medial (nasal) half of each retina, including the medial half of the **macula,** cross the midline and enter the **optic tract** of the opposite side, while the fibers from the lateral (temporal) half of each retina, including the lateral half of the macula, pass posteriorly in the optic tract of the same side. Most of the fibers of the optic tract terminate by synapsing with nerve cells in the **lateral geniculate body**, which is a small projection from the posterior part of the thalamus. New fibers pass to the **pretectal nucleus** and **superior colliculus** of the midbrain and are concerned with the light reflexes (see below).

The axons from the lateral geniculate body pass posteriorly as the **optic radiation** and terminate in the **visual cortex (area 17)** of the cerebral hemisphere (Fig. 18-2). This cortex occupies the upper and lower lips of the calcarine sulcus on the medial surface of the cerebral hemisphere. The visual association cortex (areas 18 and 19) is responsible for recognition of objects and perception of color. Note that the macula lutea is represented on the posterior part of area 17, and the periphery of the retina is represented anteriorly.

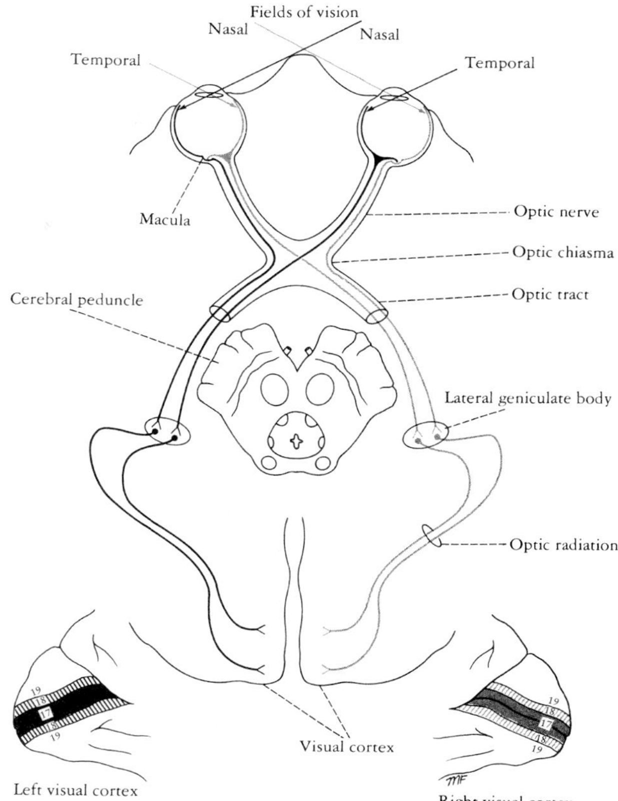

Figure 18–2 Optic pathway.

Visual Reflexes

DIRECT AND CONSENSUAL LIGHT REFLEXES

If a light is shone into one eye, the pupils of both eyes normally constrict. The constriction of the pupil on which the light is shone is called the **direct light reflex**; the constriction of the opposite pupil even though no light fell on that eye is called the **consensual light reflex** (Fig. 18-3).

The afferent impulses travel through the optic nerve, optic chiasma, and optic tract. Here a small number of fibers leave the optic tract and synapse on nerve cells in the **pretectal nucleus**, which lies close to the superior colliculus. The impulses are passed by axons of the pretectal nerve cells to the parasympathetic nuclei (**Edinger-Westphal nuclei**) of the third cranial nerve on both sides. Here the fibers synapse and the parasympathetic nerves travel through the third cranial nerve to the **ciliary ganglion** in the orbit (Fig. 18-3). Finally, postganglionic parasympathetic fibers pass through the **short ciliary nerves** to the eyeball and the **constrictor pupillae muscle** of the iris. Both pupils constrict in the consensual light reflex because the pretectal nucleus sends fibers to the parasympathetic nuclei on both sides of the midbrain (Fig. 18-3). The fibers that cross the median plane do so close to the cerebral aqueduct in the posterior commissure.

ACCOMMODATION REFLEX

When the eyes are directed from a distant to a near object, contraction of the medial recti brings about convergence of the ocular axes, the lens thickens to increase its refractive power by contraction of the ciliary muscle, and the pupils constrict to restrict the light waves to the thickest central part of the lens. The afferent impulses travel through the optic nerve, the optic chiasma, the optic tract, the lateral geniculate body, and the optic radiation to the visual cortex. The visual cortex is connected to the eye field of the frontal cortex (Fig. 18-3). From here, cortical fibers descend through the internal capsule to the oculomotor nuclei in the midbrain. The oculomotor nerve travels to the medial recti muscles. Some of the descending cortical fibers synapse with the parasympathetic nuclei (Edinger-Westphal nuclei) of the third cranial nerve on both sides. Here the fibers synapse and the parasympathetic nerves travel through the third cranial nerve to the ciliary ganglion in the orbit. Finally, postganglionic parasympathetic fibers pass through the short ciliary nerves to the **ciliary muscle** and the **constrictor pupillae muscle** of the iris (Fig. 18-3).

CORNEAL REFLEX

Light touching of the cornea or conjunctiva results in blinking of the eyelids. Afferent impulses from the cornea or conjunctiva travel through the ophthalmic division of the

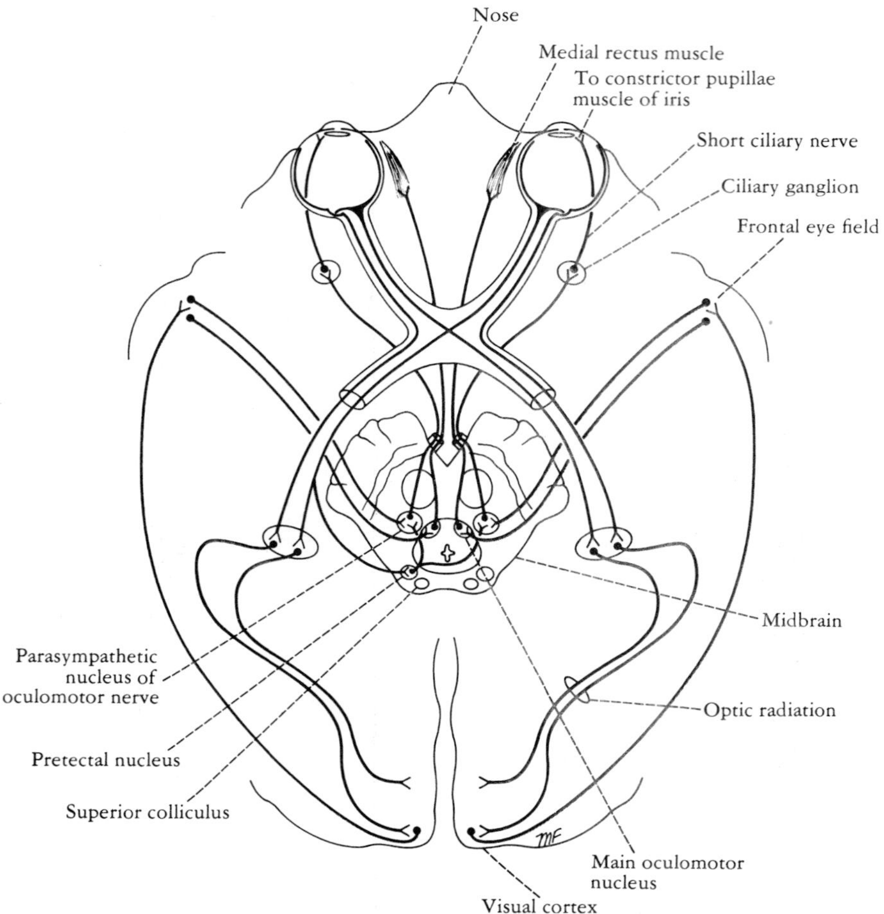

Figure 18–3 Optic pathways and the visual reflexes.

trigeminal nerve to the sensory nucleus of the trigeminal nerve. Internuncial neurons connect with the motor nucleus of the facial nerve on both sides through the medial longitudinal fasciculus. The facial nerve and its branches supply the orbicularis oculi muscle, which causes closure of the eyelids.

A summary of the distribution of the optic nerve is seen in Table 18-2, p 191.

Clinical Notes

Visual Field Defects Associated with Lesions of the Optic Pathways

The various visual field defects are summarized in Figure 18-4. Note that circumferential blindness may be due to hysteria or optic neuritis. Total blindness of one eye would follow complete section of one optic nerve. Lesions of the optic tract and optic radiation produce the same hemianopia for both eyes, i.e., homonymous hemianopia. Bitemporal hemianopia is a loss of the lateral halves of the fields of vision of both eyes. This condition is commonly caused by a tumor of the pituitary gland exerting pressure on the optic chiasma.

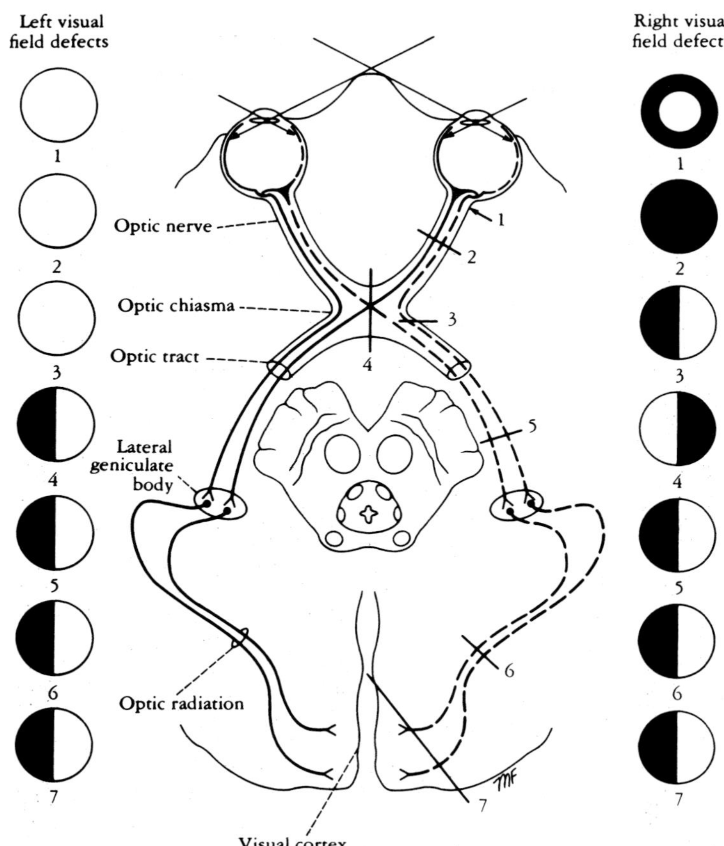

Figure 18–4 Visual field defects associated with lesions of the optic pathways. 1. Right-sided circumferential blindness due to retrobulbar neuritis. 2. Total blindness of right eye due to division of right optic nerve. 3. Right nasal hemianopia due to partial lesion of right side of optic chiasma. 4. Bitemporal hemianopia due to complete lesion of optic chiasma. 5. Left temporal hemianopia and right nasal hemianopia due to lesion of right optic tract. 6. Left temporal and right nasal hemianopia due to lesion of right optic radiation. 7. Left temporal and right nasal hemianopia due to lesion of right visual cortex.

OCULOMOTOR NERVE (CRANIAL NERVE III)

The oculomotor nerve is entirely motor in function.

Oculomotor Nuclei

The oculomotor nerve has two motor nuclei: (1) the main motor nucleus and (2) the accessory parasympathetic nucleus.

The **main oculomotor nucleus** is situated in the anterior part of the gray matter that surrounds the **cerebral aqueduct of the midbrain** (Fig. 18-5). It lies at the level of the superior colliculus. The nucleus consists of groups of nerve cells that supply all the extrinsic muscles of the eye except the superior oblique and the lateral rectus. The outgoing nerve fibers pass anteriorly through the red nucleus and emerge on the anterior surface of the midbrain in the **interpeduncular fossa**. The main oculomotor nucleus receives corticonuclear fibers from both cerebral hemispheres. It receives tectobulbar fibers from the superior colliculus and through this route receives information from the visual cortex. It also receives fibers from the medial longitudinal fasciculus, by which it is connected to the nuclei of the fourth, sixth, and eighth cranial nerves.

The **accessory parasympathetic nucleus (Edinger-Westphal nucleus)** is situated posterior to the main oculomotor nucleus (Fig. 18-5). The axons of the nerve cells, which are preganglionic, accompany the other oculomotor fibers to the orbit. Here they synapse in the **ciliary ganglion** and postganglionic fibers pass through the **short ciliary nerves** to the constrictor pupillae of the iris and the ciliary muscles. The accessory parasympathetic nucleus receives corticonuclear fibers for the accommodation reflex and fibers from the pretectal nucleus for the direct and consensual light reflexes.

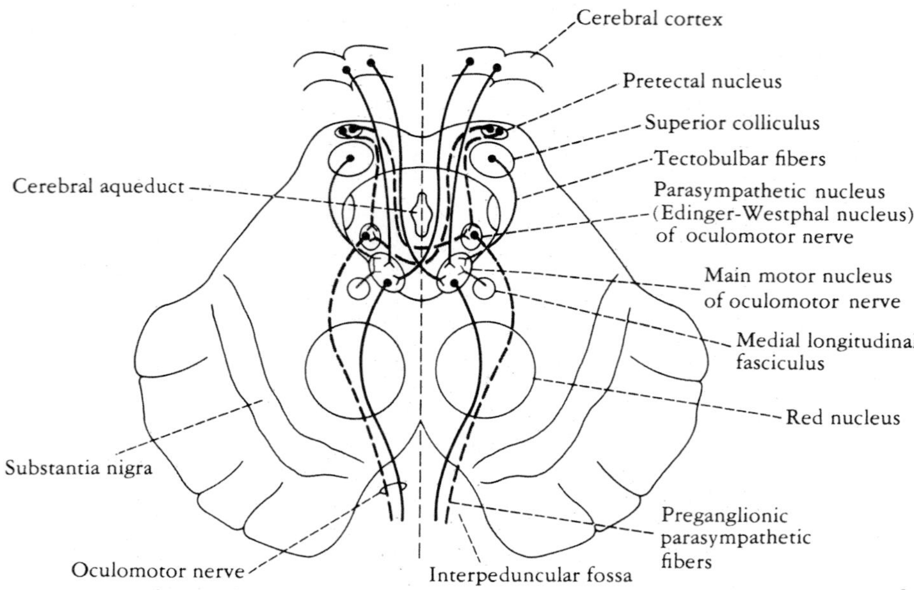

Figure 18–5 Oculomotor nuclei and their central connections.

Oculomotor Nerve

The oculomotor nerve emerges on the anterior surface of the midbrain. It passes forward between the posterior cerebral and the superior cerebellar arteries. It then continues into the middle cranial fossa in the lateral wall of the cavernous sinus. Here, it divides into a superior and an inferior ramus, which enter the orbital cavity through the superior orbital fissure.

The oculomotor nerve supplies the following extrinsic muscles of the eye: levator palpebrae superioris, superior rectus, medial rectus, inferior rectus, and inferior oblique. It also supplies through its branch to the ciliary ganglion and the short ciliary nerves parasympathetic nerve fibers to the following intrinsic muscles: the constrictor pupillae of the iris and the ciliary muscles.

The oculomotor nerve is therefore entirely motor and is responsible for lifting the upper eyelid; turning the eye upward, downward, and medially; constricting the pupil; and accommodating the eye. A summary of the distribution of the oculomotor nerve is seen in Table 18-2, p 191.

Clinical Notes

The small diameter of the oculomotor nerve and its relatively long course within the skull make the nerve prone to damage in head injuries. Other conditions commonly affecting the oculomotor nerve include diabetes, aneurysm, tumors, and vascular disease. See lesions of the oculomotor nerve in the midbrain (Benedikt's syndrome).

Complete Oculomotor Paralysis

In complete oculomotor paralysis the eye cannot be moved upward, downward, or inward. At rest the eye looks laterally (external strabismus) owing to the activity of the lateral rectus and downward owing to the activity of the superior oblique. The patient has diplopia. There is ptosis of the upper eyelid due to paralysis of the levator palpebrae superioris. The pupil is widely dilated and nonreactive to light due to the paralysis of the sphincter pupillae and the unopposed action of the dilator pupillae (supplied by the sympathetic). Accommodation is impossible.

Incomplete Oculomotor Paralysis

Incomplete lesions of the oculomotor nerve are common and may spare the extraocular muscles or the intraocular muscles. The condition in which innervation of the extraocular muscles is spared but there is selective loss of the autonomic innervation of the sphincter pupillae and ciliary muscle is called **internal ophthalmoplegia**. The condition in which the sphincter pupillae and the ciliary muscle are spared but there is paralysis of the extraocular muscles is called **external ophthalmoplegia**.

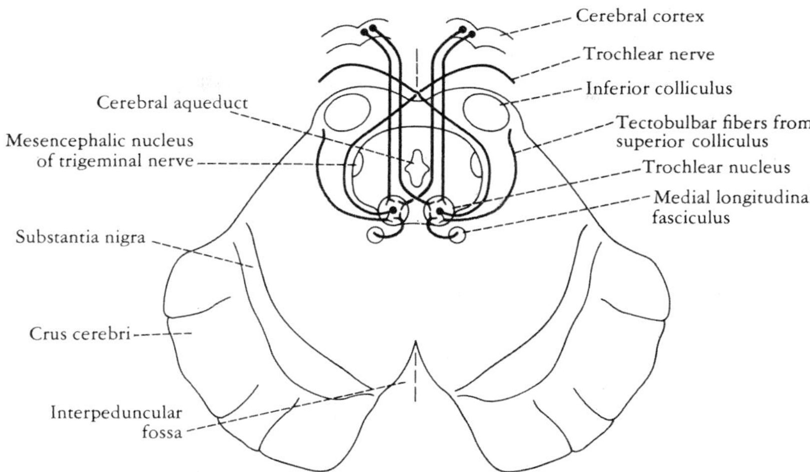

Figure 18–6 Trochlear nerve nucleus and its central connections.

TROCHLEAR NERVE (CRANIAL NERVE IV)

The trochlear nerve is entirely motor in function.

Trochlear Nucleus

The trochlear nucleus is situated in the anterior part of the gray matter that surrounds the cerebral aqueduct of the midbrain (Fig. 18-6). It lies inferior to the oculomotor nucleus at the level of the inferior colliculus. The nerve fibers, after leaving the nucleus, pass posteriorly around the central gray matter to reach the posterior surface of the midbrain.

The trochlear nucleus receives corticonuclear fibers from both cerebral hemispheres. It receives the tectobulbar fibers, which connect it to the visual cortex through the superior colliculus. It also receives fibers from the medial longitudinal fasciculus, by which it is connected to the nuclei of the third, sixth, and eighth cranial nerves.

Trochlear Nerve

The trochlear nerve, the most slender of the cranial nerves and the only one to leave the posterior surface of the brainstem, emerges from the midbrain and **immediately decussates with the nerve of the opposite side**. The trochlear nerve passes forward through the middle cranial fossa in the lateral wall of the cavernous sinus and enters the orbit through the superior orbital fissure. The nerve supplies the superior oblique muscle of the eyeball. The trochlear nerve is entirely motor and assists in turning the eye downward and laterally. A summary of the distribution of the trochlear nerve is seen in Table 18-2, p. 191.

CLINICAL NOTES

The trochlear nerve is the most slender of the cranial nerves and its long course around the midbrain close to the edge of the tentorium cerebelli makes this nerve very prone to damage in head injuries. Other conditions commonly affecting the trochlear nerve include diabetes mellitus, tumors, cavernous sinus thrombosis, aneurysm of the internal carotid artery , and vascular lesions of the dorsal part of the midbrain.

TROCHLEAR NERVE PARALYSIS

In trochlear nerve paralysis, the patient complains of double vision when looking straight downward. This is because the superior oblique is paralyzed, and the eye turns medially as well as downward. The patient has great difficulty in turning the eye downward and laterally.

REVIEW QUESTIONS

Directions: Each of the numbered items or incomplete statements in this section is followed by answers or by completions of the statement. Select the ONE lettered answer or completion that is BEST in each case.

1. Which of the following statements concerning the cranial nerves is (are) correct?
   (a) All the cranial nerves are only distributed to structures in the head and neck
   (b) Most of the cranial nerves do not leave the skull
   (c) All motor neurons of the cranial nerve nuclei receive descending motor fibers from both cerebral hemispheres.
   (d) The corticonuclear fibers pass through the midbrain lateral to the corticospinal fibers to the lower limb.
   (e) The facial, glossopharyngeal, and vagus nerves are both sensory and motor in function.

2. Which of the following statements concerning the cranial nerves is (are) correct?
   (a) The nerve cells of somatic and branchiomotor nuclei are upper motor neurons
   (b) The general visceral motor nuclei form the cranial outflow of the parasympathetic part of the autonomic nervous system
   (c) Special visceral afferent components of a cranial nerve are concerned with hearing, balance, and vision
   (d) The general visceral motor nuclei of the cranial nerves do not receive afferent fibers from the hypothalamus.
   (e) The oculomotor, trochlear, and hypoglossal nerves are not entirely motor in function.
3. Which of the following statements concerning the oculomotor nerve is correct?
   (a) The nerve has three nuclei
   (b) It contains both motor and sensory fibers
   (c) The nuclei lie in the midbrain at the level of the superior colliculus
   (d) The nerve fibers pass posteriorly around the red nucleus
   (e) The somatic motor nucleus receives corticobulbar fibers only from the contralateral cerebral cortex

For questions 4-7 study Figure 18-7, showing the optic pathway.

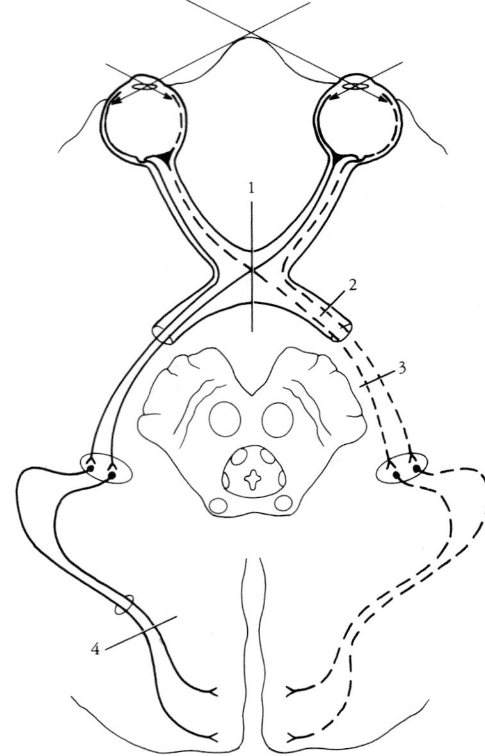

Figure 18–7 Optic pathway.

4. Lesion number 1 will result in the visual defect known as:
   (a) bitemporal hemianopia
   (b) binasal hemianopia
   (c) left temporal hemianopia and right nasal hemianopia
   (d) right nasal hemianopia (only)
   (e) left nasal hemianopia (only)
5. Lesion number 2 will result in the visual defect known as:
   (a) binasal hemianopia
   (b) left temporal hemianopia and right nasal hemianopia
   (c) right nasal hemianopia (only)
   (d) left nasal hemianopia (only)
   (e) bitemporal hemianopia
6. Lesion number 3 will result in the visual defect known as:
   (a) right-sided circumferential blindness
   (b) total blindness in both eyes
   (c) bitemporal hemianopia
   (d) right nasal hemianopia
   (e) left temporal hemianopia and right nasal hemianopia
7. Lesion number 4 will result in the visual defect known as:
   (a) bitemporal hemianopia
   (b) right nasal hemianopia (only)
   (c) right temporal and left nasal hemianopia
   (d) left nasal hemianopia (only)
   (e) left temporal hemianopia and right nasal hemianopia

Directions: Each of the numbered items in this section is followed by answers that are positively phrased. Select the ONE lettered answer that is an EXCEPTION.

8. The following statements concerning the sensory nuclei of cranial nerves are correct **except:**
   (a) Some of the afferent fibers to the nuclei are derived from nerve cells situated in ganglia outside the brain
   (b) The axons of the nuclei cross the midline of the brain
   (c) With the exception of the olfactory input, all ascending fibers from the nuclei synapse with nerve cells in the thalamus
   (d) Most of the information from the cranial nerve nuclei ultimately terminates in the postcentral gyrus of the cerebral cortex
   (e) There are only somatic sensory nuclei associated with the cranial nerves
9. The following statements concerning the olfactory nerve are correct **except:**
   (a) The receptor cells lie in the mucous membrane in the lower part of the nasal cavity
   (b) The axons of the olfactory nerves synapse with mitral cells in the olfactory bulbs
   (c) The lateral olfactory stria carries the axons of the mitral cells to the olfactory area of the cortex
   (d) The periamygdaloid and prepiriform areas form the primary olfactory cortex

(e) The entorhinal area (area 28) of the parahippocampal gyrus forms the secondary olfactory cortex

10. The following statements concerning the optic nerve are correct **except:**
(a) The axons arise from the ganglionic layer of the retina
(b) At the optic chiasma, the fibers from the lateral half of each retina cross the midline and enter the optic tract of the opposite side
(c) The optic nerve leaves the orbital cavity through the optic canal
(d) The optic nerve is surrounded by the three meninges and an extension of the subarachnoid space into the orbital cavity
(e) The optic nerve is made up of myelinated axons but the sheaths are formed from oligodendrocytes and not Schwann cells

11. The following statements concerning the optic tract are correct **except:**
(a) Most of the fibers in the optic tract terminate in the lateral geniculate body
(b) A few fibers of the optic tract pass to the pretectal nucleus and are concerned with light reflexes
(c) The optic tract emerges from the optic chiasma and passes posterolaterally around the cerebral peduncle
(d) Nerve fibers originating in the macula do not enter the optic tract
(e) The optic tract does not contain postganglionic sympathetic nerve fibers derived from the superior cervical sympathetic ganglion

12. The following statements concerning the optic radiation are correct **except:**
(a) It is located in the posterior part of the internal capsule
(b) It contains axons derived from nerve cells in the lateral geniculate body
(c) The axons pass directly to the area of Wernicke
(d) The axons terminate in area 17 of the cerebral cortex
(e) The optic radiation lies lateral to the posterior portion of the lateral ventricle

13. The following statements concerning the direct light reflex are correct **except:**
(a) The nerve impulses travel through the optic nerve, the optic chiasma, and the optic tract
(b) The pretectal nucleus is an important relay station
(c) The Edinger-Westphal nuclei on both sides of the midbrain are stimulated
(d) The preganglionic nerve fibers pass through the short ciliary nerves
(e) The ciliary ganglia of both eyes are stimulated

14. The following statements concerning the consensual light reflex are correct **except:**
(a) The parasympathetic nuclei of both oculomotor nerves are involved
(b) The optic radiation is involved with this reflex
(c) The nerve fibers from the pretectal nuclei cross the midline close to the cerebral aqueduct
(d) With an Argyll Robertson pupil the pretectal fibers passing to the oculomotor nucleus are destroyed by syphilis
(e) With the consensual light reflex, both pupils constrict even though the light is shone into only one eye

15. The cerebral cortex plays no role in the following reflexes **except:**
(a) Consensual light reflex
(b) Corneal reflex
(c) Pupillary light reflex
(d) Accommodation reflex
(e) Visual body reflex

16. Light waves of the nasal field of vision of the left eye are projected to the following structures **except:**
(a) Left lateral geniculate body
(b) Left pretectal nucleus
(c) Right lateral geniculate body
(d) Both banks of the left calcarine fissure
(e) Cortical areas 17, 18, and 19 of the left cerebral hemisphere

17. The following statements concerning the oculomotor nerve are correct **except:**
(a) The motor nucleus receives tectobulbar fibers from the superior colliculus
(b) The nerve may be found in the interpeduncular fossa
(c) The motor nucleus is connected to the nuclei of the fourth, sixth, and eighth cranial nerves
(d) The nerve passes into the orbital cavity through the inferior orbital fissure
(e) The motor nucleus receives nerve fibers from the medial longitudinal fasciculus

18. The following statements concerning the function of the oculomotor nerve are correct **except:**
(a) It accommodates the eye
(b) It raises the upper eyelid
(c) It innervates the lateral rectus muscle and thus turns the eye laterally
(d) It turns the eye downward
(e) It constricts the pupil

19. The following statements concerning the trochlear nerve are correct **except:**
(a) It supplies the superior oblique muscle
(b) It immediately decussates with the nerve of the opposite side on emerging from the brain
(c) The nucleus is located in the midbrain at the level of the inferior colliculus
(d) The nucleus receives corticobulbar fibers from both cerebral hemispheres
(e) It is a large nerve that is rarely damaged in patients with head injuries

20. The following statements concerning a lesion of the trochlear nerve are correct **except:**
(a) The patient's eye tends to turn medially
(b) The nerve lesion is of the upper motor neuron type
(c) The nerve lesion is of the lower motor neuron type
(d) The patient has great difficulty in turning the eye downward and laterally
(e) The patient complains of double vision

Directions: Read the case history then answer the question. A 58-year-old woman is seen by a neurologist because of trouble reading the newspaper. She said that the print starts to tilt and she begins to see double. She also stated that she has difficulty walking down steps because she cannot easily look downward with her left eye. On physical examination, the patient was found to have weakness of the movement of the left eye, both downward and laterally.

21. The following facts may explain the signs and symptoms **except:**
    (a) A small hemorrhage or thrombosis of an artery in the midbrain at the level of the inferior colliculus has occurred
    (b) The left trochlear nerve is damaged by pressure from an expanding tumor
    (c) Since the trochlear nerves decussate on emergence from the midbrain, the right trochlear nucleus is the site of the lesion
    (d) The difficulty with reading and the diplopia cannot be explained by paralysis of the left superior oblique muscle
    (e) The difficulty with walking down steps can be explained by paralysis of the left superior oblique muscle

ANSWERS AND EXPLANATIONS

1. E. A. All the cranial nerves are distributed in the head and neck except the tenth, which also supplies structures in the thorax and abdomen. B. All the cranial nerves have branches which leave the cranial cavity. C. All motor neurons of the cranial nerve nuclei receive descending motor fibers from both cerebral hemispheres, except those of the facial nerve nucleus that supply the muscles of the lower part of the face and those of the hypoglossal nucleus that supply the genioglossus muscle. These exceptional motor neurons only receive descending fibers from the cortex of the opposite cerebral hemisphere. D. The descending corticonuclear (corticobulbar) fibers pass through the crus cerebri of the midbrain along with the corticospinal fibers; the corticonuclear fibers are situated medial to the corticospinal fibers.
2. B. A. The nerve cells of somatic and branchiomotor nuclei are lower motor neurons. C. Special visceral afferent components of a cranial nerve are concerned with smell, and taste. D. The general visceral motor nuclei of the cranial nerves do receive afferent fibers from the hypothalamus. E. The oculomotor, trochlear, and hypoglossal nerves are entirely motor in function.
3. C. A. The nerve has two nuclei, a somatic motor nucleus and a parasympathetic autonomic motor nucleus (Edinger-Westphal nucleus). B. It contains only motor fibers. D. The nerve fibers pass anteriorly through the red nucleus. E. The somatic motor nucleus receives corticobulbar fibers from the cerebral cortex of both cerebral hemispheres
4. A
5. B
6. E
7. C
8. E. Visceral sensory nuclei are associated with cranial nerves VII, IX, and X.
9. A. The olfactory receptor cells lie in the mucous membrane in the upper part of the nasal cavity above the level of the superior concha.
10. B. At the optic chiasma, the fibers from the medial half of each retina cross the midline and enter the optic tract of the opposite side.
11. D
12. C. No nerve fibers of the optic radiation pass to the area of Wernicke.
13. D. The postganglionic fibers from the ciliary ganglion pass through the short ciliary nerves.
14. B. The optic radiation is not involved with this reflex.
15. D
16. C
17. D. The oculomotor nerve enters the orbital cavity through the superior orbital fissure.
18. C. The lateral rectus muscle is innervated by the sixth cranial nerve.
19. E. The trochlear nerve is long and slender and is commonly damaged in head injuries.
20. B. The nerve lesion involves the axons of the lower motor neuron.
21. D. The difficulty with reading and the diplopia can be explained by paralysis of the left superior oblique muscle. When a patient with paralysis of the superior oblique muscle looks straight downward, the affected eye turns medially as well as downward. Moreover, the patient has great difficulty turning that eye downward and laterally. This abnormality can be explained as follows: Contraction of the inferior rectus muscle rotates the eyeball so that the cornea is depressed downward. Because of the manner of its insertion, the inferior rectus muscle also rotates the eyeball medially. This tendency to rotate the eyeball medially is normally neutralized by simultaneous contraction of the superior oblique muscle, whose action is to rotate the eyeball laterally as well as to depress the cornea downward.

CHAPTER 19

Cranial Nerves V–VIII

CHAPTER OUTLINE

SUGGESTED PLAN FOR REVIEW OF CHAPTER 19

1. The details of all cranial nerves must be learned.
2. The trigeminal nerve and its branches are frequently involved by trauma and disease. The nerve and its nuclei provide many good questions for examiners.
3. The abducent nerve only does one thing—it supplies the lateral rectus muscle of the eye. Review the gross anatomy of the extraocular muscles of the eye with their nerve supply and understand and learn their actions on the eyeball.

SUGGESTED PLAN FOR REVIEW OF CHAPTER 19 (*continued*)

4. The facial nerve is frequently involved by disease, which may affect the lower or the upper motor neurons. Remember that the neurons in the main motor nucleus that supply the muscles of the lower part of the face receive corticobulbar fibers only from the opposite cerebral cortex.
5. The vestibulocochlear nerve is complicated, but the details should be learned.

INTRODUCTION

The trigeminal nerve (V) is the largest cranial nerve. It is called the trigeminal nerve because it has three major branches: **ophthalmic (V1), maxillary (V2),** and **mandibular (V3).** The main trunk of the trigeminal nerve leaves the ventral surface of the pons as a large sensory root and a small motor root. The sensory fibers are largely distributed to the skin of the face and the motor fibers innervate the muscles of mastication.

The abducent nerve (VI) is a small motor nerve that leaves the ventral surface of the brain between the pons and the medulla oblongata. It innervates the lateral rectus muscle of the eye.

The facial nerve (VII) has two nerve roots that leave the ventral surface of the brain between the pons and the medulla oblongata. The motor root is distributed mainly to the muscles of facial expression. The sensory root contains taste fibers from the mouth and palate and carries secretomotor fibers to the salivary glands, the nasal and palatine glands, and the lacrimal gland.

The vestibulocochlear nerve (VIII) consists of two distinct parts, the **vestibular nerve** and the **cochlear nerve**, which leave the ventral surface of the brain between the pons and the medulla oblongata. They are concerned with the transmission of afferent information from the internal ear to the central nervous system.

The purpose of this chapter is to discuss the nuclei of these cranial nerves, their central connections, and their distribution.

TRIGEMINAL NERVE (CRANIAL NERVE V)

Trigeminal Nerve Nuclei

The trigeminal nerve contains both sensory and motor fibers. It has four nuclei: (1) the main sensory nucleus, (2) the spinal nucleus, (3) the mesencephalic nucleus, and (4) the motor nucleus.

MAIN SENSORY NUCLEUS

This lies in the posterior part of the pons, lateral to the motor nucleus (Fig. 19-1). It is continuous below with the spinal nucleus.

SPINAL NUCLEUS

This is continuous superiorly with the main sensory nucleus in the pons and extends inferiorly through the medulla oblongata and the upper part of the spinal cord, as far as the second cervical segment (Fig. 19-1).

MESENCEPHALIC NUCLEUS

This is situated in the lateral part of the gray matter around the cerebral aqueduct. It extends inferiorly into the pons as far as the main sensory nucleus (Fig. 19-1).

MOTOR NUCLEUS

This is situated in the pons medial to the main sensory nucleus (Fig. 19-1).

Sensory Components of the Trigeminal Nerve

The sensations of pain, temperature, touch, and pressure from the skin of the face and mucous membranes travel along axons whose cell bodies are situated in the **trigeminal sensory ganglion**. The central processes of these cells form the sensory root of the trigeminal nerve. The fibers divide into ascending and descending branches when they enter the pons or they ascend or descend without division (Fig. 19-1). The ascending branches terminate in the main sensory nucleus and the descending branches terminate in the spinal nucleus. The sensations of touch and pressure are conveyed by nerve fibers that terminate in the main sensory nucleus. The sensations of pain and temperature pass to the spinal nucleus (Fig. 19-1). The sensory fibers from the ophthalmic division of the trigeminal nerve terminate in the inferior part of the spinal nucleus; fibers from the maxillary division terminate in the middle of the spinal nucleus; and fibers from the mandibular division end in the superior part of the spinal nucleus.

Proprioceptive impulses from the muscles of mastication and from the facial and extraocular muscles are carried by fibers in the sensory root of the trigeminal nerve that have bypassed the semilunar or trigeminal ganglion (Fig. 19-1). The fibers' cell of origin are the unipolar cells of the mesencephalic nucleus (Fig. 19-1).

The axons of the neurons in the main sensory and spinal nuclei, and the central processes of the cells in the mesen-

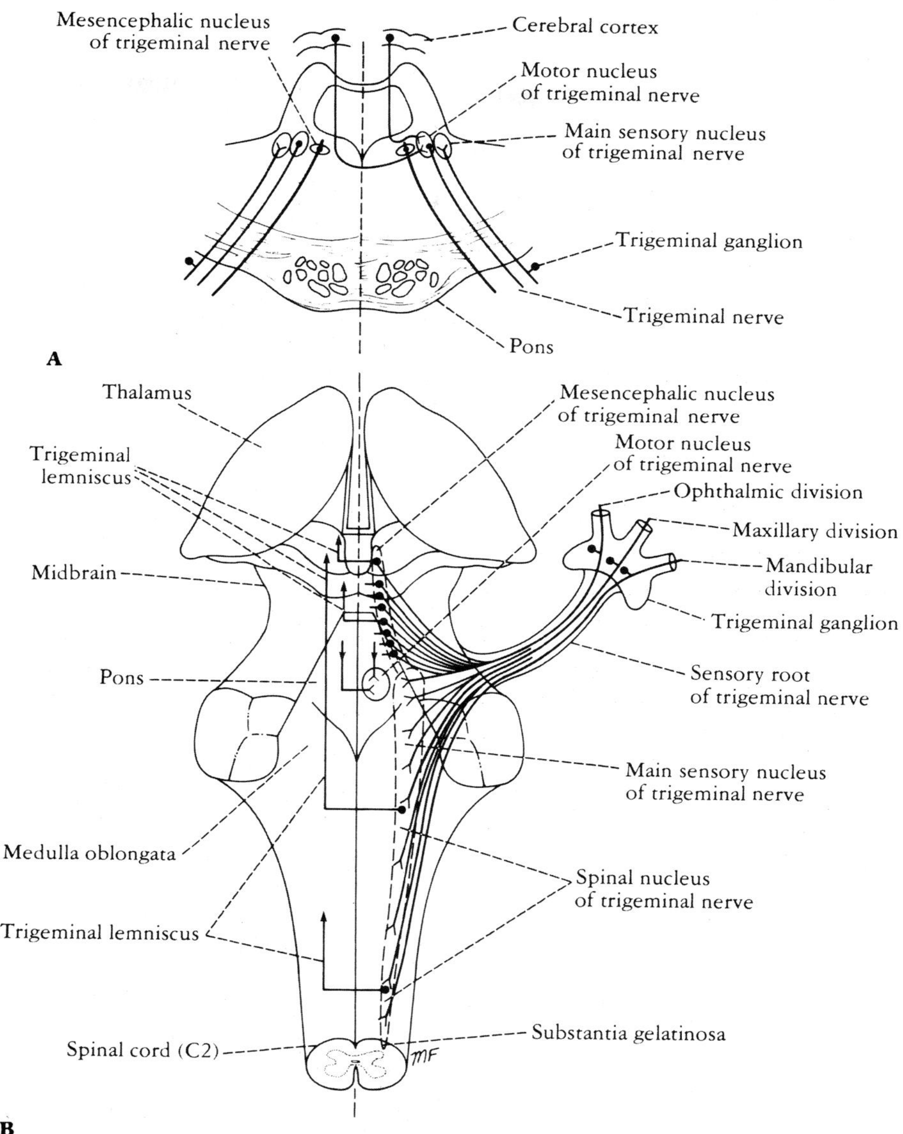

Figure 19–1 **A.** Trigeminal nerve nuclei seen in a coronal section of the pons. **B.** Trigeminal nerve nuclei in the brainstem and their central connections.

cephalic nucleus, now cross the median plane and ascend as the **trigeminal lemniscus** to terminate on nerve cells of the **ventral posteromedial nucleus of the thalamus**. The axons of these cells now travel through the internal capsule to the postcentral gyrus (areas 3, 1, and 2) of the cerebral cortex.

Motor Component of the Trigeminal Nerve

The motor nucleus receives corticonuclear fibers from both cerebral hemispheres (Fig. 19-1), fibers from the reticular formation, the red nucleus, the tectum, and the medial longitudinal fasciculus. In addition, it receives fibers from the mesencephalic nucleus, thereby forming a monosynaptic reflex arc.

The cells of the motor nucleus give rise to the axons that form the motor root. The motor nucleus supplies the **muscles of mastication,** the **tensor tympani,** the **tensor veli palatini,** and the **mylohyoid** and the **anterior belly of the digastric muscle**.

Trigeminal Nerve

The trigeminal nerve leaves the anterior aspect of the pons as a small motor root and a large sensory root. The nerve passes forward out of the posterior cranial fossa and rests on

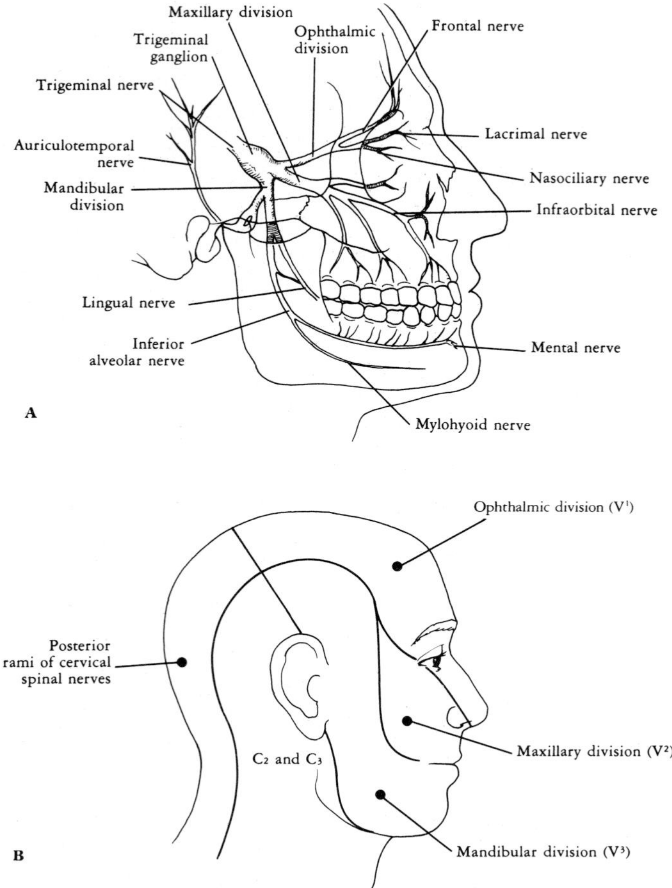

Figure 19–2 A and B. Diagrams showing the distribution of the sensory branches of the trigeminal nerve. Note that the skin area over the angle of the jaw is supplied by branches of the cervical plexus (B).

the upper surface of the apex of the petrous part of the temporal bone in the middle cranial fossa. The large sensory root now expands to form the crescent-shaped **trigeminal ganglion**, which lies within a pouch of dura mater called the **trigeminal or Meckel's cave**. The ophthalmic, maxillary, and mandibular nerves arise from the anterior border of the ganglion. The ophthalmic nerve (V1) contains only sensory fibers and leaves the skull through the superior orbital fissure to enter the orbital cavity. The maxillary nerve (V2) also contains only sensory fibers and leaves the skull through the foramen rotundum. The mandibular nerve (V3) contains both sensory and motor fibers and leaves the skull through the foramen ovale.

The sensory fibers to the skin of the face from each division supply a distinct zone (Fig. 19-2), there being little or no overlap of the dermatomes. (Compare with the overlap of the dermatomes of the spinal nerves.) As noted previously, the motor fibers in the mandibular division are mainly distributed to the muscles of mastication. A summary of the distribution of the trigeminal nerve is seen in Table 18-2, p. 191.

Clinical Notes

Trigeminal Nerve Lesions

There will be sensory loss over each zone of the face supplied by the divisions of the trigeminal nerve. In addition, in lesions of the ophthalmic division, the cornea and conjunctiva will be insensitive to touch. Motor loss will be seen if the patient is asked to clench the teeth. The masseter and temporalis muscles can be palpated and felt to harden when they contract; when the innervation is lost, they will fail to contract.

Trigeminal Neuralgia

This severe, stabbing pain over the face involves the pain fibers of the trigeminal nerve and is of unknown cause. Pain is felt most commonly over the skin areas innervated by the mandibular and maxillary divisions of the trigeminal nerve; only rarely is pain felt in the area supplied by the ophthalmic division.

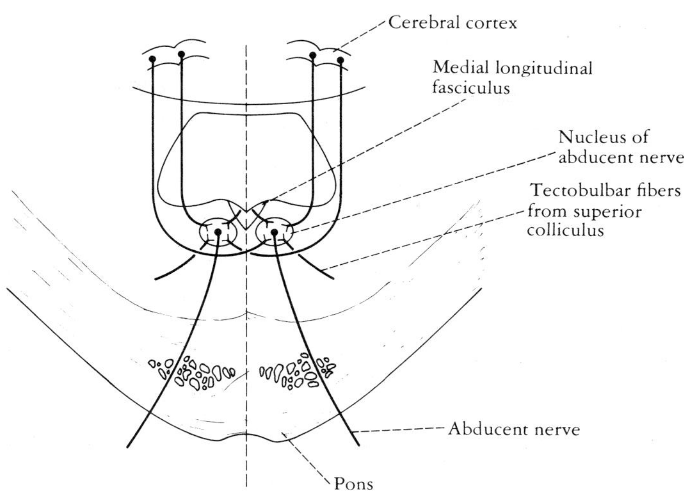

Figure 19–3 Abducent nerve nucleus and its central connections.

ABDUCENT NERVE (CRANIAL NERVE VI)

The abducent nerve is a small motor nerve that supplies the **lateral rectus muscle** of the eyeball. The motor nucleus is situated in the pons beneath the floor of the fourth ventricle, close to the midline and beneath the **colliculus facialis** (Fig. 19-3).

Abducent Nerve Nucleus

The nucleus receives afferent corticonuclear fibers from both cerebral hemispheres. It also receives the tectobulbar tract from the superior colliculus, by which the visual cortex is connected to the nucleus. In addition, it receives fibers from the medial longitudinal fasciculus, by which it is connected to the nuclei of the third, fourth, and eighth cranial nerves (Fig.19-3).

Abducent Nerve

The fibers of the abducent nerve pass anteriorly through the pons and emerge in the groove between the lower border of the pons and the medulla oblongata. It passes forward through the cavernous sinus, lying below and lateral to the internal carotid artery. The nerve then enters the orbit through the superior orbital fissure. The abducent nerve is entirely a motor nerve and supplies the lateral rectus muscle and is, therefore, responsible for turning the eye laterally. A summary of the distribution of the abducent nerve is seen in Table 18-2, p. 191.

CLINICAL NOTES

ABDUCENT NERVE LESION

The long intracranial course of this slender nerve makes it prone to damage in head injuries. A lesion of the abducent nerve causes a paralysis of the lateral rectus muscle of the eyeball and the patient is unable to turn the eye laterally. At rest the eye is turned medially (medial strabismus) by the unopposed action of the medial rectus muscle (supplied by the oculomotor nerve).

In addition to head injuries the abducent nerve may be damaged in cavernous sinus thrombosis, aneurysms of the internal carotid artery, and vascular lesions of the pons.

FACIAL NERVE (CRANIAL NERVE VII)

Facial Nerve Nuclei

The facial nerve has three nuclei: (1) the main motor nucleus, (2) the parasympathetic nuclei, and (3) the sensory nucleus.

MAIN MOTOR NUCLEUS

This nucleus lies in the reticular formation of the lower part of the pons (Fig. 19-4). The part of the nucleus that supplies the muscles of the upper part of the face receives corticonuclear fibers from both cerebral hemispheres. **The part**

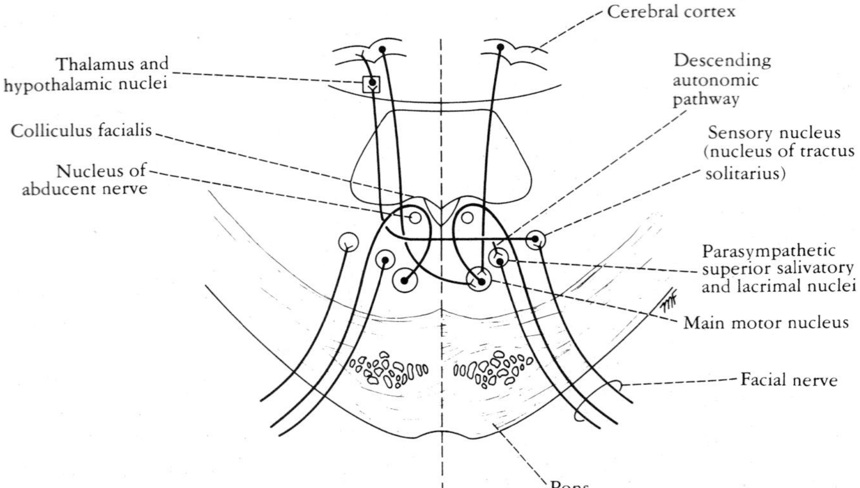

Figure 19–4 Facial nerve nuclei and their central connections.

of the nucleus that supplies the muscles of the lower part of the face receives only corticonuclear fibers from the opposite cerebral hemisphere.

These pathways explain the voluntary control of facial muscles. However, another involuntary pathway exists; it is separate and controls **mimetic or emotional changes in facial expression**. The origin and course of this upper motor neuron pathway are unknown.

PARASYMPATHETIC NUCLEI

These nuclei lie posterolateral to the main motor nucleus. They are the **superior salivatory** and **lacrimal nuclei** (Fig. 19-4). The superior salivatory nucleus receives afferent fibers from the hypothalamus through the **descending autonomic pathways**. Information concerning taste is also received from the **nucleus of the solitary tract** from the mouth cavity.

The lacrimal nucleus receives afferent fibers from the hypothalamus for emotional responses and from the sensory nuclei of the trigeminal nerve for reflex lacrimation secondary to irritation of the cornea or conjunctiva.

SENSORY NUCLEUS

This nucleus is the upper part of the **nucleus of the tractus solitarius** and lies close to the motor nucleus (Fig. 19-4). Sensations of taste travel through the peripheral axons of nerve cells situated in the **geniculate ganglion** on the seventh cranial nerve. The central processes of these cells synapse on nerve cells in the nucleus. Efferent fibers cross the median plane and ascend to the ventral posterior medial nucleus of the opposite thalamus and also a number of hypothalamic nuclei. From the thalamus, the axons of the thalamic cells pass through the internal capsule and corona radiata to end in the taste area of the cortex in the lower part of the postcentral gyrus.

Facial Nerve

The facial nerve consists of a motor and a sensory root. The fibers of the motor root first travel posteriorly around the medial side of the abducent nucleus. Then they pass around the nucleus beneath the **colliculus facialis** in the floor of the fourth ventricle and finally pass anteriorly to emerge from the brainstem (Fig. 19-4).

The sensory root (**nervus intermedius**) is formed of the central processes of the unipolar cells of the geniculate ganglion. It also contains the efferent preganglionic parasympathetic fibers from the parasympathetic nuclei.

The two roots of the facial nerve emerge from the anterior surface of the brain between the pons and the medulla oblongata. They pass laterally in the posterior cranial fossa with the vestibulocochlear nerve and enter the internal acoustic meatus in the petrous part of the temporal bone. At the bottom of the meatus, the nerve enters the facial canal and runs laterally through the inner ear. On reaching the medial wall of the tympanic cavity, the nerve expands to form the sensory **geniculate ganglion** and turns sharply backward above the promontory. At the posterior wall of the tympanic cavity the facial nerve turns downward on the medial side of the aditus of the mastoid antrum, descends behind the pyramid, and emerges from the stylomastoid foramen.

Distribution of the Facial Nerve

The **motor nucleus** supplies the muscles of facial expression, the auricular muscles, the stapedius, the posterior belly of the digastric, and the stylohyoid muscles (Fig. 19-5).

The **superior salivatory nucleus** supplies the submandibular and sublingual salivary glands and the nasal and palatine glands. The **lacrimal nucleus** supplies the lacrimal gland.

The **sensory nucleus** receives taste fibers from the anterior two-thirds of the tongue, the floor of the mouth, and the palate. A summary of the distribution of the facial nerve is seen in Table 18-2, p. 191.

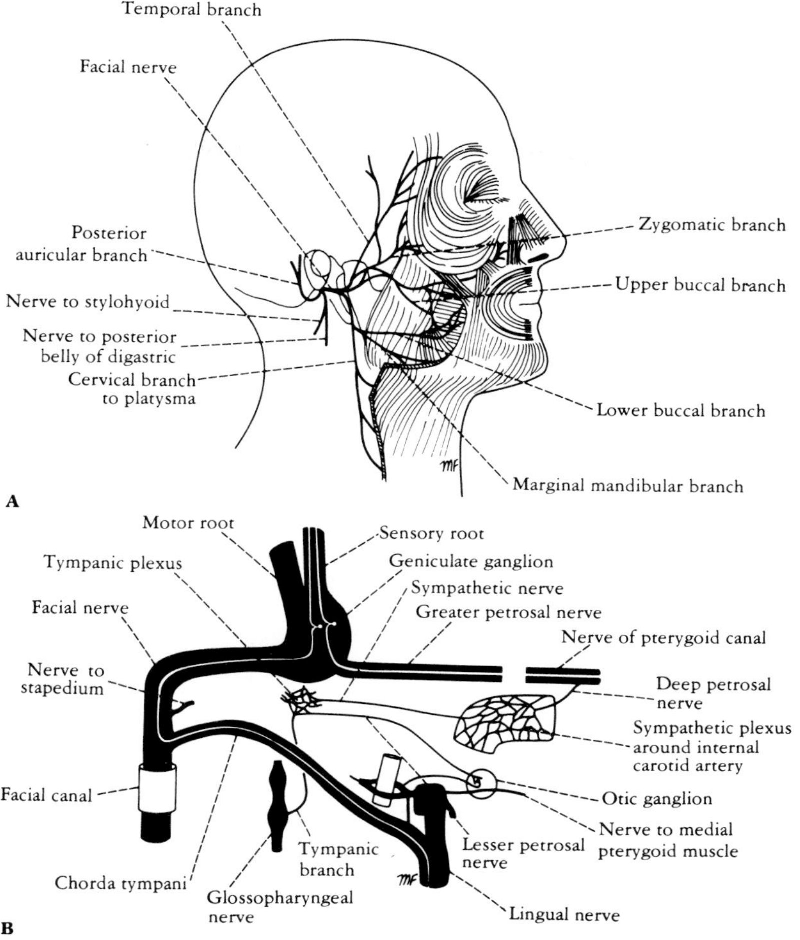

Figure 19–5 Facial nerve. **A.** Branches of the facial nerve. **B.** The branches of the facial nerve within the petrous part of the temporal bone. The taste fibers are shown in white. The glossopharyngeal nerve is also included.

Clinical Notes

Facial Nerve Lesions

Upper Motor Neuron Lesions

The part of the facial nucleus that controls the muscles of the upper part of the face receives corticonuclear fibers from both cerebral hemispheres, while the part of the nucleus that controls the muscles of the lower part of the face receives corticonuclear fibers from **only** the opposite cerebral hemisphere. Therefore it follows that with a lesion involving the upper motor neurons on one side, the muscles of the lower part of the face on the opposite side will be paralyzed. The angle of the mouth will sag on that side.

In patients with hemiplegia, the emotional movements of the face are usually preserved. This indicates that the upper motor neurons controlling these **mimetic movements** have a course separate from that of the main corticobulbar fibers. A lesion involving this separate pathway alone results in a loss of emotional movements, but voluntary movements are preserved. A more extensive lesion will produce both mimetic and voluntary facial paralysis.

Lower Motor Neuron Lesions

In lesions of the facial nerve nucleus or the facial nerve itself, all muscles of the face on the affected side will be paralyzed. The lower eyelid will droop, and the angle of the mouth will sag. Tears will flow over the lower eyelid, and saliva will dribble from the corner of the mouth. The patient will be unable to close the eye and will be unable to expose the teeth fully on the affected side.

SECREMOTOR LOSS

Secretory activity of the lacrimal, submandibular, and sublingual glands will be lost.

SENSORY LOSS

The sensation of taste for the anterior two-thirds of the tongue and the floor of the mouth will be lost.

BELL'S PALSY

Bell's palsy is a temporary dysfunction of the facial nerve as it lies within the facial canal. The swelling of the nerve within the bony canal results in a lower motor neuron type of facial paralysis. It is usually unilateral and the cause is unknown.

VESTIBULOCOCHLEAR NERVE (CRANIAL NERVE VIII)

This nerve consists of two distinct parts, the **vestibular nerve** and the **cochlear nerve**, which are concerned with the transmission of afferent information from the internal ear to the central nervous system (Fig. 19-6).

Vestibular Nerve

The vestibular nerve conducts nerve impulses from the utricle and saccule that provide information concerning the position of the head; the nerve also conducts impulses from the semicircular canals that provide information concerning movements of the head.

The nerve fibers of the vestibular nerve are the central processes of nerve cells located in the **vestibular ganglion**, which is situated in the **internal acoustic meatus**. They enter the anterior surface of the brainstem in a groove between the lower border of the pons and the upper part of the medulla oblongata (Fig. 19-6). On entering the vestibular nuclear complex, the fibers divide into short ascending and long descending fibers; a small number of fibers pass directly to the cerebellum through the inferior cerebellar peduncle, thus bypassing the vestibular nuclei.

VESTIBULAR NUCLEAR COMPLEX

This complex consists of a group of four nuclei situated beneath the floor of the fourth ventricle (Fig. 19-6): (1) the **lateral vestibular nucleus**, (2) the **superior vestibular nucleus**, (3) the **medial vestibular nucleus**, and (4) the **inferior vestibular nucleus**.

The vestibular nuclei receive afferent fibers from the **utricle**, the **saccule,** and the **semicircular canals** through the vestibular nerve and fibers from the cerebellum through the inferior cerebellar peduncle. Efferent fibers from the nuclei pass to the cerebellum through the inferior cerebellar peduncle. Efferent fibers also descend uncrossed to the spinal cord from the lateral vestibular nucleus and form the **vestibulospinal tract** (Fig. 19-6). In addition, efferent fibers pass to the nuclei of the oculomotor, trochlear, and abducent nerves through the medial longitudinal fasciculus.

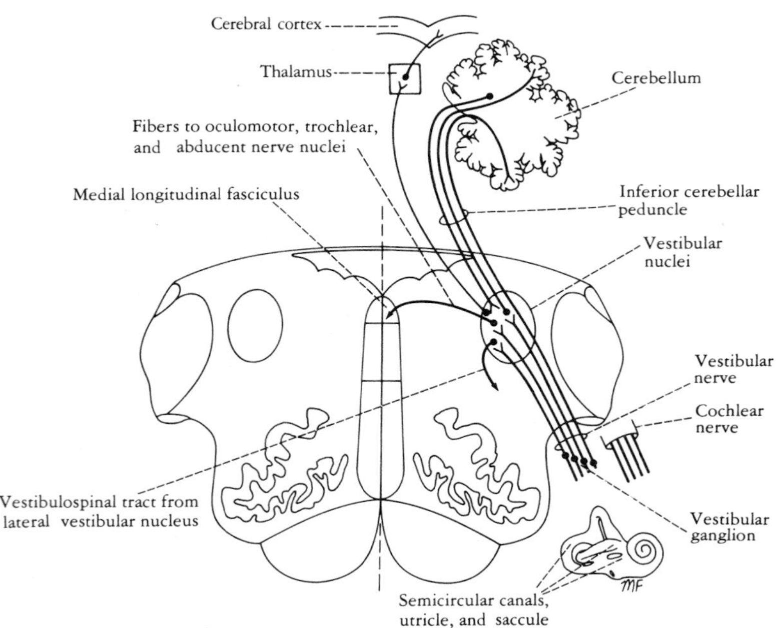

Figure 19–6 Vestibular nerve nuclei and their central connections.

As the result of these connections the movements of the head and the eyes can be coordinated, so that visual fixation on an object can be maintained. The information received from the internal ear can assist in maintaining balance, by influencing the muscle tone of the limbs and trunk.

Ascending fibers also pass upward from the vestibular nuclei to the ventral posterior nuclei of the thalamus. After relaying, axons pass to the vestibular area in the postcentral gyrus. These connections probably enable the cerebral cortex consciously to orientate the individual to space.

Cochlear Nerve

The cochlear nerve conducts nerve impulses concerned with sound from the organ of Corti in the cochlea. The fibers of the cochlear nerve are the central processes of nerve cells located in the **spiral ganglion of the cochlea.** They enter the anterior surface of the brainstem at the lower border of the pons on the lateral side of the emerging facial nerve and are separated from it by the vestibular nerve (Fig. 19-7). On entering the pons the nerve fibers divide, one branch entering the **posterior cochlear nucleus** and the other branch entering the **anterior cochlear nucleus.**

COCHLEAR NUCLEI

The anterior and posterior cochlear nuclei are situated on the surface of the inferior cerebellar peduncle. They receive afferent fibers from the cochlea through the cochlear nerve. The cochlear nuclei send axons medially to end in the **trapezoid body** and the **olivary nucleus.** Here they are relayed in the **posterior nucleus of the trapezoid body** and the **superior olivary nucleus** on the same or the opposite side. The axons now ascend through the posterior part of the pons and midbrain and form a tract known as the **lateral lemniscus** (Fig. 19-7). Each lateral lemniscus, therefore, consists of neurons from both sides. As these fibers ascend, some of them relay in small groups of nerve cells, which collectively are known as the **nucleus of the lateral lemniscus** (Fig. 19-7).

On reaching the midbrain, the fibers of the lateral lemniscus either terminate in the nucleus of the **inferior colliculus**

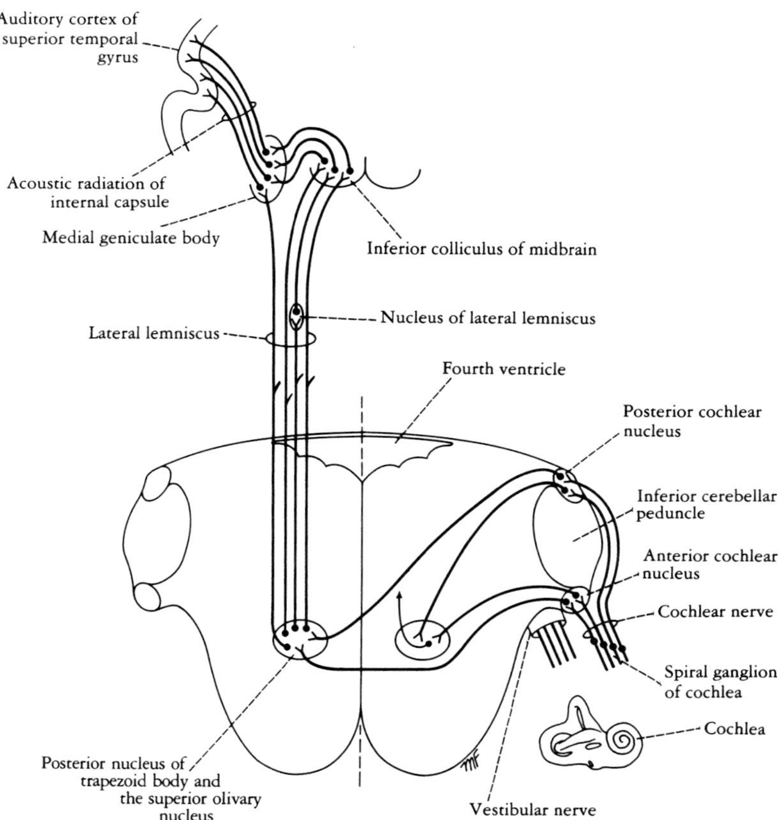

Figure 19–7 Cochlear nerve nuclei and their central connections. The descending pathways have been omitted.

or are relayed in the **medial geniculate body** and pass to the **auditory cortex** of the cerebral hemisphere through the **acoustic radiation of the internal capsule** (Fig. 19-7).

The primary auditory cortex (areas 41 and 42) includes the gyrus of Heschl on the upper surface of the superior temporal gyrus. The recognition and interpretation of sounds on the basis of past experience take place in the secondary auditory area.

Vestibulocochlear Nerve

The vestibular and cochlear parts of the nerve leave the anterior surface of the brain between the lower border of the pons and the medulla oblongata and run laterally in the posterior cranial fossa entering the internal acoustic meatus with the facial nerve. A summary of the distribution of the vestibulocochlear nerve is seen in Table 18-2, p. 191.

Clinical Notes

Vestibulocochlear Nerve Lesions

The vestibular fibers are concerned with the sense of position and movement of the head. The cochlear fibers are concerned with the sense of hearing. Disturbances of vestibular function include giddiness (vertigo) and nystagmus. Disturbances of cochlear function include deafness and tinnitus.

REVIEW QUESTIONS

Directions: Each of the numbered incomplete statements in this section is followed by completions of the statement. Select the ONE lettered completion that is BEST in each case.

For questions 1-5 study Figure 19-8, showing a transverse section through the caudal part of the pons.

1. Structure number 1 is the
   (a) nucleus of the tractus solitarius
   (b) superior salivatory nucleus
   (c) nucleus of abducent nerve
   (d) motor nucleus of facial nerve
   (e) medial longitudinal fasciculus
2. Structure number 2 is the
   (a) motor nucleus of the facial nerve
   (b) nucleus of the tractus solitarius
   (c) nucleus of the abducent nerve
   (d) mesencephalic nucleus
   (e) lacrimal nucleus
3. Structure number 3 is the
   (a) superior salivatory nucleus
   (b) main sensory nucleus of the trigeminal nerve
   (c) motor nucleus of the facial nerve
   (d) motor nucleus of the trigeminal nerve
   (e) nucleus of the abducent nerve
4. Structure number 4 is the
   (a) inferior salivatory nucleus
   (b) nucleus of the tractus solitarius
   (c) nucleus of the abducent nerve
   (d) superior salivatory nucleus
   (e) medial longitudinal fasciculus
5. Structure number 5 is the
   (a) medial longitudinal fasciculus
   (b) motor nucleus of the trigeminal nerve
   (c) mesencephalic nucleus
   (d) nucleus of abducent nerve
   (e) pontine nucleus

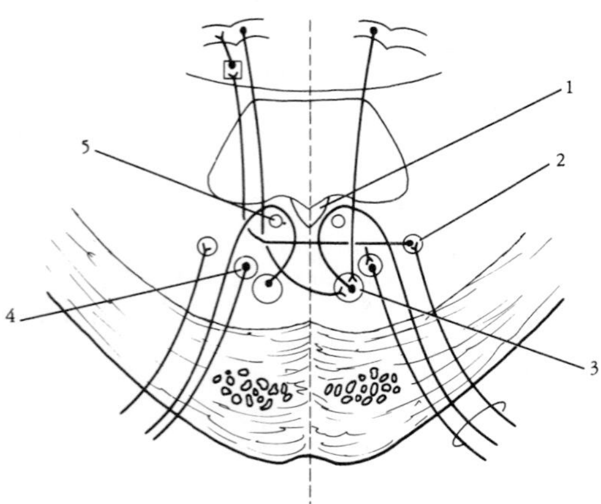

Figure 19–8 Transverse section through the caudal part of the pons.

Directions: Each of the numbered items in this section is followed by answers that are positively phrased. Select the ONE lettered answer that is an EXCEPTION.

6. The following facts concerning the trigeminal nerve and its nuclei are correct **except:**
   (a) The trigeminal nerve has a large motor root and a small sensory root
   (b) The trigeminal nerve leaves the brain on the anterior surface of the pons
   (c) The main sensory nucleus is continuous below with the spinal nucleus
   (d) The spinal nucleus extends inferiorly as far as the second cervical segment of the spinal cord
   (e) The mesencephalic nucleus receives information from the muscles of facial expression and the extraocular muscles

7. The following facts concerning the trigeminal nerve, its nuclei and their connections are correct **except:**
   (a) The afferent fibers from the muscles of mastication are the peripheral nerve processes of the unipolar cells in the mesencephalic nucleus
   (b) The trigeminal lemniscus terminates in the ventral posteromedial nucleus of the thalamus
   (c) The ascending sensory fibers from the trigeminal nuclei cross to the opposite side of the brainstem
   (d) The motor nucleus only receives fibers from the cerebral cortex of the opposite cerebral hemisphere
   (e) The motor nucleus supplies not only the muscles of mastication but also the mylohyoid and the anterior belly of the digastric muscle
8. The following statements concerning the ophthalmic division of the trigeminal nerve are correct **except:**
   (a) It contains only sensory nerve fibers
   (b) Its main branches leave the skull through the superior orbital fissure
   (c) It supplies the skin of the forehead
   (d) The dermatome overlaps for some distance that of the maxillary nerve
   (e) It supplies the skin of the nose down as far as its tip
9. The following statements concerning a lesion of the trigeminal nerve are correct **except:**
   (a) The masseter muscle cannot be felt to contract
   (b) There is loss of skin sensation over the angle of the jaw
   (c) The cornea and conjunctiva are insensitive to touch
   (d) The temporalis muscle cannot be felt to contract
   (e) There is a loss of skin sensation over the cheek
10. The following facts concerning the trigeminal ganglion are correct **except:**
   (a) The central processes of the nerve cells of the ganglion form the sensory root of the trigeminal nerve
   (b) The afferent fibers of the mesencephalic nucleus bypass the ganglion
   (c) The ganglion lies within a pouch of dura mater called the trigeminal cave
   (d) Each nerve cell body is devoid of capsular cells.
   (e) The ganglion is crescent shaped and gives rise to the ophthalmic, maxillary and mandibular nerves.
11. The following statements concerning the abducent nerve are correct **except:**
   (a) The long slender nerve is prone to injury
   (b) The nerve supplies the medial rectus muscle
   (c) The motor nucleus has the motor root of the facial nerve winding around it
   (d) The nucleus lies beneath the floor of the fourth ventricle
   (e) The nerve leaves the brainstem on its anterior surface between the pons and the medulla oblongata
12. The following statements concerning the facial nerve nuclei are correct **except:**
   (a) The motor and parasympathetic nuclei are located in the upper part of the pons
   (b) The part of the motor nucleus that supplies the muscles of the lower part of the face receives corticobulbar fibers only from the contralateral cerebral cortex
   (c) The nuclei are both motor and sensory
   (d) The parasympathetic nuclei supply the lacrimal, submandibular, and sublingual salivary glands
   (e) The sensory nucleus receives taste fibers from the anterior two-thirds of the tongue
13. The following statements concerning the facial nerve are correct **except:**
   (a) The facial nerve runs close to the middle ear and can be damaged during operations for otitis media
   (b) The facial nerve leaves the brainstem on the anterior surface between the pons and the medulla oblongata
   (c) The facial nerve accompanies the vestibulocochlear nerve into the internal acoustic meatus
   (d) The geniculate ganglion consists of nerve cells whose function is to conduct information of taste to the central nervous system
   (e) The parasympathetic nerve fibers travel with the somatic nerve fibers in the motor root of the facial nerve
14. The following statements concerning a lesion of the facial nerve are correct **except:**
   (a) In Bell's palsy the paralysis is usually unilateral and is temporary
   (b) All the muscles of the face on the affected side are paralyzed
   (c) The paralysis produced is of the upper motor neuron type
   (d) A lesion of the facial nerve produces identical signs and symptoms as a lesion of the facial motor nucleus
   (e) There is a loss of taste sensation on the anterior two-thirds of the tongue
15. The following nuclei are associated with the facial nerve **except:**
   (a) Lacrimal nucleus
   (b) Inferior salivatory nucleus
   (c) Nucleus of the tractus solitarius
   (d) Main motor nucleus
   (e) Superior salivatory nucleus
16. The following facts concerning the vestibular nuclei are correct **except:**
   (a) They are four in number
   (b) They receive afferent fibers from the utricle and saccule of the internal ear
   (c) They are connected to the third, fourth, and sixth cranial nerve nuclei by the medial longitudinal fasciculus
   (d) They do not receive afferent fibers from the semicircular canals
   (e) They are located beneath the floor of the fourth ventricle
17. The following facts concerning the cochlear nerve are correct **except:**
   (a) The nerve fibers are the central processes of nerve cells in the spiral ganglion

(b) The fibers of the lateral lemniscus terminate in the lateral geniculate body
(c) The nerve fibers end in the anterior and posterior cochlear nuclei
(d) Each lateral lemniscus consists of ascending nerve fibers concerned with the reception of sound from both ears
(e) The cochlear nerve enters the brainstem at the lower border of the pons

18. The following structures participate in the reception of sound **except:**
(a) Posterior nucleus of trapezoid body
(b) Trigeminal nerve
(c) Lateral lemniscus
(d) Medial lemniscus
(e) Facial nerve

19. The following facts concerning the reception of sound are correct **except:**
(a) The nerve impulses pass through the acoustic radiation
(b) The primary auditory cortex is areas 41 and 42
(c) The gyrus of Heschl is not involved in the reception of sound
(d) The inferior colliculus is involved in the process
(e) The cochlear nuclei send axons to the trapezoid body

Directions: Read the case history then answer the question. A 46-year-old man, who was otherwise perfectly fit, woke up one morning to find the left side of his face paralyzed. To his great concern, his left lower eyelid was drooping and the left angle of his mouth was sagging; saliva tended to dribble from the left corner of his mouth. On physical examination, the patient was unable to close the left eye completely and had difficulty exposing his teeth fully on the left side. No further abnormal signs were found.

20. The following facts concerning this patient are probably correct **except:**
(a) There is complete left-sided facial paralysis
(b) The sagging of the left corner of the mouth is due to the pull of the nonparalyzed muscles on the right side of the face
(c) The patient has left-sided Bell's palsy
(d) The dribbling from the left corner of the mouth is due to loss of tone of the cheek muscles on the left side and the tilting of the mouth
(e) The suddenness of the onset of the condition can probably be explained by a small hemorrhage into the medulla oblongata affecting the motor nucleus of the left facial nerve

ANSWERS AND EXPLANATIONS

1. E
2. B
3. C
4. D
5. D
6. A. The trigeminal nerve has a large sensory root and a small motor root.
7. D. The motor nucleus of the trigeminal nerve receives descending fibers from the cerebral cortex on both sides.
8. D. The dermatomes of the ophthalmic, maxillary, and mandibular divisions of the trigeminal nerve do not overlap.
9. B. The skin over the angle of the jaw is supplied by the great auricular nerve (C2 and C3) and not by the trigeminal nerve.
10. D. All the nerve cell bodies in the trigeminal ganglion are surrounded by capsular cells
11. B. The abducent nerve supplies the lateral rectus muscle.
12. A. The motor and parasympathetic nuclei are located in the lower part of the pons
13. E. The parasympathetic secretomotor fibers travel in the sensory root (nervus intermedius) of the facial nerve.
14. C. The paralysis produced by a lesion of the facial nerve is of the lower motor neuron type.
15. B. The inferior salivatory nucleus controls the secretions of the parotid salivary gland and is part of the glossopharyngeal nerve group of nuclei.
16. D. They do receive afferent fibers from the semicircular canals.
17. B. The lateral geniculate body is concerned with light reflexes. The lateral lemniscus terminates in the medial geniculate body and the inferior colliculus of the midbrain.
18. D. A. The posterior nucleus of the trapezoid body is a relay station and gives origin to the axons of the lateral lemniscus. B. The trigeminal nerve supplies the tensor tympani muscle. C. The lateral lemniscus conducts nerve impulses concerned with sound from the trapezoid body to the inferior colliculus or the medial geniculate body. E. The facial nerve supplies the stapedius muscle in the middle ear, which with the tensor tympani is concerned with damping down the excessive oscillations of the middle ear ossicles.
19. C. The gyrus of Heschl forms part of the primary auditory cortex.
20. E. The facial nerve nuclei are located in the lower part of the pons and not in the medulla oblongata. This patient had left-sided Bell's palsy and recovery was complete in 3 weeks.

CHAPTER 20

Cranial Nerves IX–XII

CHAPTER OUTLINE

SUGGESTED PLAN FOR REVIEW OF CHAPTER 20

1. Learn the details of all these cranial nerves.
2. Note that the glossopharyngeal and vagus nerves form part of the cranial parasympathetic outflow (the oculomotor and the facial nerves are the other contributors).
3. Understand the lengthy distribution of the vagus nerve through the thorax and the abdomen. Realize that the abdominal part of the vagus nerve is distributed to the intestinal tract down as far as the splenic flexure of the colon. Appreciate that the branches of the vagus nerve below the stomach cannot be seen with the naked eye in dissected specimens; they run close to the sympathetic nerves along the arteries in the branches of the superior mesenteric plexus.
4. Remember that the accessory nerve has two parts, cranial and spinal. The cranial part is distributed within the branches of the vagus nerve.

SUGGESTED PLAN FOR REVIEW OF CHAPTER 20 (*continued*)

5. Appreciate that the nuclei of cranial nerves IX to XII are located very close to one another in the medulla oblongata and that consequently disease usually affects more than one of these nerves.
6. Learn the hypoglossal nerve carefully. Understand the movements of the tongue, especially those involving the genioglossus muscles. When a patient is asked to protrude the tongue, the tongue is pulled forward by the equal contraction of both the right and left genioglossus muscles, which are attached in front to the mandible. If both muscles are acting normally with equal strength, the tongue will protrude forward in the midline. If, for example, the right genioglossus is weaker than the left, then the tip of the tongue will point to the right; that is, it will be pulled forward and pushed over to the right by the stronger left muscle.

INTRODUCTION

The glossopharyngeal nerve (IX) is a sensory and a motor nerve. It receives sensations from the posterior third of the tongue, the pharynx, and the middle ear and has an afferent input from the carotid sinus and carotid body. It supplies one small muscle of the pharynx (stylopharyngeus muscle) and contains parasympathetic secretomotor fibers to the parotid salivary gland.

The vagus nerve (X) is the longest cranial nerve, having a course and distribution that extend through the neck, thorax, and abdomen. It is a sensory and a motor nerve and the fibers are distributed to the heart; great thoracic vessels; larynx, trachea, and lungs; alimentary tract from the pharynx to the splenic flexure of the colon; and the liver, kidneys, and pancreas. Many of the motor fibers form part of the parasympathetic outflow.

The accessory nerve (XI) is entirely motor in function. It is an anatomical oddity in that it has a cranial root that resembles a true cranial nerve and arises from the brain inside the skull, and a spinal root that resembles an anterior root of a spinal nerve and arises from the upper five cervical segments; the spinal root then ascends through the foramen magnum to enter the skull and accompany the cranial root. A further peculiarity is that the cranial root joins the vagus nerve outside the skull and is distributed within its branches. The spinal root, as one would expect, supplies muscles in the neck, namely, the sternocleidomastoid and the trapezius.

The hypoglossal nerve (XII) is entirely motor in function and supplies the muscles of the tongue.

The purpose of this chapter is to discuss the nuclei of these cranial nerves, their central connections, and their distribution.

GLOSSOPHARYNGEAL NERVE (CRANIAL NERVE IX)

The glossopharyngeal nerve is a motor and a sensory nerve.

Glossopharyngeal Nerve Nuclei

The glossopharyngeal nerve has three nuclei: (1) the main motor nucleus, (2) the parasympathetic nucleus, and (3) the sensory nucleus.

MAIN MOTOR NUCLEUS

This nucleus is deeply placed in the medulla oblongata and is formed by part of the nucleus ambiguus (Fig. 20-1). It receives corticonuclear fibers from both cerebral hemispheres. The efferent fibers supply the stylopharyngeus muscle.

PARASYMPATHETIC NUCLEUS

This nucleus is called the **inferior salivatory nucleus** (Fig. 20-1). It receives afferent fibers from the hypothalamus through the descending autonomic pathways. It also receives information from the olfactory system through the reticular formation and information concerning taste from the nucleus of the solitary tract from the mouth cavity.

The efferent preganglionic parasympathetic fibers reach the otic ganglion through the **tympanic branch of the glossopharyngeal nerve,** the **tympanic plexus,** and the **lesser petrosal nerve**. The postganglionic fibers pass to the parotid salivary gland.

SENSORY NUCLEUS

This nucleus is part of the **nucleus of the tractus solitarius** (Fig. 20-1). Sensations of taste from the posterior one-third of the tongue and from the pharynx travel through the peripheral axons of nerve cells situated in the ganglion on the glossopharyngeal nerve. The central processes of these cells synapse on nerve cells in the nucleus. Efferent fibers cross the median plane and ascend to the ventral group of nuclei of the opposite thalamus and also a number of hypothalamic nuclei. From the thalamus, axons pass through the internal capsule and corona radiata to end in the lower part of the postcentral gyrus.

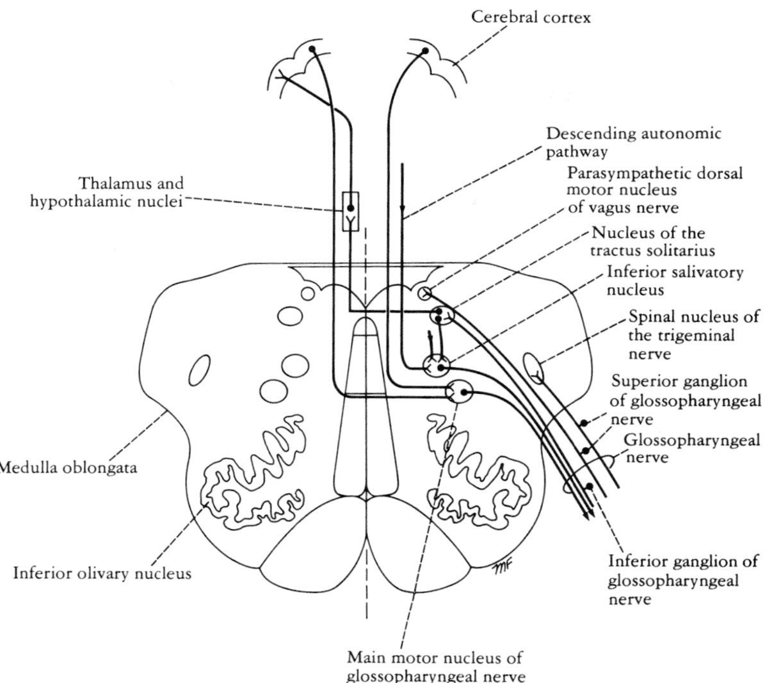

Figure 20–1 Glossopharyngeal nerve nuclei and their central connections.

Note that afferent information that concerns common sensation from the posterior one-third of the tongue, the pharynx, and the ear enters the brainstem through the superior ganglion of the glossopharyngeal nerve, but ends in the spinal nucleus of the trigeminal nerve. Afferent impulses from the carotid body and sinus also travel with the glossopharyngeal nerve. They terminate in the **nucleus of the tractus solitarius**. The carotid sinus reflex that involves the glossopharyngeal and vagus nerves assists in the regulation of arterial blood pressure.

Glossopharyngeal Nerve

The glossopharyngeal nerve emerges from the anterior surface of the medulla oblongata between the olive and the inferior cerebellar peduncle (Fig. 20-1). It passes laterally in the posterior cranial fossa and leaves the skull through the jugular foramen. The superior and inferior glossopharyngeal ganglia are situated on the nerve here. The nerve then descends through the upper part of the neck in company with the internal jugular vein and the internal carotid artery to reach the posterior border of the stylopharyngeus muscle, which it supplies. The nerve then passes forward between the superior and middle constrictor muscles to give sensory branches to the mucous membrane of the pharynx and the posterior third of the tongue. A summary of the distribution of the glossopharyngeal nerve is seen in Table 18-2, p. 191.

Clinical Notes

Glossopharyngeal Nerve Lesions

Lesions of the glossopharyngeal nerve usually also affect the vagus nerve. Bilateral corticobulbar lesions produce severe dysphagia. A neurological deficit involving the glossopharyngeal nerve can be evaluated by testing for loss of the sensation for touch or taste on the posterior third of the tongue.

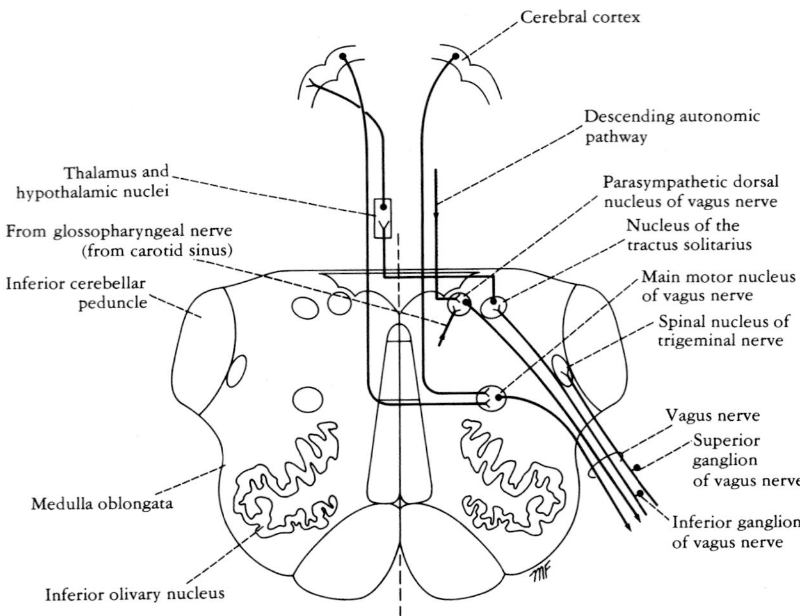

Figure 20–2 Vagus nerve nuclei and their central connections.

VAGUS NERVE (CRANIAL NERVE X)

The vagus nerve is a motor and a sensory nerve.

Vagus Nerve Nuclei

The vagus nerve has three nuclei: (1) the main motor nucleus, (2) the parasympathetic nucleus, and (3) the sensory nucleus.

MAIN MOTOR NUCLEUS

This nucleus is deeply placed in the medulla oblongata and is formed by the nucleus ambiguus (Fig. 20-2). It receives corticonuclear fibers from both cerebral hemispheres. The efferent fibers supply the constrictor muscles of the pharynx and the intrinsic muscles of the larynx.

PARASYMPATHETIC NUCLEUS

This nucleus forms the **dorsal nucleus of the vagus** and lies beneath the floor of the lower part of the fourth ventricle (Fig. 20-2). It receives afferent fibers from the hypothalamus. It also receives other afferents, including those from the glossopharyngeal nerve (carotid sinus reflex). The efferent fibers are distributed to the involuntary muscle of the bronchi, heart, esophagus, stomach, small intestine, and large intestine as far as the distal one-third of the transverse colon.

SENSORY NUCLEUS

This nucleus is the lower part of the **nucleus of the tractus solitarius**. Sensations of taste from the pharynx travel through the peripheral axons of nerve cells situated in the **inferior ganglion of the vagus nerve**. The central processes of those cells synapse on nerve cells in the nucleus (Fig. 20-2). Efferent fibers cross the median plane and ascend to the ventral group of nuclei of the opposite thalamus and also to the hypothalamus. From the thalamus, axons pass through the internal capsule and corona radiata to end in the postcentral gyrus.

Note that afferent information, concerning common sensation from the pharynx and larynx, enters the brainstem through the superior ganglion of the vagus nerve but ends in the **spinal nucleus of the trigeminal nerve**.

Vagus Nerve

The vagus nerve emerges from the anterior surface of the medulla oblongata between the olive and the inferior cerebellar peduncle (Fig. 20-2). The nerve passes laterally through the posterior cranial fossa and leaves the skull through the jugular foramen. The vagus nerve possesses two sensory ganglia, a rounded **superior ganglion**, situated on the nerve within the jugular foramen, and a cylindrical **inferior ganglion**, which lies on the nerve just below the foramen. Below the inferior ganglion, the cranial root of the accessory nerve joins the vagus nerve and is distributed mainly in its pharyngeal and recurrent laryngeal branches.

The vagus nerve descends vertically in the neck within the carotid sheath with the internal jugular vein and the internal and common carotid arteries.

The **right vagus nerve** enters the thorax and passes posterior to the root of the right lung contributing to the pulmonary plexus. It then passes on to the posterior surface of the esophagus and contributes to the **esophageal plexus**.

It enters the abdomen through the esophageal opening of the diaphragm. The posterior vagal trunk (which is the name now given to the right vagus) is distributed to the posterior surface of the stomach and by a large celiac branch to the duodenum, liver, kidneys, and small and large intestines as far as the distal third of the transverse colon. This wide distribution is accomplished through the celiac, superior mesenteric, and renal plexuses.

The **left vagus nerve** enters the thorax, crosses the left side of the aortic arch, and descends behind the root of the left lung, contributing to the **pulmonary plexus**. The left vagus then descends on the anterior surface of the esophagus, contributing to the **esophageal plexus**. It enters the abdomen through the esophageal opening of the diaphragm. The anterior vagal trunk (which is the name now given to the left vagus) divides into several branches, which are distributed to the stomach, liver, and upper part of the duodenum and head of the pancreas. A summary of the distribution of the vagus nerve is seen in Table 18-2, p. 191.

CLINICAL NOTES

VAGUS NERVE LESIONS

Lesions involving the vagus nerve commonly also involve the glossopharyngeal, accessory, and hypoglossal nerves, because they are located so close together.. The vagus nerve innervates many important organs, but the examination of this nerve depends on testing the function of the branches to the pharynx, soft palate, and larynx. The pharyngeal reflex can be tested by touching the lateral wall of the pharynx with a spatula. This should immediately cause the patient to gag; that is, the pharyngeal muscles will contract. The afferent neuron of the pharyngeal reflex runs in the glossopharyngeal nerve, and the efferent neurons run in the glossopharyngeal (to the stylopharyngeus muscle) and vagus nerves (pharyngeal constrictor muscles). Unilateral lesions of the vagus will show little or no gag reflex on that side.

The innervation of the soft palate can be tested by asking the patient to say "ah." Normally, the soft palate rises and the uvula moves backward in the midline. If there is a lesion of the right vagus nerve, for example, the uvula will be pulled upward, backward, and to the left, since the right muscles are paralyzed.

All the muscles of the larynx are supplied by the recurrent laryngeal branch of the vagus, except the cricothyroid muscle, which is supplied by the external laryngeal branch of the superior laryngeal branch of the vagus. Hoarseness or absence of the voice may occur as a symptom of vagal nerve palsy. The movements of the vocal cords can be examined by means of a laryngoscope.

ACCESSORY NERVE (CRANIAL NERVE XI)

The accessory nerve is a motor nerve that is formed by the union of a cranial and a spinal root.

Cranial Root (Part)

The cranial root is formed from the axons of nerve cells of the nucleus ambiguus (Fig. 20-3). The nucleus receives corticonuclear fibers from both cerebral hemispheres. The efferent fibers of the nucleus emerge from the anterior surface of the medulla oblongata between the olive and the inferior cerebellar peduncle. The nerve runs laterally in the posterior cranial fossa and joins the spinal root. The two roots unite and leave the skull through the jugular foramen. The roots then separate and the cranial root joins the vagus nerve and is distributed in its pharyngeal and recurrent laryngeal branches to the muscles of the soft palate, pharynx, and larynx.

Spinal Root (Part)

The spinal root is formed from axons of nerve cells in the **spinal nucleus**, which is situated in the anterior gray column of the spinal cord in the upper five cervical segments (Fig. 20-3). The spinal nucleus is thought to receive corticospinal fibers from both cerebral hemispheres.

The nerve fibers emerge from the spinal cord midway between the anterior and posterior nerve roots of the cervical spinal nerves. The fibers form a nerve trunk that ascends into the skull through the foramen magnum. The spinal root passes laterally and joins the cranial root as they pass through the jugular foramen. After a short distance, the spinal part separates from the cranial root, runs downward and laterally, and enters the deep surface of the sternocleidomastoid muscle, which it supplies. The nerve then crosses the posterior triangle of the neck and passes beneath the trapezius muscle, which it supplies.

The accessory nerve thus brings about movements of the soft palate, pharynx, and larynx and controls the movements of two large muscles in the neck. A summary of the distribution of the accessory nerve is seen in Table 18-2, p. 191.

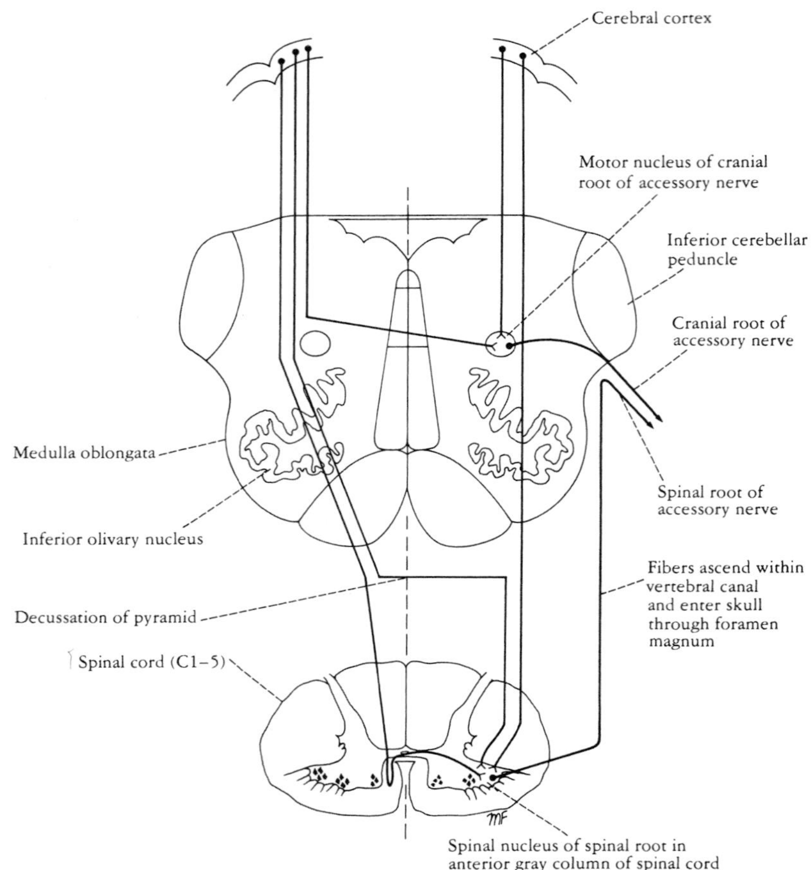

Figure 20–3 Cranial and spinal nuclei of the accessory nerve and their central connections.

CLINICAL NOTES

ACCESSORY NERVE LESIONS

The accessory nerve supplies the sternocleidomastoid and trapezius muscles by means of its spinal root. A lesion of the accessory nerve will result in paralysis of these muscles. The sternocleidomastoid muscle will atrophy and there will be weakness in turning the head to the opposite side. The trapezius muscle will also atrophy and the shoulder will droop on that side; there will also be weakness and difficulty in raising the arm above the horizontal.

HYPOGLOSSAL NERVE (CRANIAL NERVE XII)

The hypoglossal nerve is a motor nerve and supplies all the intrinsic muscles of the tongue and, in addition, the styloglossus, the hyoglossus, and the genioglossus muscles.

Hypoglossal Nucleus

The hypoglossal nucleus is situated close to the midline immediately beneath the floor of the lower part of the fourth ventricle (Fig. 20-4). It receives corticonuclear fibers from both cerebral hemispheres. However, the **cells responsible for supplying the genioglossus muscle only receive corticonuclear fibers from the opposite cerebral hemisphere**.

The hypoglossal nerve fibers emerge on the anterior surface of the medulla oblongata between the pyramid and the olive (Fig. 20-4). They cross the posterior cranial fossa and leave the skull through the hypoglossal canal. The nerve passes downward and forward in the neck between the internal carotid artery and the internal jugular vein until it reaches the lower border of the posterior belly of the digas-

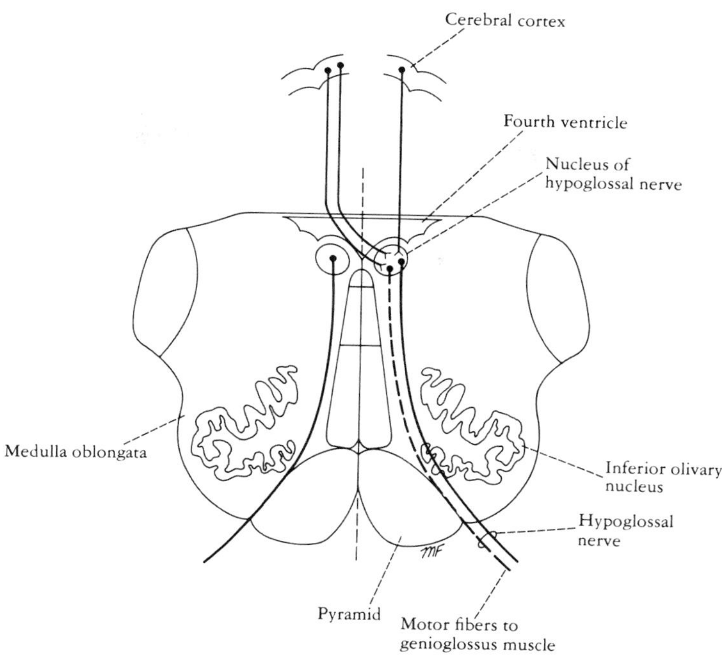

Figure 20–4 Hypoglossal nucleus and its central connections.

tric muscle. Here, it turns forward and crosses the internal and external carotid arteries and the loop of the lingual artery. It passes deep to the posterior margin of the mylohyoid muscle and sends branches to the muscles of the tongue. The hypoglossal nerve thus controls the movements and shape of the tongue.

In the upper part of its course, the hypoglossal nerve is joined by C1 fibers from the cervical plexus. These delicate cervical nerves use the hypoglossal nerve trunk for support and later leave the hypoglossal nerve to supply the geniohyoid and thyrohyoid muscles. A summary of the distribution of the hypoglossal nerve is seen in Table 18-2, p. 191.

CLINICAL NOTES

HYPOGLOSSAL NERVE LESIONS

In lesions of the hypoglossal nerve, the tongue deviates toward the paralyzed side. The tongue will be smaller on the side of the lesion, owing to muscle atrophy. The greater part of the hypoglossal nucleus receives corticonuclear fibers from both cerebral hemispheres. However, the part of the nucleus that supplies the genioglossus receives corticonuclear fibers only from the opposite cerebral hemisphere. If a patient has a lesion of the corticonuclear fibers, there will be no atrophy of the tongue and on protrusion the tongue will deviate to the side opposite the lesion. (Note that the genioglossus is the muscle that pulls the tongue forward.)

REVIEW QUESTIONS

Directions: Each of the numbered items in this section is followed by answers that are positively phrased. Select the ONE lettered answer that is an EXCEPTION.

1. The following statements concerning the glossopharyngeal nerve are correct **except:**
   (a) The nerve emerges from the brainstem between the olive and the inferior cerebellar peduncle
   (b) The nerve possesses superior and inferior sensory ganglia
   (c) The main motor nucleus is situated in the medulla oblongata and forms part of the nucleus ambiguus
   (d) The parasympathetic nucleus controls the sublingual salivary gland
   (e) The sensory nucleus forms part of the nucleus of the tractus solitarius
2. The following statements concerning the sensory input of the glossopharyngeal nerve are correct **except:**
   (a) The sensory nucleus receives the sensations of taste from the anterior one-third of the tongue

(b) Common sensation impulses from the posterior one-third of the tongue end in the spinal nucleus of the trigeminal nerve
(c) Impulses from the carotid sinus end in the nucleus of the tractus solitarius and are connected to the dorsal motor nucleus of the vagus nerve
(d) Impulses from the carotid body end in the nucleus of the tractus solitarius
(e) Lesions of the sensory input result in loss of taste sensation on the pharyngeal wall

3. The following statements concerning the vagus nerve are correct **except:**
(a) It forms part of the cranial parasympathetic outflow
(b) It possesses no sensory ganglia
(c) It innervates the alimentary tract from the pharynx down as far as the splenic flexure of the colon
(d) The nerve leaves the skull through the jugular foramen
(e) The nerve leaves the medulla oblongata between the olive and the inferior cerebellar peduncle

4. The following statements concerning a lesion of the vagus nerve are correct **except:**
(a) The pharyngeal gag reflex is lost
(b) The soft palate deviates to the contralateral side when the patient says "ah"
(c) There is no loss of taste sensation from the anterior two-thirds of the tongue
(d) The pupil dilates on the side of the lesion
(e) Hoarseness or absence of the voice may be a symptom

5. The following statements concerning the spinal part of the accessory nerve are correct.**except:**
(a) It arises from the first three cervical segments of the spinal cord
(b) It enters the skull through the foramen magnum
(c) It joins the cranial part of the accessory nerve in the posterior cranial fossa
(d) It supplies the sternocleidomastoid and trapezius muscles
(e) It can be injured in the posterior triangle of the neck

6. The following statements concerning the cranial part of the accessory nerve are correct **except:**
(a) It is entirely motor in function
(b) It leaves the medulla oblongata between the olive and the inferior cerebellar peduncle
(c) It joins the vagus nerve and is distributed in its branches to the pharynx and larynx
(d) It leaves the skull through the jugular foramen
(e) The axons do not arise from nerve cells in the nucleus ambiguus

7. The following statements concerning the hypoglossal nerve nucleus are correct **except:**
(a) It is located beneath the floor of the fourth ventricle
(b) It is separate from the nucleus ambiguus
(c) It receives corticonuclear fibers from both cerebral hemispheres
(d) It is connected to the vagal nucleus by the medial longitudinal fasciculus
(e) The neurons of the nucleus that supply the genioglossus muscle receive only corticobulbar fibers from the cerebral cortex of the contralateral side

8. The following statements concerning the hypoglossal nerve are correct **except:**
(a) It supplies all the intrinsic muscles of the tongue
(b) In lesions of the nerve, the tip of the tongue deviates to the same side when the tongue is protruded from the mouth
(c) It supplies the palatoglossus muscle
(d) It leaves the anterior surface of the brain between the pyramid and the olive
(e) It supplies the styloglossus and the hyoglossus muscles

9. The following statements concerning the nerve supply to the muscles of the head and neck are correct **except:**
(a) The main motor nucleus of the vagus nerve supplies the constrictor muscles of the pharynx
(b) The motor nucleus of the glossopharyngeal nerve supplies the stylopharyngeus muscle
(c) The hypoglossal nerve supplies the geniohyoid muscle
(d) The spinal part of the accessory nerve supplies the sternocleidomastoid muscle
(e) The cranial part of the accessory nerve supplies the muscles of the soft palate

Directions: Read the case history then answer the question. An 18-year-old man was seen in the emergency department following a stab wound at the front of the neck. The knife entrance wound was located on the right side of the neck just lateral to the tip of the greater cornu of the hyoid bone. During the physical examination, the patient was asked to protrude his tongue forward in the midline; this was found to be impossible and the tongue deviated to the right.

10. The following comments relating to this case are correct **except:**
(a) When a normal patient is instructed to protrude the tongue forward in the midline, both the right and left genioglossus muscles contract equally
(b) The left genioglossus muscle in this patient is normal
(c) The right genioglossus muscle is paralyzed in this patient
(d) The right hypoglossal nerve is severed where it turns forward and medially and crosses the internal and external carotid arteries
(e) The left hypoglossal nerve is damaged

ANSWERS AND EXPLANATIONS

1. D. The parasympathetic nucleus of the glossopharyngeal nerve controls the parotid salivary gland.
2. A. The sensory nucleus of the glossopharyngeal nerve receives the sensations of taste from the posterior one-third of the tongue (the taste sensation from the anterior two-thirds of the tongue is served by the facial nerve).
3. B. The vagus nerve possesses a superior and an inferior sensory ganglion.
4. D. The iris is innervated by sympathetic nerves, which cause pupillary dilation, and the oculomotor nerve (parasympathetic), which causes pupillary constriction.
5. A. The spinal part of the accessory nerve arises from the first five cervical segments of the spinal cord.
6. E. The axons of the cranial part of the accessory nerve arise from the nerve cells of the nucleus ambiguus.
7. D. The hypoglossal nerve nucleus is not connected to the vagal nucleus by the medial longitudinal fasciculus.
8. C. The palatoglossus muscle is supplied by the cranial part of the accessory nerve through the pharyngeal branches of the vagus nerve.
9. C. The geniohyoid muscle is supplied by C1 spinal nerve; it travels with the hypoglossal nerve in the neck.
10. E. The knife severed the right hypoglossal nerve in this patient, resulting in paralysis of the right genioglossus muscle.

CHAPTER 21

Autonomic Nervous System

CHAPTER OUTLINE

SUGGESTED PLAN FOR REVIEW OF CHAPTER 21

1. The autonomic nervous system and the endocrine system control the internal environment of the body. The autonomic system is a difficult but important system to learn. Read the chapter slowly and commit the basic information to memory. Physiologists, pharmacologists, and clinicians require this information.

SUGGESTED PLAN FOR REVIEW OF CHAPTER 21 (*continued*)

2. Know precisely what is meant by the terms sympathetic and parasympathetic outflows.
3. Recognize that both the sympathetic and parasympathetic parts of the autonomic nervous system have afferent and efferent fibers and higher centers of control. Appreciate that parts of the autonomic system are present in both the peripheral and central parts of the nervous system.
4. Be able to make a simple drawing of a transverse section of the spinal cord in the thoracic region showing the sympathetic outflow, the rami, and the ganglionated sympathetic trunk.
5. Be able to define (a) gray ramus, (b) white ramus, (c) splanchnic nerve, and (d) sympathetic plexus. Understand the innervation of the suprarenal medulla.
6. Know the positions of the main parasympathetic ganglia in the head and neck.
7. Learn about neurotransmitters, ganglion blocking agents, and blocking agents concerned with cholinergic and adrenergic receptors.
8. Be able to compare the structure and functions of the sympathetic and parasympathetic parts of the autonomic system.
9. Understand the control of the autonomic nervous system and the role played by the hypothalamus.
10. Learn in detail the examples of autonomic innervations given in this chapter. These are commonly used by examiners to construct good questions.

INTRODUCTION

The autonomic nervous system, along with the endocrine system, exerts control over the functions of many organs and tissues in the body.

The autonomic nervous system, like the somatic nervous system, has afferent, connector, and efferent neurons. The afferent impulses originate in visceral receptors and travel via afferent pathways to the central nervous system where they are integrated through connector neurons at different levels and then leave via efferent pathways to visceral effector organs.

The efferent pathways of the autonomic system are made up of preganglionic and postganglionic neurons. The cell bodies of the preganglionic neurons are situated in the lateral gray column of the spinal cord and in the motor nuclei of the third, seventh, ninth, and tenth cranial nerves. The axons of these neurons synapse with the postganglionic neurons that are collected together to form ganglia outside the central nervous system.

The control exerted by the autonomic system is widespread since one preganglionic axon may synapse with several postganglionic neurons. Large collections of afferent and efferent nerve fibers and their associated ganglia form autonomic plexuses in the thorax, abdomen, and pelvis.

The visceral receptors include chemoreceptors, baroreceptors, and osmoreceptors. Pain receptors are present in viscera, and certain types of stimuli, such as stretching or lack of oxygen, can cause extreme pain.

BASIC ANATOMY OF THE AUTONOMIC NERVOUS SYSTEM

The autonomic nervous system innervates involuntary structures such as the heart, smooth muscles, and glands. The system is distributed throughout the central and peripheral nervous systems; is divided into two parts, the **sympathetic** and the **parasympathetic**; and, as emphasized above, consists of both afferent and efferent fibers. This division between sympathetic and parasympathetic is made on the basis of anatomical differences, differences in the neurotransmitters, and differences in the physiological effects.

SYMPATHETIC PART OF THE AUTONOMIC NERVOUS SYSTEM

The sympathetic system is the larger of the two parts of the autonomic system and is widely distributed throughout the body, innervating the heart and lungs, the muscle in the walls of many blood vessels, the hair follicles and the sweat glands, and many abdominopelvic viscera.

The function of the sympathetic system is to prepare the body for an emergency. The heart rate is increased, arterioles of the skin and intestine are constricted, those of skeletal muscle are dilated, and blood pressure is raised. There is a redistribution of blood so that it leaves the skin and gastrointestinal tract and passes to the brain, heart, and skeletal muscle. In addition, the sympathetic nerves dilate the pupils; inhibit smooth muscle of the bronchi, intestine, and bladder wall; and close the sphincters. The hair is made to stand on end, and sweating occurs.

The sympathetic system consists of the efferent outflow from the spinal cord, two ganglionated sympathetic trunks, important branches, plexuses, and regional ganglia.

Efferent Nerve Fibers (Sympathetic Outflow)

The lateral gray columns (horns) of the spinal cord from the first thoracic segment to the second lumbar segment (sometimes third lumbar segment) possess the cell bodies of the sympathetic connector neurons (Fig. 21-1). The myelinated axons of these cells leave the cord in the anterior nerve roots and pass via the **white rami communicantes** (the white rami are white because the nerve fibers are covered with white myelin) to the **paravertebral ganglia** of the **sympathetic trunk**. Once these fibers (preganglionic) reach the ganglia in the sympathetic trunk, they are distributed as follows:

1. They synapse with an excitor neuron in the ganglion (Fig. 21-2). The gap between the two neurons is bridged by the neurotransmitter **acetylcholine**. The postganglionic nonmyelinated axons leave the ganglion and pass to the thoracic spinal nerves as **gray rami communicantes**. They are distributed in branches of the spinal nerves to smooth muscle in the blood vessel walls, sweat glands, and arrector pili muscles of the skin.
2. They travel cephalad in the sympathetic trunk to synapse in ganglia in the cervical region (Fig. 21-2). The postganglionic nerve fibers pass via gray rami communicantes to join the cervical spinal nerves. Many of the preganglionic fibers entering the lower part of the sympathetic trunk from the lower thoracic and upper two lumbar segments of the spinal cord travel caudal to synapse in ganglia in the lower lumbar and sacral regions. Here again, the postganglionic nerve fibers pass via gray rami communicantes to join the lumbar, sacral, and coccygeal spinal nerves (Fig. 21-2).
3. They may pass through the ganglia of the sympathetic trunk without synapsing. These myelinated fibers leave the sympathetic trunk as the **greater splanchnic, lesser splanchnic,** and **lowest or least splanchnic nerves**. The greater splanchnic nerve is formed from branches from the fifth to the ninth thoracic ganglia. It descends obliquely on the sides of the bodies of the thoracic vertebrae and pierces the crus of the diaphragm to synapse with excitor cells in the ganglia of the celiac plexus, the **renal plexus**, and the **suprarenal medulla**. The lesser splanchnic nerve is formed from branches of the tenth and eleventh thoracic ganglia. It descends with the greater splanchnic nerve and pierces the diaphragm to join excitor cells in ganglia in the lower part of the **celiac plexus**. The lowest splanchnic nerve (when present) arises from the twelfth thoracic ganglion, pierces the diaphragm, and synapses with excitor neurons in the ganglia of the **renal plexus**. The splanchnic nerves, therefore, are formed of preganglionic fibers. The postganglionic fibers arise from the excitor cells in the peripheral plexuses and are distributed to the smooth muscle and glands of the viscera. A few preganglionic fibers, traveling in the greater splanchnic nerve, end directly on the cells of the **suprarenal medulla**.

Afferent Nerve Fibers

The afferent myelinated nerve fibers travel from the viscera through the sympathetic ganglia without synapsing. They pass to the spinal nerve via white rami communicantes and reach their cell bodies in the posterior root ganglion of the corresponding spinal nerve (Fig. 21-1). The central axons then enter the spinal cord and may

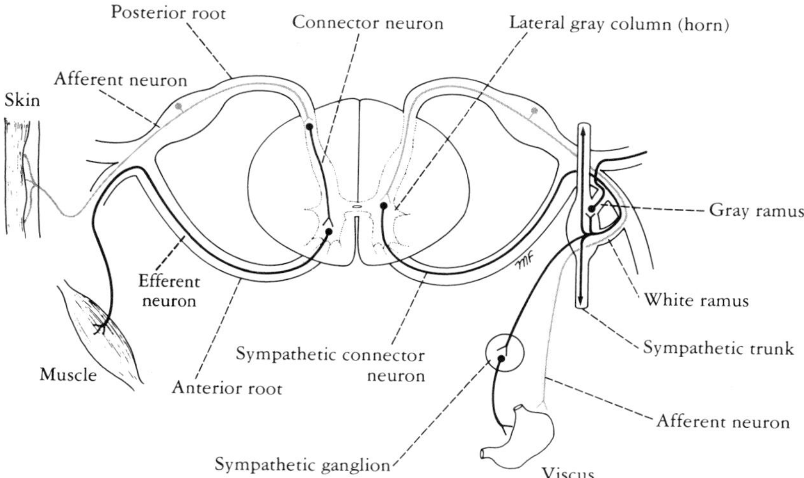

Figure 21–1 Arrangement of the somatic part of the nervous system (left) and the autonomic part of the nervous system (right).

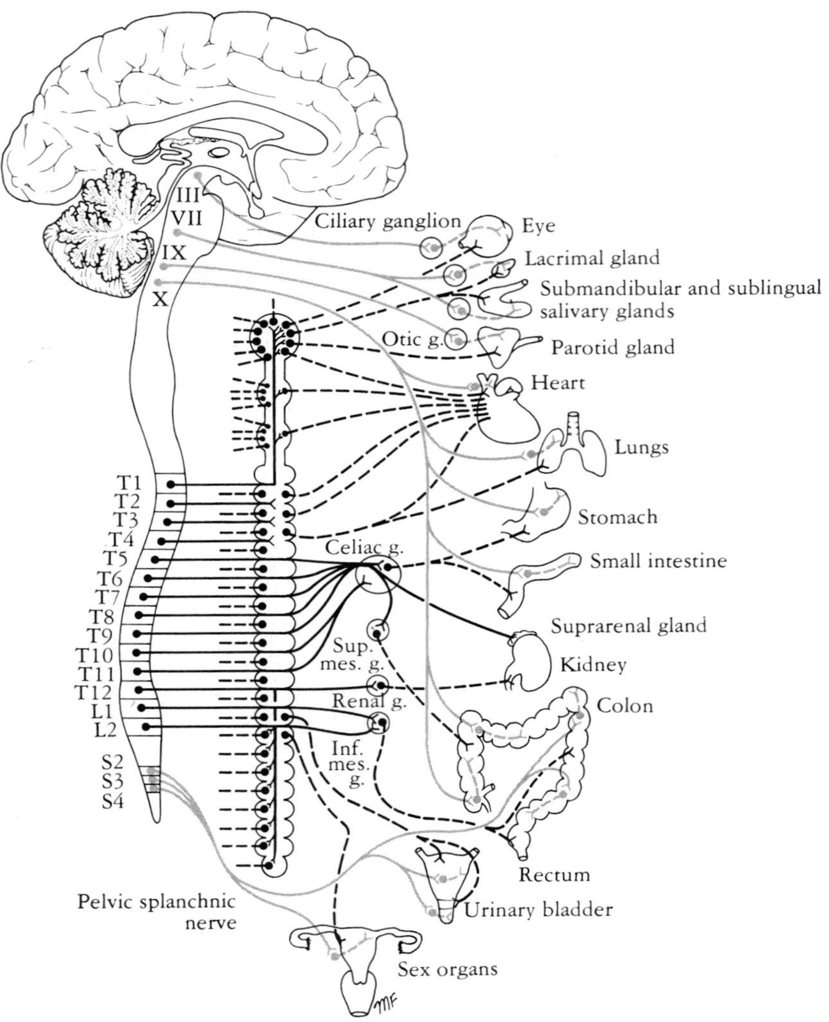

Figure 21–2 Efferent part of the autonomic nervous system.

form the afferent component of a local reflex arc or ascend to higher centers, such as the hypothalamus.

The Sympathetic Trunks

The sympathetic trunks are two ganglionated nerve trunks that extend the whole length of the vertebral column (Fig. 21-2). In the neck each trunk has 3 ganglia, in the thorax there are 11 or 12, in the lumbar region 4 or 5, and in the pelvis 4 or 5.

PARASYMPATHETIC PART OF THE AUTONOMIC NERVOUS SYSTEM

The activities of the parasympathetic part of the autonomic system are directed toward conserving and restoring energy. The heart rate is slowed, pupils are constricted, peristalsis is increased and glandular activity is augmented, sphincters are opened, and the bladder wall is contracted.

Efferent Nerve Fibers (Craniosacral Outflow)

The connector nerve cells of this part of the system are located in the brainstem and the sacral segments of the spinal cord (Fig. 21-2). Those nerve cells located in the brainstem form parts of the nuclei of origin of the following cranial nerves: the **oculomotor** (parasympathetic or Edinger-Westphal nucleus), the **facial** (superior salivatory nucleus and lacrimatory nucleus), the **glossopharyngeal** (inferior salivatory nucleus), and the **vagus** nerves (dorsal nucleus of vagus). The axons of these connector nerve cells emerge from the brain contained in the cranial nerves.

The sacral connector nerve cells are found in the gray matter of the **second, third, and fourth sacral segments of the cord**. These cells are not sufficiently numerous to form a lateral gray horn, as do the sympathetic connector neurons in the thoracolumbar region. The myelinated axons leave the spinal cord in the anterior nerve roots of the corresponding spinal nerves. They then leave the sacral nerves and form the **pelvic splanchnic nerves** (Fig. 21-2).

All the myelinated efferent fibers described so far are preganglionic, and they synapse with excitor neurons in the peripheral ganglia, which are usually situated close to the viscera they innervate. Here again acetylcholine is the transmitter. The cranial preganglionic fibers relay in the **ciliary, pterygopalatine, submandibular,** and **otic ganglia** (Fig. 21-2). The preganglionic fibers in the pelvic splanchnic nerves relay in ganglia in the **hypogastric plexuses**. In certain situations, the ganglion cells are diffusely arranged in nerve plexuses such as the **cardiac plexus,** the **pulmonary plexus**, and in the **myenteric** and **mucosal plexuses** of the gastrointestinal tract. The pelvic splanchnic nerves synapse in ganglia in the hypogastric plexuses. The postganglionic fibers are nonmyelinated and short.

Afferent Nerve Fibers

The afferent myelinated fibers leave the viscera and reach their cell bodies in the sensory ganglia of cranial nerves or in posterior root ganglia of the sacral spinal nerves. The central axons then enter the central nervous system and form regional reflex arcs or ascend to higher centers, such as the hypothalamus. Once the afferent fibers gain entrance to the spinal cord or brain, they are thought to travel alongside, or to be mixed with, the somatic afferent fibers.

THE LARGE AUTONOMIC PLEXUSES

Large collections of sympathetic and parasympathetic efferent nerve fibers and their associated ganglia, together with visceral afferent fibers, form autonomic nerve plexuses in the thorax, abdomen, and pelvis. Branches from these plexuses innervate the viscera. In the abdomen the plexuses are associated with the aorta and its branches and the subdivisions of these autonomic plexuses are named according to the branch of the aorta along which they are lying: cardiac, pulmonary, celiac, superior mesenteric, inferior mesenteric, aortic, and superior and inferior hypogastric plexus.

AUTONOMIC GANGLIA

The autonomic ganglion is the site where preganglionic fibers synapse on postganglionic neurons. Ganglia are situated along the course of efferent nerve fibers of the autonomic nervous system. Sympathetic ganglia form part of the sympathetic trunk or are prevertebral in position (e.g., celiac ganglia). Parasympathetic ganglia, on the other hand, are situated close to or within the walls of the viscera.

Preganglionic fibers are myelinated, small, and relatively slow-conducting B fibers. The postganglionic fibers are unmyelinated, smaller, and slower-conducting C fibers.

The presence of small interneurons within autonomic ganglia has now been recognized. These cells exhibit catecholamine fluorescence and are referred to as **small intensely fluorescent (SIF)** cells. In some ganglia these interneurons receive preganglionic cholinergic fibers so that they may modulate ganglionic transmission. In other ganglia they receive collateral branches and may serve some integrative function. Many SIF cells contain **dopamine** which is thought to be their transmitter.

Preganglionic Transmitters

The synaptic transmitter that excites the postganglionic neurons in both sympathetic and parasympathetic ganglia is **acetylcholine** (Fig. 21-3). The action of **acetylcholine** in autonomic ganglia is terminated by acetylcholinesterase. Many of the small ganglionic interneurons contain **dopamine**, which is thought to act as a transmitter. **Nicotinic** and **muscarinic** receptors are present on the dendrites and cell bodies of the postganglionic neurons. Their existence allows the postsynaptic membrane potential to be altered and ganglionic transmission modulated.

Ganglion Blocking Agents

There are two types of ganglion blocking agents, depolarizing and nonpolarizing. **Nicotine** acts as a blocking agent in high concentrations, by first stimulating the postganglionic neuron and causing depolarization, and then by maintaining depolarization of the excitable membrane. **Hexamethonium** and **tetraethylammonium** block ganglia by competing with acetylcholine at the receptor sites (Fig. 21-3).

POSTGANGLIONIC NERVE ENDINGS

Postganglionic fibers terminate on the effector cells without special discrete endings. The axons run between the gland cells and the smooth and cardiac muscle cells and lose their covering of Schwann cells. At sites where transmission occurs, clusters of vesicles are present within the axoplasm. If the site on the axon is at some distance from the effector cell, transmission time may be slow. The diffusion of transmitter through large extracellular distances permits a given nerve to have an action on a large number of effector cells.

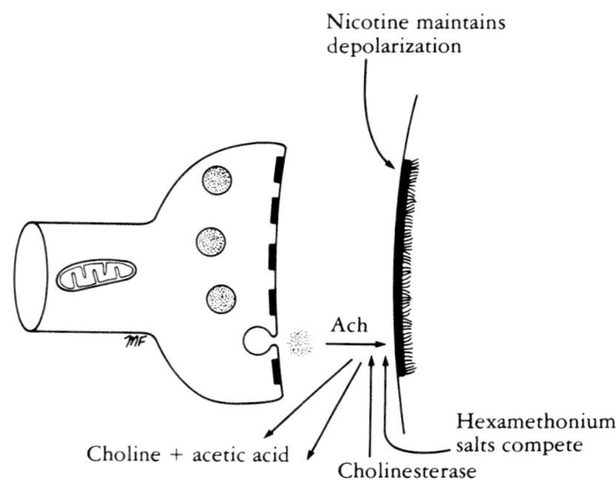

Figure 21–3 Diagram showing the liberation of acetylcholine (Ach) at an autonomic synapse.

Postganglionic Transmitters

Parasympathetic postganglionic nerve endings liberate **acetylcholine** as their transmitter substance. The acetylcholine traverses the synaptic cleft and binds reversibly with the cholinergic receptor on the postsynaptic membrane. Within 2 to 3 msec it is hydrolyzed into acetic acid and choline by the enzyme **acetylcholinesterase,** which is located on the surface of the nerve and receptor membranes. The choline is reabsorbed into the nerve ending and used again for synthesis of acetylcholine.

Most sympathetic postganglionic nerve endings liberate **norepinephrine** as their transmitter substance. In addition, some sympathetic postganglionic nerve endings, particularly those that end on cells of sweat glands, release acetylcholine.

Sympathetic endings that use norepinephrine are called **adrenergic endings**. There are two kinds of receptors in the effector organs, called **alpha** and **beta receptors**.

Two subgroups of alpha receptors (alpha-1 and alpha-2 receptors) and two subgroups of beta receptors (beta-1 and beta-2 receptors) have been described. Norepinephrine has a greater effect on alpha receptors than on beta receptors. **Phenylephrine** is a pure alpha stimulator. The bronchodilating drugs, such as **metaproterenol** and **albuterol**, mainly act on beta-2 receptors. As a general rule, alpha receptor sites are associated with most of the excitatory functions of the sympathetic system (e.g., smooth muscle contraction, vasoconstriction, diaphoresis), whereas the beta receptor sites are associated with most of the inhibitory functions (e.g., smooth muscle relaxation). Beta-2 receptors are mainly in the lung, and stimulation results in bronchodilation. Beta-1 receptors are in the myocardium, where they are associated with excitation.

The action of norepinephrine on the receptor site of the effector cell is terminated by reuptake into the nerve terminal where it is stored in presynaptic vesicles for reuse. Some of the norepinephrine escapes from the synaptic cleft into the general circulation and is subsequently metabolised in the liver.

Blocking of Cholinergic Receptors

In the case of the parasympathetic and the sympathetic postganglionic nerve endings that liberate acetylcholine as the transmitter substance, the receptors on the effector cells are **muscarinic**. This means that the action can be blocked by **atropine**. Atropine competitively antagonizes the muscarinic action by occupying the cholinergic receptor sites on the effector cells.

Blocking of Adrenergic Receptors

Phenoxybenzamine is an example of a drug that is capable of blocking alpha-norepinephrine receptors; the beta-norepinephrine receptors can be blocked by agents such as **propranolol.** The synthesis and storage of norepinephrine at sympathetic endings can be inhibited by **reserpine.**

HIGHER CONTROL OF THE AUTONOMIC NERVOUS SYSTEM

The sympathetic outflow in the spinal cord (T1–L2[3]) and the parasympathetic craniosacral outflow (cranial nuclei III, VII, IX, and X; spinal S2, S3, and S4) are controlled by the hypothalamus. The hypothalamus appears to integrate the autonomic and neuroendocrine systems, thus preserving body homeostasis. It receives signals from all parts of the nervous system, afferent input from the viscera, and information concerning the hormone levels in the blood. This input is integrated within the hypothalamus and transmitted to the lower autonomic centers in the brainstem and spinal cord by descending tracts of the reticular formation. In a similar manner, **releasing factors** or **release-inhibiting factors** are liberated into the circulation, affecting hormone levels and endocrine secretions and thus influencing organ activity.

Stimulation of different parts of the cerebral cortex and the limbic system can produce autonomic effects that are brought about through the hypothalamus.

It is a known fact that during infancy, as a result of the process of learning, the sphincters of the bladder and rectum are brought under voluntary control. It is also recognized that many of the physical responses to an emotional reaction are brought about by the autonomic nervous system. These changes can be explained by the connections that exist between the cerebral cortex, the limbic system, and the hypothalamus.

FUNCTIONS OF THE AUTONOMIC NERVOUS SYSTEM

The autonomic nervous system, along with the endocrine system, maintains body homeostasis. The endocrine control is slower and exerts its influence by means of bloodborne hormones.

The sympathetic and parasympathetic components of the autonomic system cooperate in maintaining the stability of the internal environment. The sympathetic part prepares and mobilizes the body in an emergency, when there is sudden severe exercise, fear, or rage. The parasympathetic part aims at conserving and storing energy, for example, in the promotion of digestion and the absorption of food by increasing secretions of the glands of the gastrointestinal tract and stimulating peristalsis.

The sympathetic and parasympathetic parts of the system usually have antagonistic control over a viscus. For example, the sympathetic activity will increase the heart rate, whereas the parasympathetic activity will slow the heart rate. The sympathetic activity will make the bronchial smooth muscle relax but the muscle is contracted by parasympathetic activity.

It should be pointed out, however, that many viscera do not possess this fine dual control from the autonomic system; for example, the arrector pili muscles of hair follicles have sympathetic innervation only.

The autonomic system should not be regarded as an isolated portion of the nervous system, for we know that it can play a role with somatic activity in expressing emotion, and that certain autonomic activities, such as micturition, can be brought under voluntary control.

For important anatomical, physiological, and pharmacological differences between the sympathetic and the parasympathetic parts of the autonomic system, see Table 21-1.

Note that the sympathetic part of the system has a widespread action on the body, as the result of the preganglionic fibers synapsing on many postganglionic neurons and the suprarenal medulla releasing norepinephrine and epinephrine into the bloodstream. The parasympathetic part has a more discrete control, since the preganglionic fibers synapse on only a few postganglionic neurons and there is no comparable organ to the suprarenal medulla.

The effects of the autonomic nervous system on body organs are summarized in Table 21-2.

SOME IMPORTANT AUTONOMIC INNERVATIONS

Eye

UPPER LID

The smooth muscle fibers of the levator palpebrae superioris are innervated by sympathetic postganglionic fibers from the superior cervical sympathetic ganglion (Fig. 21-4).

IRIS

The sphincter pupillae is supplied by parasympathetic fibers from the parasympathetic nucleus (Edinger-Westphal nucleus) of the oculomotor nerve (Fig. 21-4). After synapsing in the **ciliary ganglion**, the postganglionic fibers pass forward to the eyeball in the **short ciliary nerves** to supply the sphincter pupillae. (Note that the ciliary muscle of the eye is also supplied by the same nerves.)

The dilator pupillae is supplied by postganglionic fibers from the superior cervical sympathetic ganglion (Fig. 21-4).

Table 21–1 Comparison of Anatomical, Physiological, and Pharmacological Characteristics of the Sympathetic and Parasympathetic Parts of the Autonomic Nervous System

	Sympathetic	Parasympathetic
Action	Prepares body for emergency	Conserves and restores energy
Outflow	T1–L2 (3)	Cranial nerves III, VII, IX, and X; S2, S3, and S4
Preganglionic fibers	Myelinated	Myelinated
Ganglia	Paravertebral (sympathetic trunks); prevertebral (e.g., celiac, superior mesenteric, inferior mesenteric)	Small ganglia close to viscera (e.g., otic, ciliary) or ganglion cells in plexuses (e.g., cardiac, pulmonary)
Neurotransmitter within ganglia	Acetylcholine	Acetylcholine
Ganglion blocking agents	Hexamethonium and tetraethylammonium by competing with acetylcholine	Hexamethonium and tetraethylammonium by competing with acetylcholine
Postganglionic fibers	Long, nonmyelinated	Short, nonmyelinated
Characteristic activity	Widespread due to many postganglionic fibers and liberation of epinephrine and norepinephrine from suprarenal medulla	Discrete action with few postganglionic fibers
Neurotransmitter at postganglionic endings	Norepinephrine at most endings and acetylcholine at few endings (sweat glands)	Acetylcholine at all endings
Blocking agents on receptors of effector cells	Alpha-adrenergic receptors—phenoxybenzamine; beta-adrenergic receptors—propranolol	Atropine, scopolamine
Agents inhibiting synthesis and storage of neurotransmitter at postganglionic endings	Reserpine	
Agents inhibiting hydrolysis of neurotransmitter at site of effector cells		Acetylcholinesterase blockers (e.g., neostigmine)
Drugs mimicking autonomic activity	Sympathomimetic drugs Phenylephrine: alpha receptors Metaproterenol and albuterol: beta receptors	Parasympathomimetic drugs Pilocarpine Methacholine
Higher control	Hypothalamus	Hypothalamus

Table 21–2 Effects of Autonomic Nervous System on Organs of the Body

Organ		Sympathetic Action	Parasympathetic Action
Eye	Pupil	Dilates	Constricts
	Ciliary muscle	Relaxes	Contracts
Glands	Lacrimal, parotid, submandibular, sublingual, nasal	Reduces secretion by causing vasoconstriction of blood vessels	Increases secretion
	Sweat	Increases secretion	
Heart	Cardiac muscle	Increases force of contraction	Decreases force of contraction
	Coronary arteries (mainly controlled by local metabolic factors)	Dilates (beta receptors), constricts (alpha receptors)	
Lung	Bronchial muscle	Relaxes (dilates bronchi)	Contracts (constricts bronchi),
	Bronchial secretion		increases secretion
	Bronchial arteries	Constricts	Dilates
Gastrointestinal tract	Muscle in walls	Decreases peristalsis	Increases peristalsis
	Muscle in sphincters	Contracts	Relaxes
	Glands	Reduces secretion by vasoconstriction of blood vessels	Increases secretion
Liver		Breaks down glycogen into glucose	
Gallbladder		Relaxes	Contracts
Kidney		Decreases output due to constriction of arteries	
Urinary bladder	Bladder wall (detrusor)	Relaxes	Contracts
	Sphincter vesicae	Contracts	Relaxes
Erectile tissue of penis and clitoris			Relaxes, causes erection
Ejaculation		Contracts smooth muscle of vas deferens, seminal vesicles, and prostate	
Systemic arteries			
Skin		Constricts	
Abdominal		Constricts	
Muscle		Constricts (alpha receptors), dilates (beta receptors), dilates (cholinergic)	
Arrector pili muscles		Contracts	
Suprarenal			
Cortex		Stimulates	
Medulla		Liberates epinephrine and norepinephrine	

The fibers reach the eyeball in the short and the long ciliary nerves.

LACRIMAL GLAND

The parasympathetic secretomotor nerves originate in the **lacrimatory nucleus** of the facial nerve (Fig. 21-5). The preganglionic fibers reach the **pterygopalatine ganglion** through the **great petrosal nerve** and the **nerve of the pterygoid canal**. The postganglionic fibers join the **maxillary nerve** and travel in its **zygomatic branch**, the **zygomaticotemporal nerve**, and the **lacrimal nerve** to reach the lacrimal gland.

The sympathetic postganglionic fibers arise from the superior cervical sympathetic ganglion and travel to the lacrimal gland in the plexus of the internal carotid artery, the **deep petrosal nerve**, the **nerve of the pterygoid canal**, the **maxillary nerve**, the **zygomatic nerve**, the **zygomaticotemporal nerve**, and finally the **lacrimal nerve**.

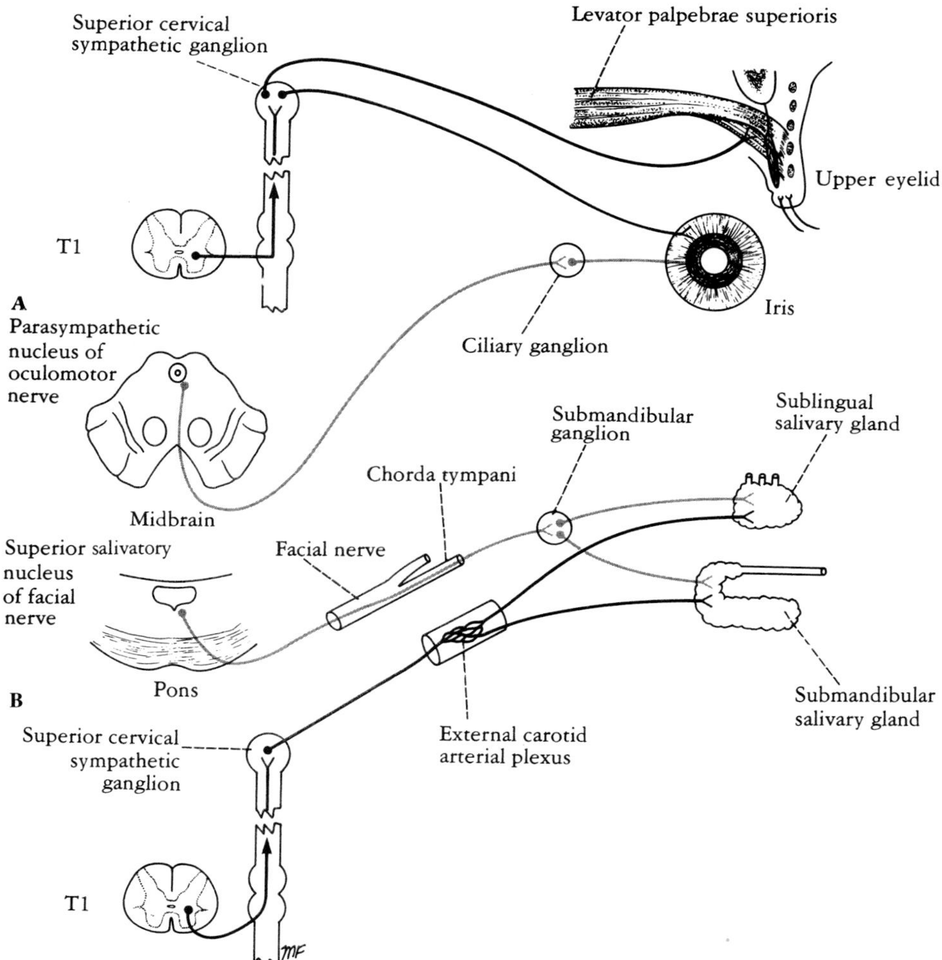

Figure 21–4 Autonomic innervation of the upper eyelid and iris (**A**) and the sublingual and submandibular salivary glands (**B**).

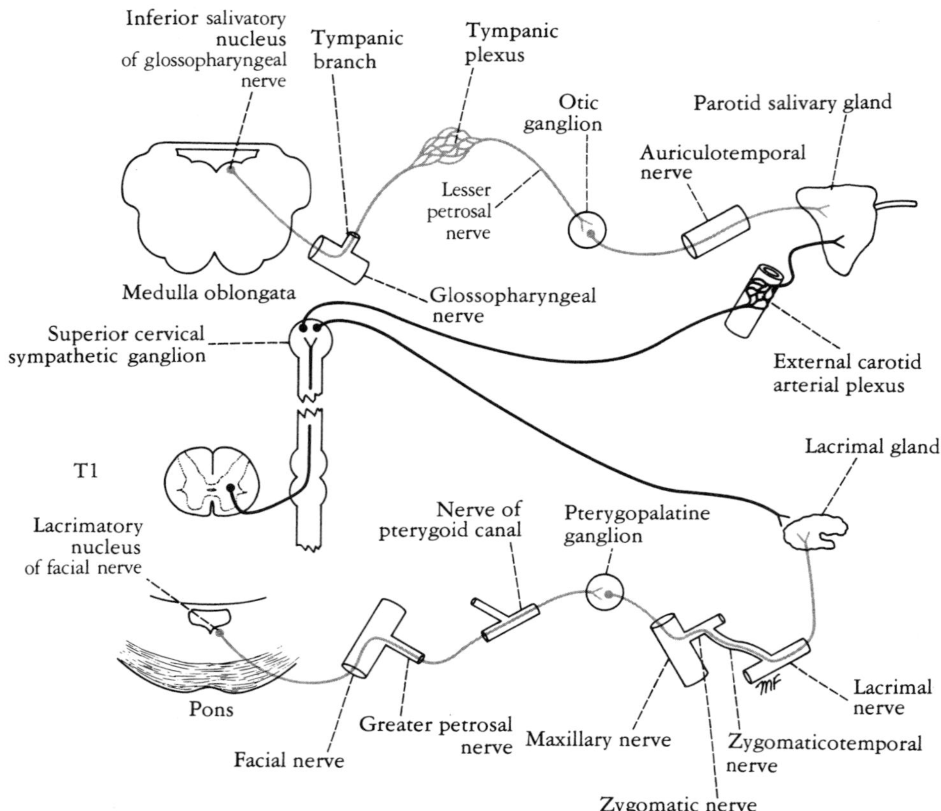

Figure 21–5 Autonomic innervation of the parotid salivary gland and the lacrimal gland.

Clinical Notes

Horner's Syndrome

This syndrome consists of (1) constriction of the pupil, (2) slight drooping of the eyelid (ptosis), (3) enophthalmos, (4) vasodilation of skin arterioles, and (5) loss of sweating (anhydrosis), all resulting from an interruption of the sympathetic nerve supply to the head and neck. The lesions responsible include multiple sclerosis and syringomyelia.

Argyll Robertson Pupil

This condition is characterized by a small pupil that is of fixed size and that does not react to light but does contract with accommodation. It is usually caused by a neurosyphilitic lesion interrupting the fibers that run from the pretectal nucleus to the parasympathetic nuclei (Edinger-Westphal nuclei) of the oculomotor nerve on both sides.

SALIVARY GLANDS

Submandibular and Sublingual Glands

Parasympathetic secretomotor fibers originate in the **superior salivatory nucleus** of the facial nerve (Fig. 21-4). The preganglionic fibers pass to the **submandibular ganglion** and other small ganglia close to the duct through the **chorda tympani nerve** and the **lingual nerve**. The postganglionic fibers pass to the glands.

Sympathetic postganglionic fibers arise from the superior cervical sympathetic ganglion and reach the glands along the arterial supply; they are vasoconstrictor in function.

Parotid Gland

Parasympathetic secretomotor fibers from the **inferior salivatory nucleus** of the glossopharyngeal nerve supply the gland (Fig. 21-5). The preganglionic fibers pass to the **otic ganglion** through the **tympanic branch of the glossopharyngeal nerve** and the **lesser petrosal nerve**. Postganglionic fibers pass to the gland through the auriculotemporal nerve.

Sympathetic postganglionic fibers arise from the superior cervical sympathetic ganglion and reach the gland along the external carotid artery.

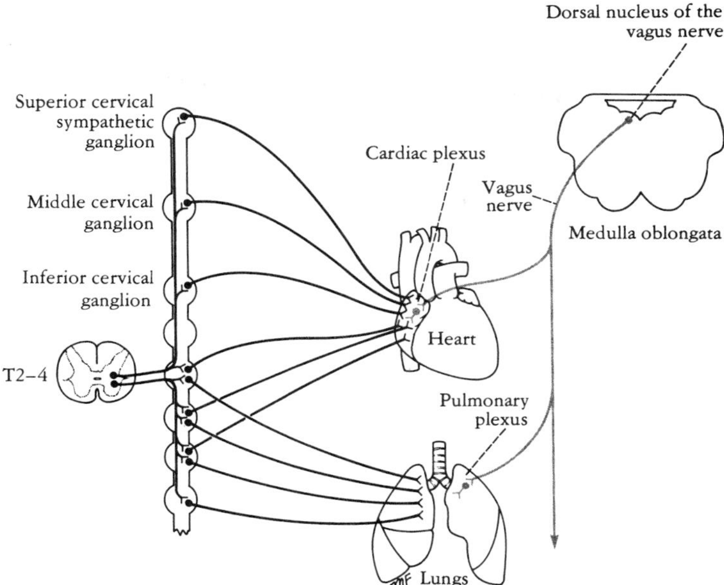

Figure 21–6 Autonomic innervation of the heart and lungs.

Heart

The sympathetic postganglionic fibers pass from the cervical and upper thoracic portions of the sympathetic trunks (Fig. 21-6). Postganglionic fibers reach the heart by way of the **superior, middle, and inferior cardiac branches** of the cervical portion of the sympathetic trunk and a number of **cardiac branches** from the thoracic portion of the sympathetic trunk. The fibers pass through the **cardiac plexuses** and terminate on the **sinoatrial node** and the **atrioventricular node**, on cardiac muscle fibers, and on coronary arteries. Activation of these fibers results in cardiac acceleration, increased force of contraction of the cardiac muscle, and dilation of the coronary arteries.

The parasympathetic preganglionic fibers originate in the **dorsal nucleus of the vagus nerve** and descend into the thorax in the **vagus nerves**. The fibers end by synapsing in the **cardiac plexuses**. The postganglionic fibers terminate on the **sinoatrial** and **atrioventricular nodes** and on the coronary arteries. Activation of these nerves results in a reduction in the rate and force of contraction of the heart and a constriction of the coronary arteries.

Further examples of autonomic innervations are shown in Table 21-2.

Clinical Notes

Referred Visceral Pain

Most viscera are innervated only by autonomic nerves. It therefore follows that visceral pain is conducted along afferent autonomic nerves. Visceral pain is diffuse and poorly localized, whereas somatic pain is intense and discretely localized. Visceral pain frequently is referred to skin areas that are innervated by the same segments of the spinal cord as the painful viscus

Cardiac Pain

Pain originating in the heart as the result of acute myocardial ischemia is caused by oxygen deficiency and the accumulation of metabolites, which stimulate the sensory nerve endings in the myocardium. The afferent nerve fibers ascend to the central nervous system through the cardiac branches of the sympathetic trunk and enter the spinal cord through the posterior roots of the upper four thoracic nerves.

The pain is **not felt in the heart**, but is referred to the skin areas supplied by the corresponding spinal nerves. The skin areas supplied by the upper four intercostal nerves and by the intercostobrachial nerve (T2) are therefore affected. The intercostobrachial nerve communicates with the medial cutaneous nerve of the arm and is distributed to skin on the medial side of the upper part of the arm. A certain amount of spread of nervous information must occur within the central nervous system, for the pain is sometimes felt in the neck and the jaw.

REVIEW QUESTIONS

Directions: Each of the numbered items or incomplete statements in this section is followed by answers or by completions of the statement. Select the ONE lettered answer or completion that is BEST in each case.

1. The parotid salivary gland receives its parasympathetic innervation from the following nerve?
   (a) vagus
   (b) facial
   (c) glossopharyngeal
   (d) oculomotor
   (e) great auricular
2. The innervation of the constrictor pupillae involves the following autonomic ganglion?
   (a) parotid ganglion
   (b) otic ganglion
   (c) pterygopalatine ganglion
   (d) ciliary ganglion
   (e) submandibular ganglion
3. The facial nerve has a nucleus known as the:
   (a) dorsal motor nucleus
   (b) lacrimatory nucleus
   (c) Edinger-Westphal nucleus
   (d) inferior salivatory nucleus
   (e) spinal nucleus
4. The glossopharyngeal nerve has a nucleus known as the:
   (a) inferior salivatory nucleus
   (b) superior salivatory nucleus
   (c) lacrimatory nucleus
   (d) Edinger-Westphal nucleus
   (e) spinal nucleus
5. The oculomotor nerve has a nucleus known as the:
   (a) superior salivatory nucleus
   (b) Edinger-Westphal nucleus
   (c) spinal nucleus
   (d) lacrimatory nucleus
   (e) sensory nucleus
6. The vagus nerve has a nucleus known as the:
   (a) ventral motor nucleus
   (b) superior salivatory nucleus
   (c) inferior salivatory nucleus
   (d) cardiac nucleus
   (e) dorsal nucleus
7. Which of the following statements concerning the autonomic system is correct?
   (a) White rami communicantes contain myelinated afferent fibers
   (b) Gray rami communicantes contain postganglionic parasympathetic nerve fibers
   (c) The greater splanchnic nerve is formed of nonmyelinated nerve fibers
   (d) The lesser splanchnic nerve arises from the fifth to the ninth ganglia of the thoracic part of the sympathetic trunk
   (e) The lowest splanchnic nerve, when present, arises from the fourth and fifth ganglia of the thoracic part of the sympathetic trunk
8. Norepinephrine is secreted by which of the following nerve endings?
   (a) Preganglionic sympathetic nerve fibers
   (b) Postganglionic parasympathetic nerve fibers
   (c) Preganglionic sympathetic nerve fibers to the suprarenal medulla
   (d) Preganglionic parasympathetic nerve fibers
   (e) Postganglionic sympathetic nerve fibers
9. Which of the following statements concerning the innervation of the submandibular salivary gland is correct?
   (a) The parasympathetic preganglionic nerve fibers synapse in the otic ganglion
   (b) The secretomotor fibers originate in the superior salivatory nucleus of the facial nerve
   (c) The parasympathetic control is in the inferior salivatory nucleus of the glossopharyngeal nerve
   (d) The sympathetic preganglionic nerve fibers arise from the fifth thoracic segment of the spinal cord
   (e) The sympathetic nerves to the gland have no effect on the blood supply to the gland
10. Which of the following concern parasympathetic outflow in the spinal cord?
    (a) T1–L2
    (b) L4, L5, and S1, S2, and S3
    (c) L2, L3, and L4
    (d) S2, S3, and S4
    (e) L1 and L2
11. Which of the following statements concerning the action of anticholinesterase drugs is correct?
    (a) They prevent the release of acetylcholine at the nerve endings
    (b) They bring about the hydrolysis of acetylcholine inhibitors
    (c) They increase the release of acetylcholine at the nerve endings
    (d) They inhibit the breakdown of acetylcholine
    (e) They mimic the action of acetylcholine at the receptor site

Directions: Each of the numbered items in this section is followed by answers that are positively phrased. Select the ONE lettered answer that is an EXCEPTION.

12. The following statements concerning the autonomic nervous system are correct **except:**
    (a) It is confined to the peripheral part of the nervous system
    (b) The sympathetic part of the system prepares the body for an emergency
    (c) Stimulation of the sympathetic innervation to the urinary bladder wall causes it to relax
    (d) Stimulation of the parasympathetic causes an increase in the peristaltic waves of the gut
    (e) The parasympathetic outflow is present in cranial nerves III, VII, IX, and X
13. The following general statements concerning the autonomic nervous system are correct **except:**
    (a) It innervates involuntary structures
    (b) It has afferent, connector, and efferent neurons

(c) The afferent impulses originate in visceral receptors
(d) The visceral afferent receptors include chemoreceptors, baroreceptors, and osmoreceptors
(e) The pain receptors can be stimulated by oxygen excess

14. The following statements concerning a lesion of the sympathetic innervation of the head and neck (Horner's syndrome) are correct **except:**
(a) The patient has vasodilation of the arteries of the facial skin
(b) The pupil is constricted
(c) There is enophthalmos
(d) There is profuse sweating of the facial skin
(e) There is ptosis of the upper eyelid

15. The following statements concerning the autonomic innervation of the heart are correct **except:**
(a) The sympathetic nerves cause cardiac acceleration, and increased force of contraction of the cardiac muscle
(b) The action of norepinephrine at sympathetic postganglionic nerve endings is terminated by monoamine oxidase
(c) The sympathetic nerves cause dilation of the coronary arteries
(d) The sympathetic preganglionic fibers originate in the upper four thoracic ganglia of the sympathetic trunk
(e) The postganglionic parasympathetic fibers terminate on the sinoatrial and atrioventricular nodes

16. The following statements concerning the sympathetic receptors are correct **except:**
(a) There are two kinds of receptors present
(b) Norepinephrine has a greater effect on alpha receptors than on beta receptors
(c) Beta receptors are predominant in the bronchial walls
(d) Metaproterenol is a strong stimulant of alpha receptors
(e) Phenylephrine stimulates alpha receptors

17. The following statements concerning autonomic postganglionic endings that liberate acetylcholine are correct **except:**
(a) The receptors on the effector organs are muscarinic
(b) The action of acetylcholine at these endings is blocked by atropine
(c) Atropine blocks the release of acetylcholine
(d) Atropine occupies the cholinergic receptor sites
(e) Acetylcholine is stored in presynaptic vesicles

18. The sympathetic nerves have the following action on the smooth muscle in the organs named below **except:**
(a) In the bronchus the muscle is relaxed
(b) In the prostate the muscle is relaxed
(c) In the pyloric sphincter it contracts
(d) In systemic arteries it contracts
(e) In the gallbladder it relaxes

Directions: Read the case history then answer the question. A 17-year-old boy was peddling drugs on a street corner when a rival dealer in a passing car shot him in the abdomen. The boy was rushed to the nearest hospital. On examination, he was found to have an entrance wound in the lower part of the left side of the abdomen, but there was no exit wound. Radiographs showed the bullet lodged in the vertebral canal at the level of the second lumbar vertebra. After the patient recovered from surgery, in which numerous small-bowel perforations were repaired, a careful neurological examination revealed he also had a complete lesion of the cauda equina.

19. The following facts concerning this patient are correct **except:**
(a) The urinary bladder receives its sympathetic innervation from the first and second lumbar segments of the spinal cord
(b) The preganglionic sympathetic nerves that descend in the anterior root of the first lumbar nerve were left intact and not sectioned by the bullet
(c) The urinary bladder receives its parasympathetic innervation from the first sacral segment of the spinal cord
(d) The preganglionic parasympathetic nerve fibers were sectioned where they descend in the vertebral canal within the anterior roots of the second, third, and fourth sacral nerves
(e) The patient has an autonomous bladder that fills to capacity and then overflows with no reflex control

ANSWERS AND EXPLANATIONS

1. C
2. D
3. B
4. A
5. B
6. E
7. A. B. Gray rami communicantes contain nonmyelinated postganglionic sympathetic nerve fibers. C. The greater splanchnic nerve is formed of myelinated preganglionic sympathetic nerve fibers. D. The lesser splanchnic nerve arises from the tenth and eleventh ganglia of the thoracic part of the sympathetic trunk. E. The lowest splanchnic nerve, when present, arises from the twelfth ganglion of the thoracic part of the sympathetic trunk.

8. E. A. Preganglionic sympathetic nerve fibers liberate acetylcholine at their endings. B. Postganglionic parasympathetic nerve fibers liberate acetylcholine at their endings. C. Preganglionic sympathetic nerve fibers to the suprarenal medulla liberate acetylcholine at their endings. D. Preganglionic parasympathetic nerve fibers liberate acetylcholine at their nerve endings.
9. B
10. D
11. D
12. A.The autonomic nervous system is widely distributed throughout the central and peripheral parts of the nervous system.
13. E. Pain receptors can be stimulated by lack of oxygen.
14. D. Because of the loss of sympathetic activity, the sweat glands of the facial skin will be inactive.
15. B. The action of norepinephrine at sympathetic postganglionic endings is terminated by reuptake into the nerve endings.
16. D. Metaproterenol is a strong stimulant of beta receptors.
17. C. Atropine does not block the release of acetylcholine, but it occupies the cholinergic receptor sites.
18. B
19. C. The urinary bladder receives its parasympathetic innervation from the second, third, and fourth sacral segments of the spinal cord. Sectioning of the preganglionic nerve fibers by the bullet, where they descend in the vertebral canal within the anterior roots of the second, third, and fourth sacral nerves, deprived the bladder of its parasympathetic innervation, and the patient cannot voluntarily empty the urinary bladder. Moreover, the break in the local reflex arc prevents the bladder from reflexly emptying automatically when filled. However, the patient will be able to activate micturition by powerful contraction of the abdominal muscles, assisted by manual pressure on the lower anterior abdominal wall.

CHAPTER 22

Meninges

CHAPTER OUTLINE

SUGGESTED PLAN FOR REVIEW OF CHAPTER 22

1. Understand the structure and arrangement of the dura mater, arachnoid mater, and pia mater.
2. Learn the vertebral level at which each of the meninges terminates inferiorly in the child and the adult.
3. Be able to define (a) subarachnoid space, (b) falx cerebri, (c) tentorium cerebelli, and (d) diaphragma sellae.
4. Know the structure of a venous sinus. How do the layers of the dura mater contribute to its walls?
5. Learn the location of the superior sagittal sinus, the inferior sagittal sinus, the straight sinus, the transverse sinus, and the sigmoid sinus.
6. Learn the location and general shape of the cavernous sinus. Know the names of the structures that pass through the sinus and the structures that lie within its lateral wall. What is the connection between this sinus and infections of the face? This sinus is a common source of questions.
7. Be able to define a cistern, an arachnoid villus, and an arachnoid granulation.

INTRODUCTION

The brain and spinal cord are enclosed within three concentric membranous sheaths, the meninges. The outermost is thick, tough, and fibrous and is called the **dura mater**; the middle membrane is thin and delicate and is known as the arachnoid mater; and the innermost is delicate and vascular and closely applied to the surfaces of the brain and spinal cord and is known as the **pia mater**.

The three meninges, together with the bones of the skull and the vertebral column, protect the nervous tissue from mechanical forces applied from the exterior. Further protection is afforded by the cerebrospinal fluid, which lies in the subarachnoid space between the arachnoid mater and the pia mater.

The purpose of this chapter is to give a brief overview of the arrangement of the meninges.

MENINGES OF THE SPINAL CORD

The meninges of the spinal cord have already been described in Chapter 6.

MENINGES OF THE BRAIN

The brain, like the spinal cord, has a covering of dura mater, arachnoid mater, and pia mater.

DURA MATER

The dura mater of the brain is formed of two layers, the endosteal layer and the meningeal layer. These are closely united except along certain lines, where they separate to form **venous sinuses**.

Endosteal Layer

The endosteal layer is the periosteum covering the inner surface of the skull. At the foramen magnum it does **not** become continuous with the dura mater of the spinal cord. Around the margins of all the foramina in the skull it becomes continuous with the **periosteum** on the outside of the skull. At the sutures, it is continuous with the **sutural ligaments**. It is most strongly adherent to the bones over the base of the skull.

Meningeal Layer

The meningeal layer is the dura mater proper. It is a dense, strong fibrous membrane covering the brain and is continuous through the foramen magnum with the dura mater of the spinal cord. It provides tubular sheaths for the cranial nerves as the latter pass through the foramina in the skull. Outside the skull, the sheaths fuse with the epineurium of the nerves.

The meningeal layer gives rise to four septa, which divide the cranial cavity into spaces that lodge the subdivisions of the brain (Figs. 22-1 and 22-2). The function of these septa is to restrict the displacement of the brain during head movements.

FALX CEREBRI

The falx cerebri is a sickle-shaped fold of dura mater that lies in the midline between the two cerebral hemispheres (Figs. 22-1 and 22-2). It is attached in front to the crista galli and posteriorly to the upper surface of the **tentorium cerebelli** and the internal surface of the skull. The **superior sagittal sinus** runs in its upper fixed border and the **inferior sagittal sinus** runs in its lower free margin; the

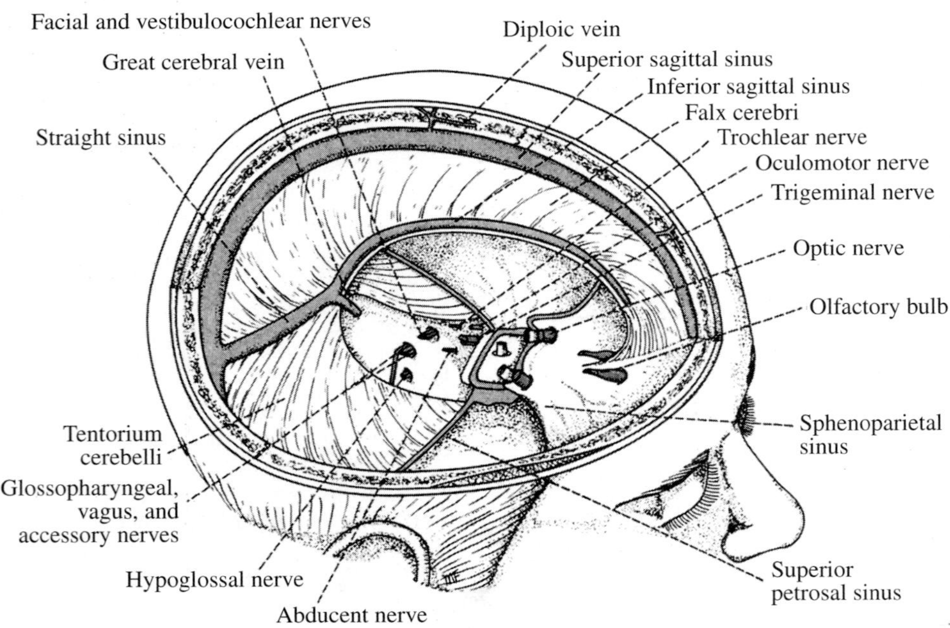

Figure 22–1 Interior of the skull, showing the dura mater and its contained venous sinuses.

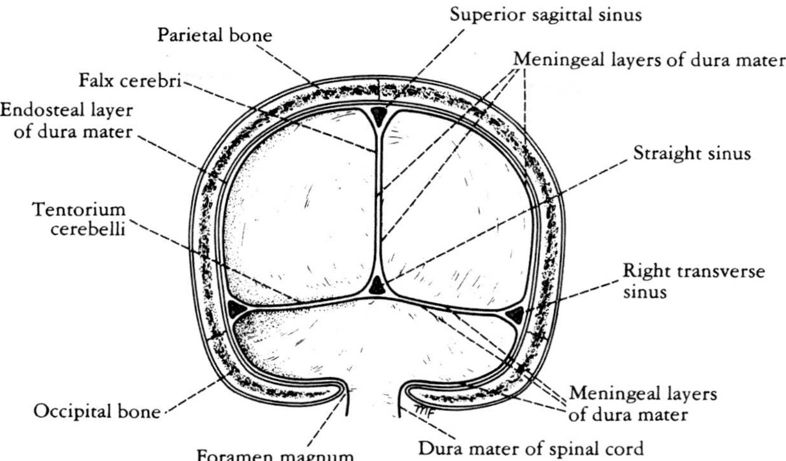

Figure 22–2 Falx cerebri and the tentorium cerebelli as seen on coronal section of the skull. Note the continuity between the meningeal layer of the dura mater within the skull and the dura mater of the spinal cord at the foramen magnum.

straight sinus runs along its attachment to the tentorium cerebelli.

TENTORIUM CEREBELLI

The tentorium cerebelli is a crescent-shaped fold of dura mater placed between the upper surface of the cerebellum and the occipital lobes of the cerebral hemispheres (Figs. 22-1, 22-2, and 22-3). In the anterior edge there is a gap, the **tentorial notch**, for the passage of the midbrain. The fixed border is attached to the posterior clinoid processes, the petrous part of the temporal bone, and the inner surface of the occipital bone. The free border is attached to the anterior clinoid process on each side. At the point where the two borders cross, the third and fourth cranial nerves pass forward to enter the lateral wall of the cavernous sinus.

The falx cerebri and the falx cerebelli are attached to the upper and lower surfaces of the tentorium, respectively. The **straight sinus** runs along its attachment to the falx cerebri, the **superior petrosal sinus** runs along its attachment to the petrous bone, and the **transverse sinus** runs along its attachment to the occipital bone.

Close to the apex of the petrous part of the temporal bone, the lower layer of the tentorium is pouched forward beneath the superior petrosal sinus to form a **recess for the trigeminal nerve and the trigeminal ganglion**.

FALX CEREBELLI

The falx cerebelli is a small, vertical fold of dura mater that projects forward between the two cerebellar hemispheres. Its posterior fixed margin contains the **occipital sinus**.

DIAPHRAGMA SELLAE

The diaphragma sellae is a small, circular fold of dura mater that forms the roof of the sella turcica (Fig. 22-3). A small hole in its center is for the passage of the stalk of the **hypophysis cerebri**.

Dural Nerve Supply

The dural nerve supply is mainly derived from branches of the **trigeminal nerve**, the **upper three cervical nerves**, the **cervical part of the sympathetic trunk**, and the **vagus nerve**.

Dural Arterial Supply

Numerous arteries supply the dura mater from the **internal carotid, ascending pharyngeal, occipital,** and **vertebral arteries**. From the clinical standpoint, the most important is the **middle meningeal artery**, which is commonly damaged in head injuries.

Middle Meningeal Artery

The middle meningeal artery arises from the maxillary artery in the infratemporal fossa. It enters the cranial cavity through the foramen spinosum and then lies between the meningeal and endosteal layers of dura. The artery then runs forward and laterally in a groove on the upper surface of the squamous part of the temporal bone. The anterior (frontal) branch deeply grooves or tunnels the anterior-inferior angle of the parietal bone, and its course corresponds roughly to the line of the underlying precentral gyrus of the brain. The posterior (parietal) branch curves backward and supplies the posterior part of the dura mater.

Dural Venous Drainage

The middle meningeal vein follows the branches of the middle meningeal artery and drains into the pterygoid venous plexus or the sphenoparietal sinus. The veins lie lateral to the arteries.

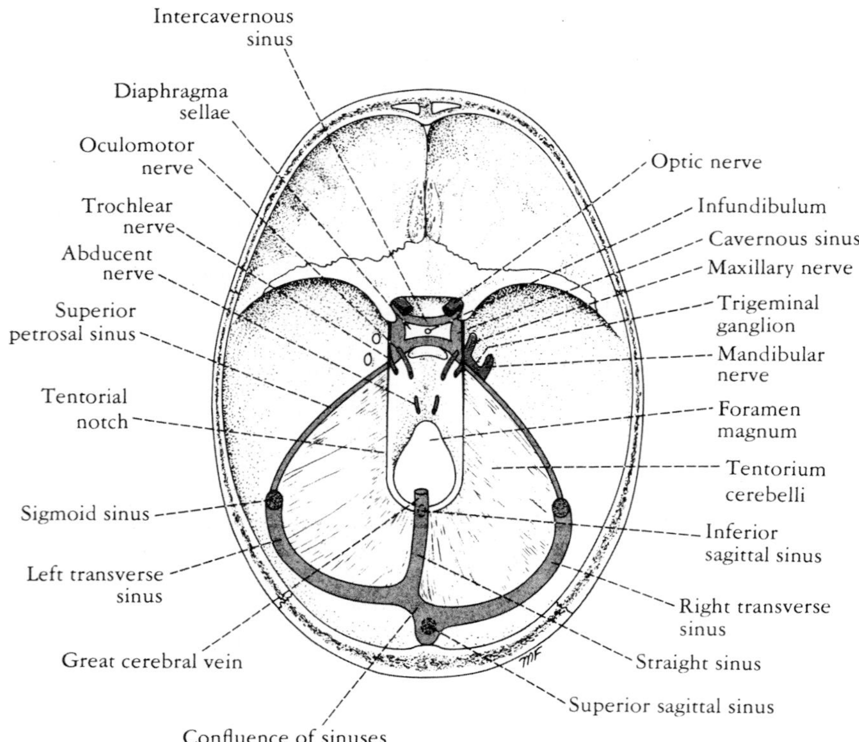

Figure 22–3 Superior view of the diaphragma sellae and tentorium cerebelli. Note the position of the cranial nerves and venous sinuses.

Clinical Notes

Dural Headache

The dura mater possesses numerous sensory endings that are sensitive to stretching. Stretching the dura above the level of the tentorium cerebelli can result in referred pain along the trigeminal nerve to an area of skin on the same side of the head. Stretching the dura below the tentorium results in pain referred to the back of the neck and the back of the scalp along the course of the greater occipital nerve.

Epidural Hemorrhage

A minor blow to the side of the head, resulting in fracture of the skull, can sever the anterior division of the middle meningeal artery or vein. The arterial hemorrhage strips the meningeal layer of dura from the internal surface of the skull, the intracranial pressure rises, and the enlarging blood clot exerts local pressure on the underlying motor area in the precentral gyrus.

DURAL VENOUS SINUSES

The venous sinuses of the cranial cavity are situated between the layers of the dura mater (Figs. 22-3 and 22-4). They receive blood from the brain, from the diploë of the skull, from the orbit, and from the internal ear; they also receive the cerebrospinal fluid from the subarachnoid space through the **arachnoid villi.** The blood in the dural sinuses ultimately drains into the internal jugular veins in the neck. The dural sinuses are lined by endothelium, and their walls are devoid of muscular tissue. They contain no valves. **Emissary veins**, which are also valveless, connect the dural venous sinuses with the **diploic veins** of the skull and with the veins of the scalp.

Superior Sagittal Sinus

The superior sagittal sinus lies in the upper fixed border of the falx cerebri (Figs. 22-1 and 22-2). It begins anteriorly at the foramen cecum, where it occasionally receives a vein from the nasal cavity. It runs posteriorly, and at the internal occipital protuberance it usually becomes continuous with the right **transverse sinus**. On each side the sinus communicates with two or three irregularly shaped **venous lacu-**

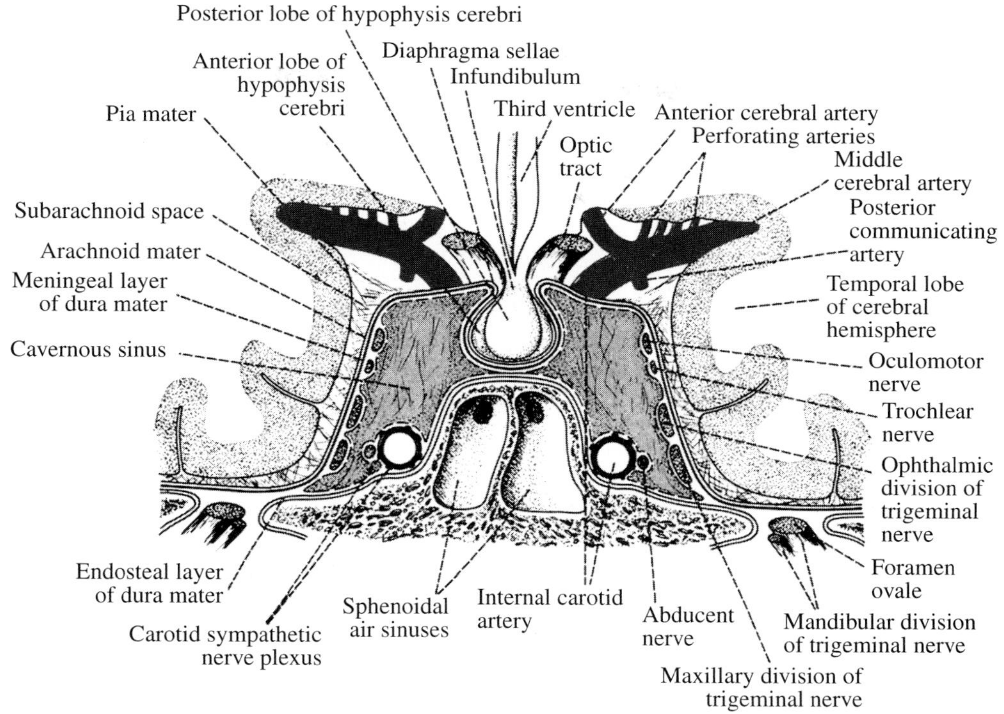

Figure 22–4 Coronal section through the body of the sphenoid bone, showing the hypophysis cerebri and cavernous sinuses. Note the position of the internal carotid artery and the cranial nerves.

nae. Numerous arachnoid villi and granulations project into the lacunae.

The superior sagittal sinus receives in its course the **superior cerebral veins**. At the internal occipital protuberance it is dilated to form the **confluence of the sinuses** and receives the **occipital sinus**.

Inferior Sagittal Sinus

The inferior sagittal sinus lies in the lower free margin of the falx cerebri (Figs. 22-1 and 22-2). It runs backward and joins the **great cerebral vein** to form the straight sinus. It receives cerebral veins from the medial surface of the cerebral hemispheres.

Straight Sinus

The straight sinus lies at the junction of the falx cerebri with the tentorium cerebelli (Fig. 22-1). It is formed by the union of the **inferior sagittal sinus** with the **great cerebral vein**. It drains usually into the left transverse sinus. It receives some of the superior cerebellar veins.

Transverse Sinus

The transverse sinuses are paired structures (Figs. 22-2 and 22-3). The right sinus begins at the internal occipital protuberance as a continuation of the superior sagittal sinus. The left sinus is usually a continuation of the straight sinus. Each sinus runs forward along the attached margin of the tentorium cerebelli. They end on each side by becoming the **sigmoid sinus**. The transverse sinuses receive the **superior petrosal sinuses** and the **inferior cerebral** and the **cerebellar veins**.

Sigmoid Sinus

The sigmoid sinuses are a direct continuation of the transverse sinuses (Fig. 22-3). Each sinus curves downward behind the mastoid antrum and leaves the skull through the posterior part of the jugular foramen to become the internal jugular vein.

Occipital Sinus

The occipital sinus lies in the attached margin of the falx cerebelli. It begins near the foramen magnum, where it communicates with the **vertebral veins** and drains into the confluence of sinuses.

Cavernous Sinuses

The cavernous sinuses are situated in the middle cranial fossa on each side of the body of the sphenoid bone (Fig. 22-4) and extend from the superior orbital fissure in front to the apex of the petrous part of the temporal bone behind. The sinus receives the inferior ophthalmic vein, the sphenoparietal sinus, the central vein of the retina, and the cerebral veins. The cavernous sinus drains into the transverse sinus through the superior petrosal sinus.

The **internal carotid artery**, surrounded by its **sympathetic nerve plexus**, runs forward through the sinus (Fig. 22-4). The **abducent nerve** also passes through the sinus. The **third and fourth cranial nerves** and the ophthalmic and maxillary divisions of the trigeminal nerve run forward in the lateral wall of the sinus (Fig. 22-4).

CLINICAL NOTES

CAVERNOUS SINUS THROMBOSIS

The anterior facial vein, the ophthalmic veins, and the cavernous sinus are in direct communication. Infection of the facial skin alongside the nose, ethmoidal sinusitis, and infection of the orbital contents can lead to thrombosis of the veins and ultimately cavernous sinus thrombosis, which is a life-threatening condition.

Intercavernous Sinuses

The intercavernous sinuses connect the two cavernous sinuses through the sella turcica (Fig. 22-3).

Superior and Inferior Petrosal Sinuses

The superior and inferior petrosal sinuses are small sinuses situated on the superior and inferior borders of the petrous part of the temporal bone on each side of the skull. Each superior sinus drains the cavernous sinus into the transverse sinus, and each inferior sinus drains the cavernous sinus into the internal jugular vein.

ARACHNOID MATER

The arachnoid mater is a delicate, impermeable membrane covering the brain and lying between the pia mater internally and the dura mater externally. It is separated from the dura by a potential space, the **subdural space,** filled by a film of fluid; it is separated from the pia by the **subarachnoid space**, which is filled with **cerebrospinal fluid**. The outer and inner surfaces of the arachnoid are covered with flattened mesothelial cells.

The arachnoid bridges over the sulci on the surface of the brain, and in certain situations the arachnoid and pia are widely separated to form the **subarachnoid cisternae**. The **cisterna cerebellomedullaris** lies between the inferior surface of the cerebellum and the roof of the fourth ventricle. The **cisterna interpeduncularis** lies between the two cerebral peduncles. All the cisternae are in free communication with one another, and with the remainder of the subarachnoid space.

The arachnoid projects into the venous sinuses (especially the superior sagittal sinus) to form **arachnoid villi** and **arachnoid granulations**. These are sites where the cerebrospinal fluid diffuses into the bloodstream.

The subarachnoid space is filled with cerebrospinal fluid and contains the cerebral arteries and the cranial nerves. At certain sites there are extensions of the subarachnoid space.

PIA MATER

The pia mater is a vascular membrane that closely covers the surface of the brain and descends into the sulci. As a two-layered fold, called the **tela choroidea**, it projects into the ventricles to form the **choroid plexuses**.

REVIEW QUESTIONS

Directions: Each of the incomplete statements in this section is followed by completions of the statement. Select the ONE lettered completion that is BEST in each case.

For questions 1-5 study Figure 22-5 of the interior of the skull, showing the dura mater and venous sinuses.

1. Structure number 1 is the:
   (a) falx cerebri
   (b) straight sinus
   (c) superior sagittal sinus
   (d) tentorium cerebelli
   (e) diploe of the skull
2. Structure number 2 is the:
   (a) straight sinus
   (b) superior sagittal sinus
   (c) falx cerebri
   (d) inferior sagittal sinus
   (e) middle cerebral vein
3. Structure number 3 is the:
   (a) lesser wing of the sphenoid bone
   (b) sphenoparietal sinus
   (c) middle meningeal artery
   (d) falx cerebelli
   (e) superior petrosal sinus

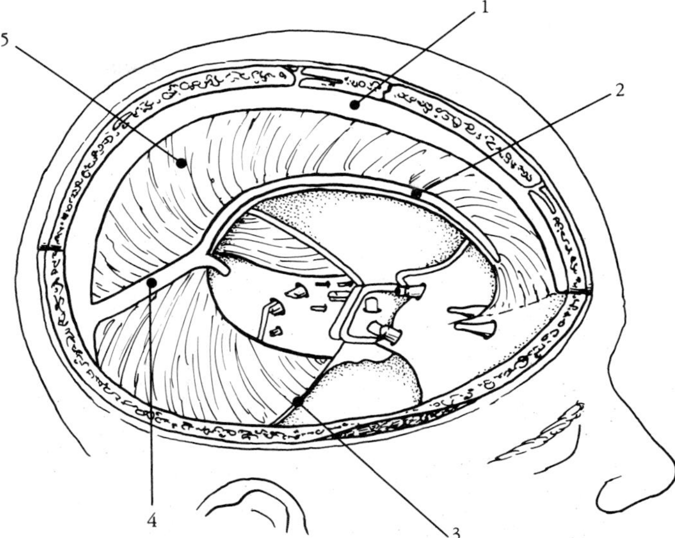

Figure 22–5 Interior of the skull, showing the dura mater and the venous sinuses

4. Structure number 4 is the:
   (a) falx cerebri
   (b) tentorium cerebelli
   (c) great cerebral vein
   (d) straight sinus
   (e) falx cerebelli
5. Structure number 5 is the:
   (a) falx cerebelli
   (b) falx cerebri
   (c) tentorium cerebelli
   (d) endosteum lining the skull
   (e) sutural ligaments
6. The pia mater that covers the brain is:
   (a) an avascular membrane
   (b) not present in the sulci of the cerebral hemispheres
   (c) separated from the substance of the brain at certain sites to form important cisternae
   (d) projected into the ventricles of the brain to form the choroid plexuses
   (e) not continuous with that covering the spinal cord

Directions: Each of the numbered items in this section is followed by answers that are positively phrased. Select the ONE lettered answer that is an EXCEPTION.

7. The following statements concerning the dura mater of the brain are correct **except:**
   (a) The meningeal layer of dura is continuous through the foramen magnum with the dura mater covering the spinal cord
   (b) The endosteal layer of dura mater is continuous through the foramina in the skull with the periosteum outside the skull
   (c) The cranial venous sinuses are located between the endosteal and meningeal layers of dura mater
   (d) Each cranial nerve pierces the meningeal layer of dura inside the skull before it leaves the skull
   (e) The meningeal layer of dura extends through the optic canal to fuse with the sclera of the eyeball
8. The following statements concerning the falx cerebri are correct **except:**
   (a) It is a sickle-shaped fold of the meningeal layer of dura mater
   (b) It is attached anteriorly to the crista galli of the ethmoid bone
   (c) The straight sinus runs along its lower free border
   (d) The superior sagittal sinus runs along its upper fixed border
   (e) It is attached to the tentorium cerebelli
9. The following statements concerning the tentorium cerebelli are correct **except:**
   (a) The tentorial notch allows the passage of the midbrain
   (b) The free border is attached anteriorly to the posterior clinoid processes
   (c) It separates the occipital lobes of the brain from the cerebellum
   (d) The transverse venous sinus lies in its attached lateral border
   (e) The superior petrosal sinus runs along its attached border to the petrous part of the temporal bone
10. The following statements concerning the blood supply to the dura mater within the skull are correct **except:**
   (a) The arteries include branches of the internal carotid, maxillary, and vertebral arteries
   (b) The middle meningeal artery arises from the maxillary artery
   (c) The middle meningeal artery enters the skull through the foramen spinosum
   (d) The middle meningeal artery runs between the bone and the endosteal layer of dura
   (e) The anterior branch of the middle meningeal artery grooves the anterior inferior angle of the parietal bone and it is here that it is commonly injured

11. The following general statements concerning the dural venous sinuses are correct **except:**
    (a) They possess no valves
    (b) They have thick muscular walls
    (c) They receive blood from the brain and the internal ear
    (d) They are connected to the scalp veins by valveless emissary veins
    (e) They drain cerebrospinal fluid through the arachnoid granulations
12. The following statements concerning the cavernous venous sinus are correct **except:**
    (a) It is situated in the middle cranial fossa
    (b) It receives the central vein of the retina and the inferior ophthalmic vein
    (c) The internal carotid artery and the trochlear nerve run through the sinus
    (d) The oculomotor and the ophthalmic and maxillary divisions of the trigeminal nerves run forward in its lateral wall
    (e) It is drained posteriorly into the transverse sinus through the superior petrosal sinus
13. The following nerves supply the dura mater with sensory fibers **except:**
    (a) The upper three cervical nerves
    (b) The ophthalmic division of the trigeminal nerve
    (c) The vestibulocochlear nerve
    (d) The maxillary division of the trigeminal nerve
    (e) The mandibular division of the trigeminal nerve
14. The following statements concerning the sigmoid sinus are correct **except:**
    (a) It is a direct continuation of the transverse sinus
    (b) It is a continuation of the posterior end of the cavernous sinus
    (c) It lies in the posterior cranial fossa
    (d) It is related anteriorly to the mastoid antrum
    (e) It leaves the skull by passing through the jugular foramen to become the internal jugular vein
15. The following statements concerning the arachnoid mater are correct **except:**
    (a) It is a delicate membrane
    (b) It does not extend through foramina in the skull to provide sheaths for the cranial nerves
    (c) It is separated from the dura mater by a film of fluid in the subdural space
    (d) Beneath it lies the subarachnoid space filled with cerebrospinal fluid
    (e) It is an impermeable membrane
16. The following statements concerning the subarachnoid space are correct **except:**
    (a) It extends inferiorly as far as the fourth sacral vertebra
    (b) It contains the cerebral arteries
    (c) The cranial nerves lie within the subarachnoid space
    (d) It contains the cerebral veins
    (e) It dips into the sulci of the cerebral hemispheres
17. The following structures restrict the movements of the brain within the skull **except:**
    (a) The falx cerebri
    (b) The falx cerebelli
    (c) The petrous part of the temporal bone
    (d) The tentorium cerebelli
    (e) The diaphragma sellae
18. The following statements concerning the meninges of the brain are correct **except:**
    (a) At the sutures the sutural ligaments connect the endosteal layer of the dura to the periosteum outside the skull
    (b) The sympathetic nerves do not supply the meninges
    (c) The fibrous tissue in the walls of the dural venous sinuses resists the outside pressure of the cerebrospinal fluid
    (d) The inner and outer surfaces of the arachnoid mater are covered with mesothelial cells
    (e) The meninges can be the site of inflammation
19. The following general statements concerning the subarachnoid cisternae are correct **except:**
    (a) There is a cisterna between the cerebral peduncles of the midbrain
    (b) The cisterna cerebellomedullaris lies between the inferior surface of the cerebellum and the roof of the fourth ventricle
    (c) The foramina of Magendie and Luschka open into the cisterna cerebellomedullaris
    (d) They form important reservoirs for the cerebrospinal fluid
    (e) One unique characteristic about the cisternae is that they have no communication with one another
20. The following general statements concerning the arachnoid mater are correct **except:**
    (a) The membrane dips into the sulci on the surface of the brain
    (b) The arachnoid villi project into the venous blood as minute outpouchings of the subarachnoid space
    (c) Groups of arachnoid villi are known as arachnoid granulations
    (d) The superior sagittal sinus possesses large numbers of arachnoid granulations
    (e) The arachnoid mater and the subarachnoid space extend forward into the orbital cavity to the back of the optic disc of the eye

Directions: Read the case history then answer the question. A 33-year-old unconscious man was admitted to the emergency department. While crossing a road, he had been hit on the right side of the head by a car. Within an hour, his state of unconsciousness deepened. On examination, he was found to have a large doughlike swelling over the right side of his head. He also had the signs of left-sided hemiplegia. Later, a right-sided, fixed, dilated pupil developed. A lateral radiograph showed a hairline fracture that extended downward and forward across the anterior-inferior angle of the right parietal bone.

21. Which of the following statements concerning this patient does not explain the signs and symptoms?
    (a) The initial loss of consciousness is probably due to cerebral trauma
    (b) The location of the fracture line over the anterior-inferior angle of the right parietal bone suggests damage to the right middle meningeal artery
    (c) The left-sided hemiplegia is probably caused by pressure on the right precentral gyrus
    (d) The right-sided, fixed, dilated pupil is explained by pressure on the right oculomotor nerve. The hippocampal gyrus sometimes herniates through the tentorial notch, causing pressure on the oculomotor nerve
    (e) Tearing of the right middle meningeal artery can result in a right-sided subdural hemorrhage

ANSWERS AND EXPLANATIONS

1. C
2. D
3. E
4. D
5. B
6. D
7. D. The meningeal layer of the dura mater extends through each foramina in the skull and provides a short sheath for the cranial nerves; the sheath fuses with the epineurium of each cranial nerve outside the skull.
8. C. The straight sinus runs along the border of the falx cerebri that is attached to the upper surface of the tentorium cerebelli. The inferior sagittal sinus runs along the lower free border of the falx cerebri.
9. B. The free border of the tentorium cerebelli is attached anteriorly to the anterior clinoid processes.
10. D. The middle meningeal artery inside the skull runs between the meningeal and endosteal layers of the dura mater. Hemorrhage from this artery is called an extradural hemorrhage because the blood will lie outside the true meningeal layer of the dura.
11. B. Dural venous sinuses have thick fibrous walls but the walls contain no muscle.
12. C. The cavernous sinus has running through its cavity (covered with endothelium) the internal carotid artery and its sympathetic plexus and the abducent nerve.
13. C
14. B
15. B. The arachnoid mater, along with the dura and pia, extend through each foramen, providing the cranial nerves with a short sheath; the meninges end by fusing with the epineurium of each cranial nerve.
16. A. The subarachnoid space extends inferiorly around the spinal cord and cauda equina as far as the second sacral vertebra.
17. E. The diaphragma sellae covers the sella turcica and protects the underlying hypophysis cerebri.
18. B. The sympathetic nerves do supply the dura mater and are distributed to the meningeal arteries.
19. E. All the subarachnoid cisternae communicate with each other via the subarachnoid space.
20. A. The arachnoid mater bridges over the sulci on the surface of the brain.
21. E. Tearing of the anterior branch of the middle meningeal artery can occur as the result of fracture of the anterior-inferior angle of the parietal bone. An extradural hemorrhage, not a subdural hemorrhage, then takes place. The location of the artery in a groove or tunnel in the bone between the meningeal layer of the dura and the endosteal layer of the dura (i.e., the periosteum of the skull) results in the blood under pressure accumulating outside the meningeal layer of dura.

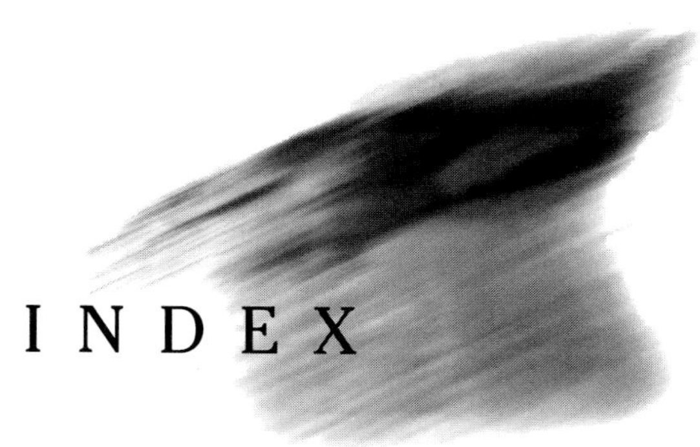

INDEX

Page numbers in *italics* denote figures; those followed by a b or t denote boxes and tables, respectively.